PALLIATIVE CARE

Transforming the Care of Serious Illness

EDITORS

DIANE E. MEIER, M.D.
STEPHEN L. ISAACS, J.D.
ROBERT G. HUGHES, Ph.D.

FOREWORD BY
RISA LAVIZZO-MOUREY

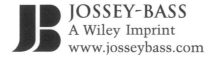

JOSSEY-BASS
A Wiley Imprint
www.josseybass.com

Published by Jossey-Bass
A Wiley Imprint
989 Market Street, San Francisco, CA 94103-1741—www.josseybass.com

Jossey-Bass books and products are available through most bookstores. To contact Jossey-Bass directly call our Customer Care Department within the U.S. at 800-956-7739, outside the U.S. at 317-572-3986, or fax 317-572-4002.

Jossey-Bass also publishes its books in a variety of electronic formats. Some content that appears in print may not be available in electronic books.

Library of Congress Cataloging-in-Publication Data

Transforming palliative care : transforming the care of serious illness / editors, Diane E. Meier, Stephen L. Isaacs, and Robert G. Hughes ; foreword by Risa Lavizzo-Mourey. – 1st ed.
   p. ; cm. – (Robert Wood Johnson Foundation series on health policy)
  Articles previously published in various sources.
  Includes bibliographical references and index.
  ISBN 978-0-470-52717-7 (pbk.)
 1. Palliative treatment. I. Meier, Diane E. II. Isaacs, Stephen L. III. Hughes, Robert G., Ph. D. IV. Series: Robert Wood Johnson Foundation series on health policy.
  [DNLM: 1. Palliative Care–trends–United States–Collected Works. 2. Patient Care–ethics–United States–Collected Works. 3. Hospice Care–United States–Collected Works.
4. Terminal Care–United States–Collected Works. WB 310 T772 2009]
  R726.8.T73 2009
  616′.029–dc22

                                                      2009026290

Printed in the United States of America
FIRST EDITION

PB Printing   10 9 8 7 6 5 4 3

CONTENTS

FOREWORD

In the late 1970s and early 1980s, when I was a physician in training, the field of palliative care did not exist. More often than not, a very sick or dying patient was viewed as a failure—a failure of technology and know-how to cure disease, or at least to extend life. Too often I observed one of two equally inadequate responses to this perceived failure: apply more technology, more intensively, or withdraw completely, physically and emotionally. Performing heroic measures—chemotherapy, surgery, artificial life support—even when there was no hope for cure or significantly prolonging life was the standard of care.

Between 1989 and 1994, the Robert Wood Johnson Foundation funded a large study called SUPPORT—the Study to Understand Prognoses and Preferences for Outcomes and Risks of Treatment—to improve the care given to seriously ill hospitalized patients by having patients and their loved ones discuss their wishes for treatment (or lack of treatment) with specially trained nurses, who would relay that information to the physicians and nurses in charge of the patients' care. The evaluation of SUPPORT showed that despite the program's work to improve communication among patients, family members, and those entrusted with their care, all too often these patients were subjected to aggressive life-prolonging treatment and spent their last days and weeks in significant pain and discomfort.

The failure of SUPPORT led the Robert Wood Johnson Foundation to embark on a multiyear, multifaceted effort to improve the care given to people with serious illness—an effort that was undertaken in loose collaboration with the Open Society Institute's Project on Death in America.

Together, the two foundations were instrumental in nurturing the field of palliative care, which is the subject of this book, the fourth in a series that highlights and examines fields that the Robert Wood Johnson Foundation has nurtured over many years. Transforming Palliative Care is about the field itself, not the Foundation's role in developing it. Like its predecessor volumes in The Robert Wood Johnson Foundation Health Policy Series—*Generalist Medicine and the U.S. Health System* (2004), *School Health Services and Programs* (2006), and *Tobacco Control Policy* (2006), *Palliative Care: Transforming the Care of Serious Illness* begins with a comprehensive review of the field. We are honored that Diane E. Meier, who co-edited this volume with Stephen L. Isaacs and Robert G. Hughes, wrote the introductory chapter. Dr. Meier's leadership in and contribution to the field of palliative care were recognized by her selection as a recipient of a 2008 MacArthur Foundation "genius award." Dr. Meier's chapter is followed by reprints of twenty-five of the most important or influential articles in the field, written by its leading practitioners and analysts.

The combination of Dr. Meier's review chapter and the reprints of key articles from books and professional journals will give readers the wherewithal to understand the evolution of palliative care and the movement for better care of the seriously ill. We hope that the wisdom contained in these pages will inform academics, students, and the American public, and that it will serve to guide policy makers in developing meaningful approaches that will lead to better bedside care for all Americans.

Risa Lavizzo-Mourey, M.D., M.B.A.
President and CEO
The Robert Wood Johnson Foundation
Princeton, New Jersey
May 2009

EDITORS' INTRODUCTION

This book is intended as an introduction and guide to palliative care and, more broadly, to the medical care of the seriously ill. Although concerns about the suffering and pain that seriously ill people and their families endure is not new—the hospice movement in the United States can be dated to the mid-1960s, and Elizabeth Kübler-Ross's seminal book, *On Death and Dying*, appeared in 1969—it was during the 1980s and 1990s that the American public began to pay serious attention. This attention has, if anything, increased during the 2000s.

Some of the heightened attention is related, no doubt, to demographics. More and more middle-aged children have been forced to watch helplessly as their parents undergo fragmented and often incomprehensible medical care from multiple specialists who communicate neither with each other nor with the patients and families they are serving. After years of roller-coaster hospitalizations, more than half of Americans still die among strangers, hooked up to a variety of machines in a hospital setting. The public's attention has been riveted by high-profile legal cases, such as that of Terry Schiavo, by the intense controversy surrounding Dr. Jack Kevorkian, and by the legalization of physician-assisted suicide in the states of Oregon and Washington.

Away from the public spotlight, physicians, nurses, social workers, ethicists, attorneys, and laypeople have been working to make sure that people with serious illnesses are able to receive the kind of care that they want and the kind of relief from pain that they need—palliative care, in short. Those practicing palliative care serve the most ancient of goals in the practice of medicine—the relief of human suffering. Palliative care provides comfort and relief of pain to seriously ill individuals in a variety of settings and at various stages of illness. Hospice, one form of palliative care, provides comfort and pain relief specifically for people who are clearly dying, whereas palliative care in general provides comfort and pain relief for anyone with a serious illness regardless of their prognosis, whether they are expected to be cured or to live for years with a chronic disease. Palliative care is offered at the same time as medical care aimed at cure or life prolongation and is appropriate for all patients in need of it, whether they will live for years or days.

Palliative care has entered the mainstream of medical practice. More than half of U.S. hospitals reported a palliative care program in 2006, and many more programs are in the planning stages. Even so, as with other so-called cognitive specialties, it faces an uphill battle, due in part to the federal government's and private insurers' unwillingness to pay sufficiently for the kinds of medical care and social services needed by seriously ill people (many of whom are elderly and frail and have multiple chronic conditions). As a consequence of such inequities in reimbursement, fewer than 2 percent of graduating U.S. medical students choose to practice in a primary care (cognitive) specialty, and most leave their training with hundreds of thousands of dollars in educational debt, virtually forcing them to pursue training in procedural subspecialties that are much more generously reimbursed by payers. The growth of the palliative care field is limited by the difficulty of recruiting and retaining the necessary workforce under such adverse financial incentives.

Nonetheless, the aging of the population makes it unavoidable that health professionals will spend more of their time caring for older people, many of whom suffer from multiple chronic conditions, and the sickest of whom require palliative care. Moreover, because palliative care improves the quality of care and reduces costs for a key population of patients—those with serious and complex illness who, while accounting for under 10 percent of patients, drive more than two-thirds of health care spending—it ought to be a central part of the solution to America's health care crisis. For these reasons, palliative care—as part of health care reform—is almost certain to rise higher on the nation's health policy agenda.

The initial chapter, by Diane E. Meier, M.D., offers a comprehensive review of the field of palliative care, covering, among other topics, the history of care of seriously ill people; the religious, legal, and ethical issues; the evolution of views regarding relief from pain; the growth and current state of the field of palliative care; and the challenges confronting it.

In selecting twenty-five of the most influential or important articles to reprint—out of literally hundreds of superb pieces that the field has generated—the editors faced what proved to be a difficult, if not impossible, task. In making our selection, we looked for "classic" articles, such as Eric J. Cassell's "The Nature of Suffering and the Goals of Medicine"; pieces written by the giants who founded the field, such as Elisabeth Kübler-Ross; and pieces that captured the most critical issues in palliative care. In making the selections, we first asked many of the field's leading experts—listed in the acknowledgments—what they considered to be the most important, influential articles in the field. We owe each of them an enormous debt of gratitude for their thoughtful responses.

After receiving the guidance of these experts, we turned to the process of winnowing the reprint list down to twenty-five, which is all that space would allow. We are fully cognizant that a number of important articles were omitted, and that three different editors would have compiled a different list. Nonetheless, we believe that the articles we have chosen to reprint offer a reasonable selection of the most important, influential articles on palliative care.

Like Dr. Risa Lavizzo-Mourey, who wrote the foreword, we too hope that this book will inform the debate about health reform and efforts to improve the delivery of long-term care to seniors. The aging of the population, the increasing number of people suffering from chronic illness, the staggering cost of medical care, the great disparities in health care, and, simply, the human considerations in caring for seriously ill people make the issues addressed in this book of the highest priority.

Diane E. Meier, M.D.
Stephen L. Isaacs, J.D.
Robert G. Hughes, Ph.D.
Editors

ACKNOWLEDGMENTS

We wish to express our gratitude to the many people whose counsel helped shape this book.

We asked some of the nation's leading experts in palliative care what they considered to be the most important issues in the field and what articles they felt had been the most significant or influential. Their collective judgment guided our thinking, and we are grateful to each of the individuals listed below for their time and thoughtfulness:

- George J. Annas
- Robert M. Arnold
- Anthony L. Back
- Andrew Billings
- Margaret L. Campbell
- Arthur L. Caplan
- Christine K. Cassel
- Nicholas A. Christakis
- Constance M. Dahlin
- Betty R. Ferrell
- Kathleen M. Foley
- Rosemary Gibson
- Bruce Jennings
- Sharon R. Kaufman
- Jean S. Kutner
- Joanne Lynn

- Stephen J. McPhee
- Alan Meisel
- Sean Morrison
- Balfour M. Mount
- Chuck Mowll
- Steven Z. Pantilat
- Holly G. Prigerson
- Timothy E. Quill
- Steven A. Schroeder
- Thomas J. Smith
- Sharyn M. Sutton
- James A. Tulsky
- Charles F. von Gunten
- David E. Weissman
- Joanne Wolfe

We are indebted to Kathleen Foley and Christine Cassel, who reviewed the article that begins the book. Their comments were extremely helpful.

We would like to recognize the contribution of staff members at the Robert Wood Johnson Foundation. Particular thanks are due to Rosemary Gibson, who as a senior program officer at the Foundation played a key role in shaping and overseeing its end-of-life programming and who reviewed the introductory chapter. We are grateful as well to David Morse for his oversight of the Robert Wood Johnson Foundation Health Policy Series and his invaluable guidance on this book; Risa Lavizzo-Mourey for her many thoughtful ideas and consistent encouragement; Roshani Desai for her fine work organizing the collaborative efforts of the three editors; Hope Woodhead and Barbara Sherwood for handling the distribution; and Hinda Feige Greenberg, Mary Beth Kren, and Barbara Sergeant for conducting literature reviews and obtaining articles for the editors to consider as reprints.

We would also like to thank Pat Crow for copyediting the article by Dr. Meier, Carolyn Shea for fact checking it, Lauren MacIntyre for entering editorial changes, and Shirley Tiangsing for transferring printed material into electronic form. At Jossey-Bass, we acknowledge the efforts of Andy Pasternack, Kelsey McGee, and Seth Schwartz. At the Center to Advance Palliative Care, we acknowledge the design and communications guidance of Lisa Morgan. Lastly, we express our appreciation to Elizabeth Dawson, research and editorial associate at Health Policy Associates, for her excellent work overseeing the editorial and production process.

D.E.M.
S.L.I.
R.G.H.

REVIEW
OF
THE PALLIATIVE CARE
FIELD

THE DEVELOPMENT, STATUS, AND FUTURE OF PALLIATIVE CARE

DIANE E. MEIER, M.D.

The constants of the human condition are birth and death. No research, no new technology, no prayer, and no divine intervention has ever changed these defining characteristics of our species, and nothing we can foresee is likely to change them. But the nature of the experience—how we are born, how we die—has changed profoundly in the last several hundred years. For most of human history, death was a near random event, due to injury, infection, starvation, or childbirth. Humans were at least as likely to die during birth, infancy, childhood, or young adulthood as they were during middle age or old age. The meaning and the ritual attached to illness and death were predicated on this fact—death was common and unpredictable; it afflicted old and young and rich and poor alike; and it played a central role in the life of the community and the family.

Between 1900 and 2000, life expectancy in the United States rose from forty-seven to seventy-seven years—equivalent to the gain in longevity between the Stone Age, more than ten thousand years ago, and 1900. A gain of this magnitude in the relatively short evolutionary time frame of a century has had dramatic effects on the human experience of illness and dying and death. Where illness and death were once central and routine community experiences, with rituals designed to heal and to reintegrate the bereaved into new roles and new relationships, modern medicine and technological innovations have removed them from their place of gravity at the close of each life and have made them seem to be accidental and almost unseemly failures, associated with the belief that they could and should have been prevented.

Yet in the last two decades Americans have begun to recognize the limitations of technology and modern medicine in meeting the needs of the chronically and seriously ill, and also to fundamentally restructure the care that people require during the last years of their lives. These developments have spawned a new field of medicine called palliative care—from the Latin *palliare,* to clothe. Palliative care focuses on the relief of suffering for patients with serious and complex illness and tries to ensure the best possible quality of life for them and their family members. It is delivered at the same time as other appropriate curative and life-prolonging treatments and is not limited to the terminally ill. In this respect, it is not limited to hospice care, a component of palliative care focused on the care of the terminally ill who have opted to stop life-prolonging treatments.

Palliative care has grown rapidly in the United States in recent years and is now poised to become a universally available approach to meeting the needs of the country's sickest and most vulnerable patients. It is a central part of the solution to America's health care crisis, since it improves the quality of care and reduces costs for a key population—those with serious, complex illnesses who, while they number less than 10 percent of patients, account for more than two-thirds of health care spending.

This chapter examines the field of palliative care. It begins by exploring why the care of seriously ill patients has become such an important issue in the United States, and why the current health care system (or lack of a system) is unable to cope with it. It then looks at past efforts to provide care for dying people, the way that treatment of pain has evolved, and the growth of hospice care. This is followed by an analysis of legal, social, and political concerns and of the research that has highlighted the problems and offered potential solutions, many of which have been tested and launched by private philanthropy. Finally, it reports on the state of palliative care in America and offers some thoughts on its future.

CARE OF THE SERIOUSLY ILL: WHY IS IT AN IMPORTANT ISSUE?

The unprecedented growth in the numbers and the needs of the chronically ill, especially the elderly; the availability and widespread use of costly medical technologies that may prolong life without restoring health or functional independence; exponential cost increases due both to larger numbers of persons turning to the health care system for help and to per-capita increases in health care spending attributable to technological advances and overuse; the crippling impact of employer-based health insurance on the American economy and the lack of government control over rising drug and device pricing; the failure to recognize and treat the pain and other distressing symptoms experienced by seriously ill people; and the consequent widespread dissatisfaction with and confusion about the medical care system—all form the context and justification for attention to medical care of the seriously ill and those approaching the end of life and the rapid recent growth of the field of palliative care.

America Is Aging, and More People Are Living with and Suffering from Years of Chronic Illness

From the standpoint of sheer numbers, the population of the United States is aging, and the odds of living a long life and dying during old age are far better than they were a hundred years ago. The average baby born in the United States today can expect to live to age seventy-eight, despite the fact that the United States is ranked forty-second in the world in life expectancy at birth, behind Jordan, Guam, and the Cayman islands.[1] If a man survives to age seventy-five, he can expect to live ten years longer, on average; a woman living to age seventy-five can expect to live twelve years longer. As a result of this dramatic increase in longevity, about 20 percent of the American population will be over age sixty-five by 2030, as compared to less than 5 percent in 1900—a demographic shift unprecedented in human history, and one for which our society is unprepared. While many people died of acute infectious illness a century ago and for millennia before then, today the leading causes of death are chronic degenerative diseases such as heart failure, emphysema, stroke, dementia, and cancer—diseases with which people may live for years, and sometimes for decades, before they die.

During the twentieth century, the location of care for the dying shifted away from the home and into hospitals and nursing homes—institutional settings where more than 70 percent of American citizens now die. The reasons for this shift are complex and include financial incentives built into the health care system that favor institutional death as well as the burden that long-term chronic care of functionally dependent loved ones places on families.

In addition, the successes of modern public health and medical care have created an expectation that all illness can be treated, if not cured, and that *ipso facto,* with enough research, death itself is preventable. Hence family members' worry that if they had just gotten another opinion, searched a little harder on the Internet, or pushed for an experimental treatment, they could have forestalled decline and death. This anxiety is part of the reason for overuse of health care services, and for costly and burdensome medical care near life's end.

The Impact of Public Health Measures and Modern Medicine on Longevity

In the mid-nineteenth century, scientists began to develop the germ theory of disease based on observations of epidemic infections from unclean drinking water. The subsequent separation of drinking water from sewage led to dramatically reduced infant, child, and maternal mortality and a gain in life expectancy at birth from under fifty years at the start of the twentieth century to nearly eighty years at present. A smaller portion of the last century's dramatic thirty-year gain in life span can be attributed to the discovery of antibiotics and the widespread use of vaccination during World War II. Most of the century's gain in life expectancy predates the recent rise in preventive and high-technology medicine, such as the control of blood pressure and smoking and the effective treatment of heart disease, stroke, and cancer (see Figure 1).

Fully 75 percent of the gain in life expectancy occurring during the twentieth century is due to decreased mortality for persons under the age of forty, resulting in a much higher likelihood of living to old age. This large gain is both the context for and a contributor to our present challenge—how to understand the meaning of serious

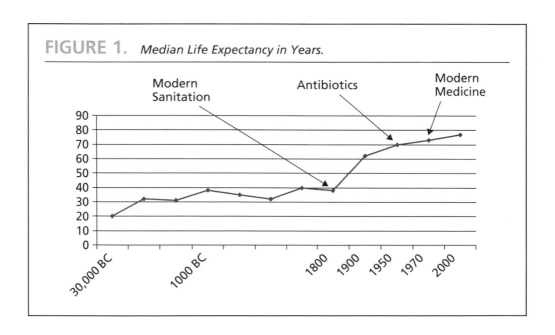

FIGURE 1. *Median Life Expectancy in Years.*

illness and death when it comes, and what our society owes us when we reach this stage in our lives.

Modern medical care and technology have also contributed to longevity in the United States. A recent study attributed roughly half of the 50 percent reduction in death from coronary heart disease during the last two decades in the United States to medical therapies and half to reductions in risk factors such as control of lipids, hypertension, and smoking.[2]

Consequences of an Aging Society The successes of public health and modern medical care have led to unprecedented growth in the number of older adults. The current generation of older people is healthier and less disabled than its predecessors, with additional gains in active life expectancy due to public health and biomedical research leading to new treatments for, and later onset of, chronic diseases.

But although the *proportion* of people with chronic disability is declining and more people are living longer and better, the sheer *number* of the elderly with chronic disability (seventy-seven million people will be over age sixty-five by 2040) means that an unprecedented number will experience prolonged functional dependency and frailty before they die. Some 57 percent of Americans age eighty and older report a severe disability.[3] The probability of needing help from another person to get through the day because of functional dependency increases with age; more than 40 percent of persons over sixty-five report at least one functional limitation, and more than 70 percent of those over age eighty require personal assistance with one or more of their everyday activities.[4] This functional impairment is due in great part to the rising prevalence of cognitive impairment after age sixty-five: more than 13 percent of the over-sixty-five population and 42 percent of those eighty-five or above have Alzheimer's disease, the most common cause of dementia (prevalence is even higher if vascular dementia is included), a number projected to rise by more than 50 percent by 2030 with the aging of the baby boom generation. Not surprisingly, and as an unintended consequence of modern medical successes, as death rates from heart disease, cancer, and stroke have declined in the last few years, Alzheimer's as a cause of death has skyrocketed, increasing by 33 percent between 2000 and 2004.

Caring for Seriously Ill People Is Very Costly

In 2007, health care spending in the United States reached $2.3 trillion (16.9 percent of the nation's gross domestic production, or GDP), and it is expected to reach $4.2 trillion by 2016 (20 percent of GDP).[5] Medicare spending (government health insurance for those over sixty-five and the disabled) is growing exponentially in tandem with the numbers, needs, and cost of care of its beneficiaries (see Figure 2).

Although nearly forty-six million Americans are uninsured, the United States spends roughly twice as much per person as other industrialized nations (more than $7,500 for every American, man, woman, and child), and those countries provide health insurance to all their citizens, and do so at under 11 percent of GDP (see Figure 3).

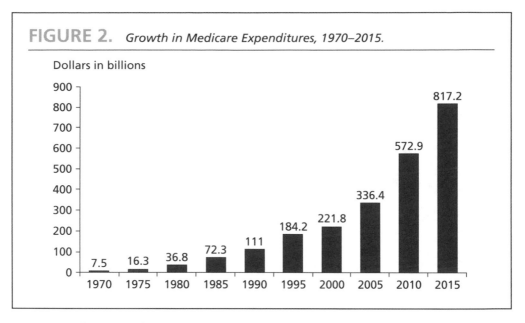

FIGURE 2. *Growth in Medicare Expenditures, 1970–2015.*

Note: Figures for 2010 and 2015 are projected.
Source: The Commonwealth Fund; Data from 2006 Medicare Trustees' Report.
Reprinted with permission.

Despite our high expenditures, a 2008 Commonwealth Fund survey of chronically ill adults in Australia, Canada, France, the Netherlands, New Zealand, the United Kingdom, and the United States found that U.S. patients are more likely to forgo needed care because of costs (54 percent), run into problems with care coordination (34 percent), and experience a significant medical error (34 percent).[6]

The primary factors driving these high costs are both intensity and pricing of service delivery—the United States uses more of the newest (and costliest) technologies and delivers various invasive procedures (such as magnetic resonance imaging and coronary bypass procedures) at a rate several times higher than other developed nations.

In addition, prices for medical care services in the United States are significantly higher than those in other countries (see Figure 4), and Americans spend five times as much per person ($486) as the OECD (Organization for Economic Cooperation and Development) median ($74) on health insurance and administrative costs.[7]

Individuals with five or more chronic illnesses are the largest consumers of health care and account for two-thirds of all Medicare spending. This patient population represents about 20 percent of all Medicare beneficiaries and is the group most likely to benefit from palliative care services (see Figure 5).

The costs associated with the number and expense of new life-prolonging technologies (such as kidney, heart, lung, and liver transplantation, implantable cardiac defibrillators, drug-eluting stents for coronary artery disease, ventricular assist devices, and new drugs to battle cancer) have risen dramatically. Medical ethicist Daniel Callahan

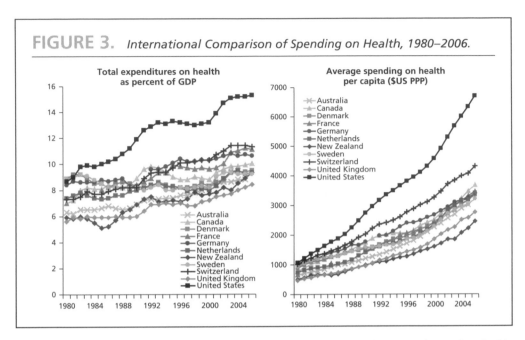

FIGURE 3. *International Comparison of Spending on Health, 1980–2006.*

Source: The Commonwealth Fund; Data from OECD Health Data 2008 (June 2008). Reprinted with permission.

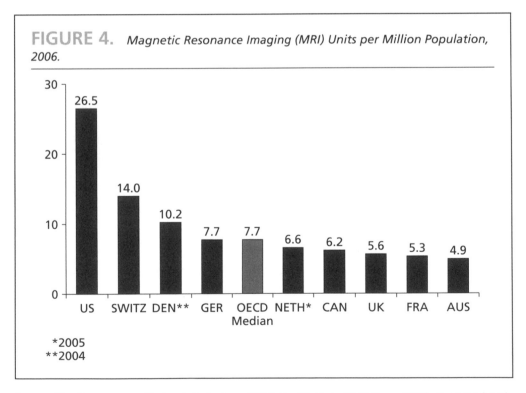

FIGURE 4. *Magnetic Resonance Imaging (MRI) Units per Million Population, 2006.*

Source: The Commonwealth Fund; Data from OECD Health Data 2008 (June 2008). Reprinted with permission.

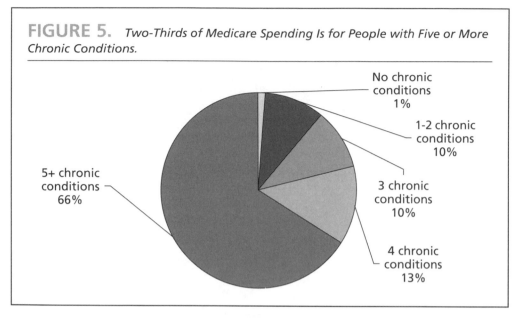

FIGURE 5. *Two-Thirds of Medicare Spending Is for People with Five or More Chronic Conditions.*

Source: The Commonwealth Fund; from G. Anderson and J. Horvath, *Chronic Conditions: Making the Case for Ongoing Care* (Baltimore, MD: Partnership for Solutions, December 2002). Reprinted with permission.

argues that the unquestioning commitment to medical progress, regardless of cost and no matter how marginal the benefit, threatens to swamp other social priorities, such as education, safe roads, clean air, and universal access to health care.[8] Despite the acknowledged critical nature of the problem, little or no social consensus exists on the distribution of our finite resources among social goods, or on the place of death as a necessary and appropriate part of a healthy life in a healthy society.

The fact is that these numbers pose a threat to American economic competitiveness in the world market, and the current world financial crisis may help create the social consensus necessary for a reexamination of the current model of health insurance in the United States and also of the built-in financial incentives favoring hospitalization, procedural care, and more specialist intervention in the system.

Dissatisfaction with Care of the Seriously Ill

Despite uniquely high per-capita expenditures, Americans with serious illness, their families, and their doctors and nurses are not satisfied with the care system. According to the 2006 *Health Confidence Survey,* dissatisfaction with the health care system, specifically how much it costs, has doubled since 1998, with 28 percent of respondents rating it fair and 31 percent rating it poor because of rapid growth in out-of-pocket expenses.[9] Of Americans responding to a national representative survey conducted by the Commonwealth Fund, 46 percent called for fundamental change and 30 percent for a complete rebuilding of the health care system; 42 percent reported experiencing inefficient, poorly coordinated, or unsafe care.[10] Among family members of Medicare decedents, substantial percentages reported inadequately treated pain (24 percent), inadequate emotional support (50 percent), and poor communication from physicians (30 percent); interestingly, the hospice care given at home was ranked excellent by more than 70 percent, compared with fewer than 50 percent of those whose family members had died in a hospital or a nursing home.[11]

EFFORTS TO COPE WITH DEATH AND PROVIDE CARE FOR THE DYING

I don't want to achieve immortality through my work.
I want to achieve it by not dying.

Woody Allen

A Brief History

In *The Hour of Our Death,* published in 1981, author Philippe Ariès described death and the history of Western attitudes toward it as both a communal and an individual act, associated with the ritual and ceremony of any major life milestone.[12] These rituals have been transformed in the last hundred years by the simultaneous decline of religious faith in many Western nations and the advent of the scientific revolution. The key components of this rite of passage are the individual's role in the acceptance of his coming death; the opportunity to say goodbye; and the period of mourning and bereavement. Ariès divides his study into four overlapping historical periods: "The Tame Death," "The Death of the Self," "The Death of the Other," and "The Invisible Death."

The Tame Death roughly corresponds with pre-Christian through the early Middle Ages. Death was central, routine, and unpredictable and was tamed through social rituals and codes of behavior. From earliest recorded history, death was a central and common part of the life and rites of the community—*"rites in the bedroom or those of the oldest liturgy express the conviction that the life of a man is not an individual destiny but a link in an unbroken chain, the biological continuation of a family or a line that begins with Adam and includes the whole human race. The community was weakened by the loss of one of its members . . . it had to recover its strength and unity by means of ceremonies . . . death was not a personal drama but an ordeal for the community, which was responsible for maintaining the continuity of the race."*

The Death of the Self begins in the Middle Ages, when mendicant Christian orders worked to convert a quasi-pagan population, with a corresponding rise in individuals' fears about their own death and an afterlife of punishment for sin. A change in attitude developed with the rise in the sense of individual fate as opposed to collective destiny—an individual destiny in an afterlife that could be secured by good behavior, prayer, simony (purchase of divine favor), and control of what happens after death through the use of wills and testaments.

The Death of the Other corresponds to the subsequent (post-Middle Ages) rise in the centrality of the family and a few intimate relationships, and the associated Romantic Movement (the deathbed scene, *ars moriendi* [the art of dying], weeping, drama). After the Middle Ages, the rise of intimate family relationships replaced the community as the primary seat of loyalty and personal survival. The rise of the family, with the associated realization that there is good and bad in each person, reduced both the conceivability and the acceptability of punishment for sin through hell and eternal damnation and encouraged a vision of permanent reunion with loved ones after death.

Arguing that death has been banished as an unacceptable and unendurable truth in our own century, Ariès describes the Invisible Death, our current phase, as a period where death is unconsciously or theoretically believed to be avoidable with enough investment in research—an expectation strengthened by the successes of public health and modern medicine in allowing, for the first time in human history, most people in Western societies to live to old age. If the presumption is that science can defeat death, each death that does occur requires explanation, is something that could theoretically have been prevented, and hence must reflect a failure—a failure of the family to find the right doctor; of the patient to take proper care of himself or herself; of the doctors to know the latest protocols; of the hospital to prevent the unpreventable; of society to invest adequately in research. Despite the fact that over 80 percent of Americans report a religious affiliation, someone or something under human control must be to blame if death is preventable.

If death is avoidable and therefore a failure, it is unsuitable for everyday life—stigmatized, hidden, and avoided in polite conversation. Since each of us still dies, each person (and the family) may come to experience his or her own dying and death as a mistake, something that could have been prevented, a personal failing, or someone else's fault—in a word, wrong.

Combining the stigma of death with the widely held belief that modern medicine and hospitals can perform miracles in the battle against death, the hospital and the nursing home have become the dominant sites for gravely ill, dying people (more than 70 percent of deaths in the United States occur in an institution). The health care institution offers families a break from the work of caring for a seriously ill person, a place to hide from prying eyes, and a respite from the shame and failure implicit in the dying process. The hospital is believed to have the professionals and the technology necessary to defeat disease and keep death at bay. The modern ritual of death involves several prolonged stays in a hospital—often in an intensive-care unit. This ritual allows the family to say to their friends and neighbors, "We did everything possible, we got the best care possible;" to keep the concrete and physically distressing aspects of the illness at a controlled and safe distance; and to avoid being labeled as a friend of death because of the acceptance of death. The physician becomes the agent of his society—battling death is the *raison d'être* of modern medicine.

Tolstoy was among the first to write about the stigma of death in his great novella *The Death of Ivan Ilych*. Ilych, a middle-class government functionary, is dying of cancer, but no one tells him the truth. His doctors and family all talk around the illness with euphemism, and the patient, desperate for genuine human relationship, experienced even greater suffering due to their denial of death's reality.

> *What tormented Ivan Ilych was the lie, this lie that for some reason they all accepted, that he was only sick and not dying, and that if he would only remain calm and take care of himself, everything would be fine; whereas he knew very well that no matter what was done the result would be only worse suffering and death. He suffered because no one was willing to admit what everyone, including himself, could see clearly. He suffered because they lied and forced him to take part in this deception. This lie that was being told on the eve of his death, that degraded the formidable and solemn act of his death . . . had become horribly painful to Ivan Ilych.*
>
> Leo Tolstoy, "The Death of Ivan Ilych"[13]

Hiding from the indecency of death extends to the mourning process. By the mid-twentieth century, the traditional community mourning rituals and codes of behavior that not only reintegrated the bereaved back into the world of the living but that also helped the group recover from the threat of death and loss in their midst—wearing black, avoiding social events—had all but disappeared in the United States and other developed nations. The loss of these codes and rituals of bereavement in the last two centuries has left us with little protection from the terror of nature and death. Hence the modern tendency to repress references to death and to suppress evidence of mourning. As Geoffrey Gorer wrote in *Death, Grief, and Mourning in Contemporary Britain*:

> *At present death and mourning are treated with much the same prudery as the sexual impulses were a century ago . . . Today it would seem to be believed, quite sincerely, that sensible rational men and women can keep their mourning under complete control by strength of will and character, so that it need be given no public expression, and, if indulged at all, in private, as furtively as if it were an analogue of masturbation.[14]*

Not only have the dying person and the grieving survivor been effectively banished from mainstream society but the reality of death itself has become taboo. It is treated as a contagious disease, something to avoid and to protect one's children from. Reaction against the stigma and the isolation of the dying that accompanied the view of death as somehow optional or preventable is the foundation of the hospice and, subsequently, palliative care movements in the United States.

Growth in the Use of Opioids for Treatment of Pain

Pain is a more terrible lord of mankind than even death himself.
Albert Schweitzer, 1922[15]

It has no future but itself.
Emily Dickinson, 1896[16]

*Pope John Paul II has issued an apostolic letter on suffering
in which he says physical, mental and moral pain pose a
mystery that can lead to spiritual growth and salvation.*
Kenneth A. Briggs, *The New York Times*, 1984

Through much of the nineteenth century, pain was viewed as God's punishment for sin and a means of spiritual purification through suffering; it was felt to have healing power in and of itself. Invoking the biblical injunction "In sorrow, thou shalt bring forth children" (Genesis 3:16) as justification, some believed that the pain of childbirth was necessary to transform women into appropriately self-sacrificing mothers. Morphine was first isolated from crude opium in 1803, though opium and its derivatives had been used for millennia. Queen Victoria began using general anesthesia during childbirth in 1853. By the late 1880s, surgical anesthesia was widespread, and an increased demand for surgery transformed hospitals from charitable asylums for the poor and the dying into purveyors of cures and the relief of suffering from disease.

The neurological underpinnings of pain were first studied in the late 1800s, and by the mid-twentieth century pain was understood as the body's warning to avoid injury. "The evolutionary purpose of pain was no longer to heal, to punish, or to ennoble, but to provide a mechanical warning of actual or potential damage to cells and tissues in a specific body area," according to the noted pain researcher Raymond Houde.[17] The twentieth century also saw the earliest efforts to measure and assess pain in humans, and to attempt quantitative study of the effectiveness of analgesics. Henry Knowles Beecher, at Harvard, wrote about the inextricable role of emotion in the experience of pain in 1959, and he, Raymond Houde, at Memorial Sloan-Kettering Cancer Center, and Cicely Saunders, at St. Christopher's Hospice in London, conducted the fundamental studies of opioid analgesia that led to modern opioid pharmacotherapy. Modern opioid pharmacology includes listening to the patient as the best source of information about pain intensity and impact. "I found that I got the same answer from just asking the patient as I did by going through a long series of testing," Houde said. It also includes keeping pain under steady control with scheduled dosing (rather than waiting for a pain crisis before offering analgesia) and having "rescue doses" available to relieve unpredictable or breakthrough pain.[18]

> *Perhaps few persons who are not physicians can realize the influence which long-continued and unendurable pain may have on both body and mind . . . Under such torments the temper changes, the most amiable grow irritable, the bravest soldier becomes a coward.*
>
> S. Weir Mitchell, M.D., 1872[19]

Understanding that chronic pain is actually harmful to the organism, as opposed to merely an unpleasant side effect of disease, was recognized as early as the 1870s and was well established by the middle of the twentieth century. John C. Liebeskind, a noted pain researcher at UCLA, provided evidence that pain actually leads to measurable immunosuppression and associated increased risk of death from cancer and other diseases. In 1943, W. K. Livingston wrote in *Pain Mechanisms,* "Pain is a sensory experience that is subjective and individual; it frequently exceeds its protective function and becomes destructive . . . If such disturbances are permitted to continue, profound and perhaps unalterable organic changes may result in the affected part . . . A vicious circle is thus created."[20]

Chronic pain is a symptom of many conditions and affects 76.2 million Americans, more than diabetes, heart disease, and cancer combined. Pain is a significant national health problem and is the leading cause of disability, suffering, and impaired quality of life.[21] It is the most common reason individuals seek medical care, accounting for up to 80 percent of doctor visits.[22] More than 25 percent of people in the United States report having had a chronic pain condition at some point in their life,[23] and the associated disability is a major liability for workers, employers, and society. More than 70 percent of cancer survivors have significant pain, and fewer than 50 percent of these report receiving adequate treatment.[24]

In hospitalized and seriously ill patients, pain has been associated with increased length of stay, longer recovery time, and poorer patient outcomes, all of which have implications for health care quality and cost.[25] A study of the experience of 9,105 seriously ill patients at five major American teaching hospitals reported moderate to severe pain in half of conscious patients during the last three days of life.[26]

Both patients and physicians agree about the extent of the problem of untreated pain. In a 1993 survey, 88 percent of physicians treating cancer patients reported that their own training in pain management was fair to poor; and 86 percent admitted that their patients were undermedicated for pain.[27] Racial minorities, the poor, patients with HIV-AIDS, women, and the elderly are all less likely than white males to receive appropriate pain treatment.[28]

Translation of the growing body of evidence that pain is bad for your health, and that relief of pain improves clinical outcomes, into routine clinical practice falls short. The multidisciplinary pain clinic has emerged as the standard of practice, utilizing a range of approaches including pharmacology, physical therapy, behavioral therapies, acupuncture, hypnosis, and family education. Many Americans cannot, however, get insurance coverage for modern comprehensive multidisciplinary pain programs, and this has reduced access to and availability of these services in many communities.[29]

DEBORAH'S STORY

Deborah, as I'll call her, is a thirty-seven-year-old mother of three young children, a practicing psychotherapist, and a breast cancer survivor. Despite state-of-the-art treatment from the best oncologists in New York City, her cancer spread to her bones, causing progressive and severe pain. Her oncologists focused on administration of chemotherapy and suggested ibuprofen and Tylenol, neither of which helped. Her pain got so bad that she was unable to take care of her kids and had to stop going to work. She spent most of her time curled on her side in bed, since the pain was much worse if she moved. She has been to the emergency room twice for the pain, but the doctors there were willing to give her only six tablets of Tylenol with codeine. When these were gone, she left messages for her oncologist, but three days later she had not received a call back. In desperation, she called her obstetrician, who referred her to a palliative care doctor. Her sister and her husband got her to the appointment and she was begun on oral morphine liquid in the office, with dose adjustments until the pain was reduced from 10 out of a possible 10 to 5 out of a possible 10 (with 0 being no pain and 10 being the worst imaginable pain). She went home with instructions for around-the-clock and rescue doses of the analgesic. Within three days, her pain was down to 2 out of a possible 10, and she was able to return to her family and work responsibilities and continue her pursuit of effective treatments for her breast cancer. Deborah wonders how she got through her illness without this kind of help, and she thinks that every patient with cancer should have not only an oncologist but also a palliative care doctor to manage all aspects of their illness.

The Hospice Movement

Origins and Growth The term "hospice"—from the Latin *hospitium,* the same linguistic root as "hospitality"—denotes a place to host, receive, and entertain guests or strangers. The term can be traced to medieval times, when it referred to a place of shelter and rest for weary or ill travelers. The original hospices, from the fourth to eleventh centuries, were houses of rest and shelter for pilgrims and crusaders traveling to and from the Holy Land; these hospices were usually kept by religious orders.

The earliest hospitals and hospices were one entity, again based in the church. St. Bartholomew's Hospital, in London, was founded in 1123 and became a secular hospital in 1546 "for the ayde and comforte of the poore, sykke, blynde, aged, and impotent persones beying not hable to helpe themselffs nor havyinh any place certeyn whereyn they may be lodged, cherysshed, or refreshed, tyll they be cured and holpen of theyre diseases and syknesse," wrote a surgeon, in a letter to Henry the Eighth.[30] During the eighteenth and nineteenth centuries, religious orders established hospices to care for the dying in France, Ireland, and London. One of these—St. Joseph's Hospice for the Dying Poor, established by the Irish Sisters of Charity—was Cicely Saunders's first exposure to hospice care.

The modern hospice movement began with a few middle-aged women determined to bring attention to the medical and emotional abandonment of the dying: Cicely Saunders in London, Florence Wald in New Haven, and Elisabeth Kübler-Ross in Chicago. Building on the grassroots work of volunteers and religious orders who stepped up to care for dying people, these three women together were able to bring professional and public attention to the societal abandonment of the dying and their families: Saunders through the establishment of St. Christopher's Hospice in London and the conduct of research and education in the clinical setting; Wald, under Saunders's tutelage, established the first American hospice, in Branford, Connecticut; and Kübler-Ross by writing the revolutionary *On Death and Dying*.[31]

Saunders, who died in 2005, was a nurse, a social worker, and a physician. She is the acknowledged founder of the modern hospice and palliative care movements. In 1967, she launched the modern hospice movement by founding St. Christopher's Hospice. She mandated the inclusion of education and research as a core component of the mission of St. Christopher's and was one of a few pioneering researchers in the effective management of pain with opioid analgesics. "It appears that many patients feel deserted by their doctors at the end. Ideally, the doctor should remain the centre of a team who work together to relieve where they cannot heal, to keep the patient's own struggle within his compass, and to bring hope and consolation to the end," she wrote.[32]

Saunders visited Yale University in 1963 and gave a lecture to medical students, nurses, social workers, and chaplains on the concept of specialized care for the dying. Her lecture included before-and-after photos of cancer patients and their families, showing dramatic differences after good symptom control. Upon the invitation of Florence Wald, then dean of Yale's School of Nursing, Saunders returned to Yale as a visiting professor in 1965. In 1968 Wald took a sabbatical at St. Christopher's, returning to America to initiate the modern American hospice movement.

> *The greatest fear of the dying and their families is the fear of pain. Sadly, this fear has often been justified. Terminal pain is frequently treated ineptly and the public myth that death from cancer involves unremitting distress is perpetuated. There are many reasons why terminal pain has been so poorly controlled. Until recently, the care of the dying has rarely been included in the training of doctors and nurses. With a few notable exceptions, medical and surgical textbooks have ignored the problems of pain control.*
>
> Cicely Saunders, 1995[33]

After studying the work of both Cicely Saunders and Elisabeth Kübler-Ross, Florence Schorske Wald established the Connecticut Hospice in 1974. This entity provided both home and inpatient care and served as a stimulus to the development of hospices across the United States. In an interview she said, "Hospice care for the terminally ill is the end piece of how to care for patients from birth on. It is a patient-family–based approach to health care that belongs in the community with natural childbirth, school-based health care, mental health care, and adult care . . . As more and more people—families of hospice patients and hospice volunteers—are exposed to this new model of how to approach end-of-life care, we are taking what was essentially a hidden scene, death, an unknown, and making it a reality. We are showing people that there are meaningful ways to cope with this very difficult situation."[34]

An international best-seller, Elisabeth Kübler-Ross's *On Death and Dying* brought attention to the Western "death-denying" culture and her theory about the five stages of grief (denial, anger, bargaining, depression, and acceptance) that a dying person typically goes through.[35] Articulating an early version of what today would be called "patient-centered care," she said in a 1975 radio interview, "The question is really, 'What does it mean to die with dignity?' To die with dignity to me means to die within your character. That means there are people who have used denial all their life long; they will most likely die in a stage of denial. There are people who have been fighters and rebels all their life long, and, by golly, they want to die that way. And to those patients, we have to help them, to say it's O.K."[36]

Financing Hospice Care A Department of Health, Education, and Welfare (HEW) task force reported in 1978 that "the hospice movement as a concept for the care of the terminally ill and their families is a viable concept and one which holds out a means of providing more humane care for Americans dying of terminal illness while possibly reducing costs. As such, it is the proper subject of federal support." This was followed by funding of a demonstration program in 1979, the creation of a Medicare hospice benefit in 1982, and the establishment of eligibility criteria in 1986 meant to control costs by trying to restrict access. Specifically, eligibility for federal reimbursement of hospice care requires that two physicians certify that the patient will die within six months "if the disease runs its normal course" and that the patient agrees to give up regular insurance coverage for life-prolonging treatments related to the terminal illness. In part as a consequence of these criteria, hospice became associated with "giving up" the fight for life in the minds of both the public and health professionals.

The Current Status of Hospice Care As the number and the needs of the chronically ill elderly have grown in the United States, the number of hospice providers grew by more than 30 percent between 1997 and 2007 (see Figure 6). In 2007, an estimated 1.4 million patients were cared for in a hospice, accounting for approximately 39 percent of all deaths in the United States, a number that has steadily increased in the last decade. Overall family satisfaction with hospice care is high, with 75 percent rating care received as excellent. Reasons for growth in hospice utilization are many and include a rise in hospice services in nursing homes, growth in the population living with advanced and end-stage chronic diseases, and greater recognition of and familiarity with the benefits of hospice care. Growth of this magnitude is accompanied by quality

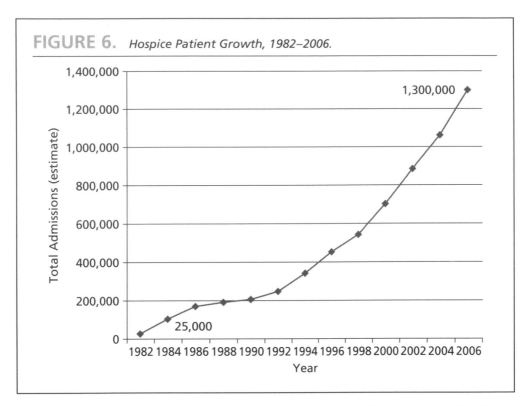

FIGURE 6. *Hospice Patient Growth, 1982–2006.*

Source: National Hospice and Palliative Care Organization; hospice data (2008). Reprinted with permission.

challenges. Much of the recent increase in hospice providers involved small for-profit hospice organizations. Delivering high-quality care to seriously ill patients with complex conditions requires some financial economies of scale that are impossible to achieve by small hospices serving few patients. Only 16.2 percent of American hospices serve more than a hundred patients per day. Despite regulatory concerns about the rise in the numbers of patients turning to hospice and the increasing length of stay for some hospice patients, recent data demonstrate substantial cost savings to Medicare (averaging $2,309 per patient) among hospice patients served for several months, depending upon the diagnosis.[37]

Referral to hospice tends to occur late in the dying process, when prognostication becomes more reliable. Length of stay in the hospice program has held steady at a median of 20.6 days, and approximately one-third of patients live for less than a week after their admission to hospice. More than half of hospice patients have terminal illnesses other than cancer and over two-thirds were over age seventy-five in 2006. About three-quarters of hospice patients die in their homes, whether they are residing in a nursing home (23 percent) or a private residence (47 percent).[38]

The Medicare Hospice Benefit and the "Failure to Die" Syndrome The link between prognosis and eligibility for hospice care has its roots in the care of patients with advanced malignancies. The typical course for such cancer patients involves an acceptable quality of life and functional status until several months before death, whereupon fatigue, weakness, and other symptoms predominate. Once a patient with metastatic solid tumor malignancy loses functional independence and becomes debilitated, a prognosis can reliably be estimated at three to four months. Although modern anticancer and supportive therapies have lengthened survival during advanced stages of illness, this link between declining function and short prognosis led to designation of the six-month criterion for eligibility for Medicare funding of hospice care.

For many cancer patients, this point of transition from functional independence to dependence remains a reasonably reliable marker of prognosis. But only 23 percent of Americans die of cancer, and for the remaining 77 percent of people who die from other diseases, functional status and debility are not good predictors of prognosis. In fact, patients in these disease categories can live for years with serious functional impairment and painful symptoms. The personal care and assistance they require can result in a substantial burden on their families and society at large. Not surprisingly, patients most likely to be referred for hospice are those placing the highest burden on family caregivers.[39]

The referral of chronically ill noncancer patients to hospice for their palliative care needs has led to what has been named the "failure to die on time" phenomenon. Because of the difficulty of predicting how long patients, especially those with noncancer diseases such as dementia and end-stage heart disease (the leading cause of death in the United States), will live, and the fact that many of these patients live longer than the six months that Medicare expects to cover, the use of the hospice benefit for patients who "fail to die on time" has received federal government scrutiny for possible fraud and misuse. Since the Medicare criteria were designed to limit access to the hospice benefit to patients who were clearly dying and to prohibit double dipping—getting high-tech expensive modern life-prolonging care while simultaneously receiving sophisticated and coordinated hospice care at home—the argument is that reimbursing hospice care for patients who live on despite their significant impairments is a misapplication of a benefit intended to care for the dying.

According to the *New York Times,* "Over the last eight years, the refusal of patients to die according to actuarial schedules has led the federal government to demand that hospices exceeding reimbursement limits repay hundreds of millions of dollars to Medicare . . . [As a result,] hundreds of hospice providers across the country are facing the catastrophic financial consequence of what would otherwise seem a positive development: their patients are living longer than expected."[40] The risk of fraud and abuse allegations and the possibility of receiving a large fine have led many hospices to reduce access for seriously ill patients with unclear prognoses. The majority of these patients are hospitalized repeatedly during the months before their death.[41]

TIMELINE

1963: Cicely Saunders lectures at Yale University.

1965: At the invitation of Florence Wald, then dean of the Yale School of Nursing, Saunders becomes a visiting faculty member of the school.

1968: Wald takes a sabbatical from Yale to work at St. Christopher's and learn about hospice.

1969: *On Death and Dying,* based on more than five hundred interviews with dying patients, is published. Written by Dr. Elisabeth Kübler-Ross, a faculty member of the University of Chicago's School of Medicine, the book identifies five stages through which many terminally ill patients progress. The book becomes an internationally known best-seller. Kübler-Ross makes a plea for home care as opposed to treatment in an institutional setting and argues that patients should have a choice and the ability to participate in the decisions that affect their destiny.

1972: Kübler-Ross testifies at the first national hearings on the subject of death with dignity, which are conducted by the Senate Special Committee on Aging. In her testimony, Kübler-Ross states, "We live in a very particular death-denying society. We isolate both the dying and the old, and it serves a purpose. They are reminders of our own mortality. We should not institutionalize people. We can give families more help with home care and visiting nurses, giving the families and the patients the spiritual, emotional, and financial help in order to facilitate the final care at home."

1974: The first American hospice, the Connecticut Hospice Institute, is established in Branford, Connecticut, by Wald and colleagues.

1975: The first comprehensive palliative medicine program is established at the Royal Victoria Hospital in Montreal by Balfour Mount. Mount coined the term "palliative care."

1976: The New Jersey Supreme Court rules, in the case of Karen Ann Quinlan, that ventilator therapy may be withdrawn from a young woman in a persistent vegetative state. The court rules that decisions to continue or withdraw life support should be guided by evidence of the patient's preferences or wishes. The Quinlan decision leads to the widespread use of hospital ethics committees and advance care planning.

1976: The International Congress on Palliative Care holds its first meeting, in Montreal.

1978: A Department of Health, Education, and Welfare task force reports that "the hospice movement as a concept for the care of the terminally ill and their families is a viable concept and one which holds out a means of providing more humane care for Americans dying of terminal illness while possibly reducing costs. As such, it is the proper subject of federal support."

Continued

Continued

1979: The federal Health Care Financing Administration initiates demonstration programs at twenty-six hospices across the country to assess the cost-effectiveness of hospice care and to help determine what a hospice is and what it should provide.

1980: The W. K. Kellogg Foundation awards a grant to the Joint Commission on Accreditation of Healthcare Organizations (JCAHO, now the Joint Commission) to investigate the status of hospice and to develop standards for hospice accreditation.

1982: Congress includes a provision to create a Medicare hospice benefit in the Tax Equity and Fiscal Responsibility Act of 1982, with a 1986 sunset provision.

1983: JCAHO initiates hospice accreditation.

1986: The Medicare hospice benefit is made permanent by Congress and hospices are given a 10 percent increase in reimbursement rates. In an effort to control costs by reducing access, criteria for eligibility for hospice care include (1) physician certification of a prognosis of under six months and (2) patient agreement to give up insurance coverage for medical care focused on cure or life-prolonging treatments.

1987: The first American academic hospital palliative care program is established by Declan Walsh at the Cleveland Clinic, designated a World Health Organization Demonstration Project in 1991 in recognition of "its unique model of a much needed service."

1990: The U. S. Supreme Court recognizes in the case of Nancy Cruzan—a young woman in a persistent vegetative state receiving artificial nutrition and hydration by feeding tube—a patient's rights to refuse unwanted treatment if his or her wishes have been expressed in a "clear and convincing" way. The decision leads to a federal law, the Patient Self-Determination Act, requiring hospitals and other health care settings to counsel patients about their right to complete an advance directive stating their wishes for future care under circumstances of cognitive impairment.

1994: Oregon's Death with Dignity Act passes on a ballot measure, legalizing access to physician-assisted suicide for patients meeting eligibility criteria.

1996: The Ninth Circuit Court of Appeals in San Francisco overrules a Washington state law against physician-assisted suicide. The Second Circuit Court of Appeals strikes down New York State's law against physician-assisted suicide. Both rulings are appealed to the Supreme Court.

1997: Congress passes legislation barring taxpayer dollars from financing physician-assisted suicide. The Supreme Court rules that mentally competent terminally ill people do not have a constitutional right to physician-assisted suicide, leaving the issue up to the states. Oregon voters reaffirm the right to physician-assisted suicide by passing for the second time the Death with Dignity Act.

1997: The Institute of Medicine issues an influential report, *Approaching Death: Improving Care at the End of Life.*

2001: The National Consensus Project for Quality Palliative Care, a foundation-funded initiative to develop guidelines and standards for palliative care clinical programs, is established. Its members consist of the five major national palliative care organizations in the United States: the American Academy of Hospice and Palliative Medicine, the Center to Advance Palliative Care, the Hospice and Palliative Nurses Association, the Last Acts Partnership, and the National Hospice and Palliative Care Organization.

2004: The National Consensus Project for Quality Palliative Care issues consensus guidelines.

2005: Terri Schiavo was a young Florida woman in a persistent vegetative state from 1990. Her husband and guardian petitioned the court to remove her feeding tube based on prior evidence of her wishes. Her parents contested this, triggering a widely publicized eight-year legal and political battle. The tube is removed in 2005, and Terri dies thirteen days later amid intense protest from right-to-life activists.

2006: In October, the American Board of Medical Specialties (ABMS) announces approval of the creation of hospice and palliative medicine as a subspecialty of ten participating member boards. The co-sponsoring boards include the American Boards of Internal Medicine, Anesthesiology, Family Medicine, Physical Medicine and Rehabilitation, Psychiatry and Neurology, Surgery, Pediatrics, Emergency Medicine, Radiology, and Obstetrics and Gynecology.

2007: Building on the National Consensus Project guidelines, the National Quality Forum establishes its *National Framework and Preferred Practices for Palliative and Hospice Care.*

2008: The first ABMS-recognized hospice and palliative medicine board-certifying examination is offered. The Accreditation Council for Graduate Medical Education approves program requirements for fellowship training in hospice and palliative medicine.

2008: The state of Washington becomes the second state to pass a ballot measure legalizing physician-assisted suicide, a measure modeled closely on Oregon's Death with Dignity Act.

In part as a consequence of this cure-versus-care mentality codified in the Medicare hospice benefit, medical care is falsely but widely understood to have two mutually exclusive goals: either to cure disease and prolong life or to provide comfort care. Consequently, the decision to focus on reducing suffering is typically made only after life-prolonging treatment has been ineffectual or disproportionately burdensome and death is imminent. The either/or nature of this choice is driven largely by the reimbursement system; that is, regular Medicare and other insurers cover curative therapies and the Medicare hospice benefit covers comfort care. The false dichotomy built into U.S. health care financing of hospice—cure *versus* care, not both—led to the phenomenon of hospice referral too late to secure its benefits and has been a spur to the growth of nonhospice palliative care in the United States in the last ten years.

SOCIAL, LEGAL, AND ETHICAL CONCERNS LEADING TO CHANGE IN THE CARE OF PERSONS WITH SERIOUS ILLNESS

The decades of the 1980s and 1990s followed the introduction of new medical technologies, the shift away from home and into hospitals for the care of serious illness, and the medicalization of serious illness and the dying process. The excesses of the "technology imperative"—if the technology exists, we must use it—led to public and legal reaction manifested by a rise in the field of medical ethics and the "right to die" movement. A number of legal cases focused debate on a series of ethical principles in conflict: the sanctity of life versus the right to control what is done to one's own body; medical paternalism versus self-determination; and distributive justice versus self-determination.

The fundamental principles that had guided the practice of medicine—relieve suffering, do no harm—were upended by the seemingly limitless ability of modern medical technology to prolong life. Almost without discussion, the primary moral principle underlying medical practice became the obligation to prolong life regardless of the toll in suffering, poor quality of life, or cost. Hence the unforgettable first day of my internship in 1977, spent subjecting an eighty-nine-year-old man with end-stage heart failure to repeated resuscitation attempts in the coronary care unit. The message was clear—my job as a physician was to prolong life for as long as possible regardless of the cost in suffering and resources, and regardless of the likelihood of benefit. Other messages, equally powerful and similarly unstated, were conveyed when no one on the team stopped to speak with the patient's eighty-seven-year-old wife after he died; no one asked me how I was handling this violent death of one of my patients on my first day as a real doctor; and there was no pause to talk about why we had done this and what the pros and cons of this kind of medical care might be. The gravity and profundity of the ending of his life were neither acknowledged nor honored.

> *Because of Nancy [Cruzan], I suspect hundreds of thousands of people can rest free, knowing that when death beckons, they can meet it face-to-face with dignity, free from the fear of unwanted and useless medical treatment. I think this is quite an accomplishment for a twenty-five-year-old kid.*
>
> Lester "Joe" Cruzan, Nancy Cruzan's father, 1990

Informed Consent and Medical Decision Making: The Right to Refuse Unwanted Medical Treatment

The indiscriminate application of life-prolonging technologies and a series of dramatic legal cases challenging this practice led to a new organizing principle—respect for patients' wishes—as a counterbalance to the medical paternalism driving efforts to prolong life, regardless of its quality or the suffering imposed by the process. The earliest attempts to put the brakes on the reflexive use of medical technology involved the affirmation of the right of people to refuse unwanted medical treatments, based on the fundamental right of persons to control what is done to their own bodies. In 1960, the Kansas Supreme Court in *Natanson v. Kline* wrote, "Anglo-American law starts with the premise of thoroughgoing self-determination." The legal principle of informed consent by which patients accept or reject an offered therapy (based on communication about and understanding of its risks, benefits, and alternatives, and on deliberation and decision in the context of personal values and preferences) grew out of this principle of patient self-determination. In essence, patients have the right to refuse unwanted medical treatment. The application of the principle of informed consent in medical decision making was articulated in a series of influential court decisions.

Case law, reinforced by state legislation, set out the current legal requirements for providing, withholding, or withdrawing life-sustaining treatments. The principles, in general, require evidence of the patient's wishes. These can be expressed directly by the patient, or, if he or she has lost the capacity to express a decision (for example, if the patient is in a coma), through the "substituted judgment" of a surrogate decision maker. Surrogates can be designated by the patient when well through a health care proxy or a durable power of attorney. Alternatively, surrogates may invoke their knowledge of the patient's wishes based on past conversations, written documents such as living wills, or, in lieu of such information, on the surrogate's assessment of what is in the best interests of the patient.

Advance Directives

Advance directives are a means for a person who can make rational decisions to anticipate and control future medical decisions under circumstances of diminished capacity. Advance directives are formal and legally recognized mechanisms to express one's wishes for future care, and include:

- Do-not-resuscitate (DNR) orders, which specify the circumstances under which a patient does not wish attempted resuscitation.

- Living wills, which contain an expression of the person's values—values that should guide decisions to provide or withhold treatment under circumstances of life-threatening illness and loss of decisional capacity.

- Health care proxies and durable powers of attorney, which designate a trusted person to make decisions about medical treatment if a patient is not able to do so. The appointed proxy or agent is supposed to represent the patient's (and not his or her own) wishes and values.

The Patient Self-Determination Act, enacted by Congress in 1990, mandates federally funded institutions (which include almost all hospitals and nursing homes) to provide state-specific written information about advance directives and to record the presence of such directives. There is no requirement for doctors or nurses to conduct these conversations, and the result in many places has been the delivery of a piece of paper (with no counseling) to the patient by an admitting clerk. Because of this, the act has had little effect on advance care planning.

SEMINAL CASE LAW ON THE RIGHT TO DIE

Karen Ann Quinlan: In 1975, this twenty-one-year-old was in a persistent vegetative state after loss of consciousness. Her parents requested the discontinuation of her ventilator after several months without improvement. The hospital refused, and legal battles ensued. The Quinlans invoked the Catholic moral theology teaching that "extraordinary means" are not required to preserve a patient's life, defined as placing an undue burden that is beyond basics needed for "ordinary" sustenance of life (air, food, water, hygiene, dignity). The New Jersey Supreme Court, quoting extensively from a 1957 address by Pope Pius XII, ruled in favor of the parents, and the ventilator was withdrawn. Quinlan lived nine more years, until 1985, with artificial nutrition and hydration via a feeding tube. This case and its aftermath led directly to the establishment of formal ethics committees in hospitals, nursing homes, and hospices, and to the development of the legal underpinnings of advance health directives.

Nancy Cruzan: In 1983, this twenty-five-year-old was thrown from her car and survived in a persistent vegetative state after resuscitation. After four years with no improvement, her parents requested removal of the feeding tube, but the hospital demanded a court order. Since food and water did not meet the extraordinary measures standard established in *Quinlan,* the Missouri courts refused to provide such an order. Their decision was upheld by the United States Supreme Court, which recognized the right of a person to refuse unwanted medical treatment and articulated a standard that "clear and convincing" evidence of the person's previously stated wishes was needed for a court to authorize withholding of medical treatment. After three friends of Cruzan's came forward with "clear and convincing" evidence of her wishes, a Missouri court gave permission to remove the tube, and it was removed in 1990. Cruzan died twelve days later, amid protests from the pro-life activist group Operation Rescue. The Cruzan case led to the development of federal law requiring that all hospitals and nursing homes inform their patients about advance directives and give them the opportunity to complete one. Almost all states have laws governing decisions to withhold or withdraw life-sustaining treatments, living wills, health care proxies, and durable powers of attorney. Nancy Cruzan's grave marker reads "Born July 20, 1957 / Departed January 11, 1983 / At Peace December 26, 1990."

Terri Schiavo: In 1990 this twenty-six-year-old suffered a cardiac arrest at home. She was resuscitated to a persistent vegetative state. Eight years later, her husband and guardian requested withdrawal of the feeding tube. Terri had no living will, and evidence of her wishes presented by her husband and others was challenged by her parents and right-to-life and disability advocacy groups. The legal and media battles lasted eight years and included fourteen appeals in Florida, five federal district court suits, Florida legislation ("Terri's Law") struck down by the Florida Supreme Court, congressional subpoenas, federal legislation, and four denials of certiorari by the United States Supreme Court. Senators Bill Frist and Rick Santorum and House Majority Leader Tom DeLay threatened contempt of Congress sanctions. Congress passed the "Palm Sunday Compromise," giving jurisdiction to the federal courts. President Bush flew to Washington from his vacation in Texas to sign the bill into law. The Supreme Court again declined to hear the case, and the tube was removed. Terri Schiavo died thirteen days later, in 2005, amid intense protest and threats from right-to-life activists.[42]

Virtually every state has passed legislation authorizing advance directives, and the prevalence of such directives among patients with serious and chronic illness has grown in recent decades, ranging from 15 to 20 percent of the general public to more than 80 percent of seriously ill adults.[43] While the prevalence of do-not-resuscitate orders has risen dramatically in recent years, it varies by disease type, ethnicity, age of patients, and care setting, suggesting a rise in acceptance of advance planning decisions prior to death in some patient populations.[44]

Unfortunately, aside from decisions not to attempt cardiopulmonary resuscitation when a patient dies, other forms of advance care planning (such as living wills) do not appear to significantly influence decisions actually made at the bedside for seriously ill patients.[45] The reasons advanced to account for this include the impossibility of anticipating the contingencies of future health status and the types of decisions that might be necessary; the common occurrence of people changing their minds in favor of continuing aggressive life-prolonging therapies as the reality of death approaches; denial and aversion of healthy people to thinking about future illness and disability; the emotional difficulty faced by duly appointed proxies when asked to make decisions (such as withdrawing a ventilator or a feeding tube) that will be perceived as the proximate cause of a loved one's death; and the failure of medical professionals to seek out or honor these directives under circumstances of life-and-death decision making. To date, the use of advance directives has been ineffective in improving quality and controlling costs.

A promising new form of advance directive called the MOLST or POLST (medical or physician orders for life-sustaining treatment) was developed in Oregon and has been adapted by other states.[46] This directive is designed for patients in their last year or two of life and allows patients and physicians to make advance decisions, reflected in physician orders, about hospitalization, DNR orders, artificial nutrition and hydration, and other treatments. It is designed to accompany the patient from setting to setting, and, at least in Oregon, has resulted in a dramatic decrease in hospitalization of terminally ill nursing home patients.[47]

The Right to Die, Assisted Suicide, and Euthanasia

Public anxieties about end-of-life care, fear of loss of control once one is in the medical care system, and rising demands for patient self-determination have led to a resurgence of millennia-old debates about the morality of suicide during terminal illness, and physician-assisted suicide in particular. Debates about euthanasia date back to at least 400 B.C., with the Hippocratic Oath, which states, "I will give no deadly medicine to anyone if asked, nor suggest any such counsel." English common law has prohibited it since the Middle Ages. Growing support for the legalization of euthanasia during the twentieth century was partially reversed with the horror caused by the Nazis' involuntary euthanasia of individuals with mental or physical disabilities. In the United States, euthanasia and the right to refuse or stop life-sustaining treatments based on common law rights to self-determination have been debated for at least the last hundred years.[48]

A heated legal and ethical debate has centered on euthanasia, a Greek word meaning "good death" and referring, generally, to a death caused by another person, sometimes described as a mercy killing. The substance of the debate on euthanasia and assisted suicide has centered on whether it was ever rational for a person to seek a hastened death, no matter how great the burden imposed by an illness; whether, by definition, a desire to die was a manifestation of treatable despair and depression; and whether it was ever ethical for a physician to, in effect, validate a patient's assessment that he or she would be better off dead.

Opponents were concerned that legalization, with its implications of societal approval of the act and concurrence that a diminished life is a societal burden and not worth living, would have a subtle coercive effect on the treatment of seriously ill patients. Opponents also noted that the requirement for a physician's agreement and active participation further stigmatized the sick person, again through the subtle message that the doctor, too, agrees that the patient would be better off dead. Organized religious groups have mounted highly effective media campaigns opposing physician-assisted suicide

Proponents have argued that the right to self-determination extends to the right to determine the timing and circumstances of one's own death, and that such a process could be safely regulated through the establishment of strict eligibility criteria and reporting transparency.[49] Public opinion polls have consistently indicated strong support for it. Gallup has been surveying the American public about euthanasia since 1936 (see Figure 7). The polls have shown that over the last sixty years, between 37 and 72 percent were in favor of mercy deaths under governmental supervision.[50]

FIGURE 7. *When a person has a disease that cannot be cured, do you think doctors should be allowed by law to end the patient's life by some painless means if the patient and his family request it?*

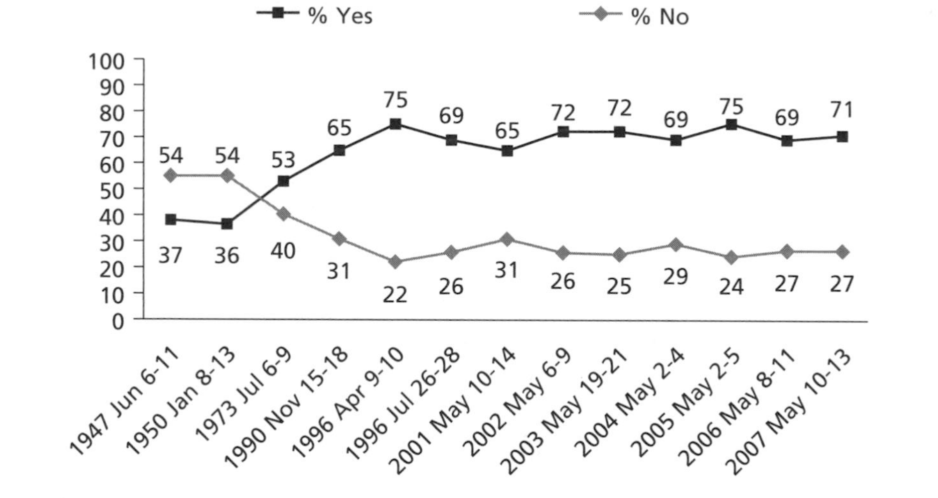

Source: The Gallup Poll, 2006. Reprinted with permission.
Note: The figure is not to scale.

The issue of physician-assisted suicide generated considerable heat in the 1980s and 1990s, after Dr. Jack Kevorkian, a Michigan pathologist, began publicly offering to help patients end their lives, using intravenous sedatives. The first person he assisted, Janet Adkins, traveled to Michigan in 1990 from the state of Washington because of an early dementia and unwillingness to live out the predictable course of a dementing illness. "I'm for absolute autonomy of the individual, and an adult, competent woman has absolute autonomy. It's her choice," Kevorkian said. He claims to have helped a total of 130 people end their lives.

After repeated efforts by the legal system, Kevorkian was imprisoned in 1999 for second-degree murder after the taped and televised voluntary euthanasia death of Thomas Youk, a fifty-two-year-old man with end-stage ventilator-dependent ALS. The public uproar and debate surrounding Kevorkian's activities led to, on the one hand, a ten-to-twenty-five-year jail term for him (he was paroled in 2007 after eight years in jail, after promising not to return to his previous activities), and, on the other, approval of a state ballot measure legalizing physician-assisted suicide, the 1994 Oregon Death with Dignity Act.[51]

Legalizing Physician-Assisted Suicide and the Oregon Death with Dignity Act

In the United States, the debate and legislative efforts have focused on physician-assisted dying (or physician-assisted suicide), where a physician provides a lethal-dose prescription to a patient with the knowledge that the patient intends to use the medicine to hasten death. Physician-assisted suicide is illegal in all states but Oregon and, after passage of a November 2008 ballot measure, Washington.[52]

Oregon's Death with Dignity Act, which passed by a 2.6 percent (31,962-vote) margin in 1994, requires a two-physician certification of a prognosis of under six months; mental competence and no evidence of impaired judgment from depression or other psychiatric illness; two requests separated by at least fifteen days, followed by a written request witnessed by two people; and counseling regarding alternatives including hospice and pain management. Eligible patients receive a prescription, but the doctor may not administer the drugs. The most common reasons for wanting the option of a physician-assisted suicide cited by the patients requesting a prescription were loss of autonomy (100 percent), decreasing ability to participate in activities that make life enjoyable (86 percent), and loss of dignity (86 percent).

Three years after the passage of the measure, a state legislative effort to strike it down was rejected by 60 percent of the voters, reaffirming the legal status of the measure. Also in 1997, Congress passed legislation barring taxpayer dollars from financing physician-assisted suicide, and the Supreme Court ruled that mentally competent terminally ill people do not have a constitutional right to physician-assisted suicide, leaving the issue up to the states. A subsequent attempt in 2001 by Attorney General John Ashcroft to suspend the medical licenses of physicians prescribing life-ending medications under Oregon law was blocked in 2002 by a federal judge, a decision affirmed by the Ninth Circuit Court of Appeals in 2004. In 2006, in *Gonzalez v. Oregon,* the Supreme Court ruled 6–3 in favor of Oregon, upholding the law.[53]

Between 1997 and 2007, 341 people ended their lives through the process set forth in the law. In 2007, 49 Death with Dignity Act patients accounted for 0.156 percent of all deaths, or 15.6 people per 10,000 deaths in Oregon. An additional 85 people received a prescription, presumably to have the reassurance that they could take control over the dying process when and if they needed to, but did not use it and died of natural causes.[54] Analyses of data from both Oregon and the Netherlands (where for over twenty years physicians who provide voluntary euthanasia by lethal injection to seriously ill patients following strict guidelines have not been prosecuted) suggest that fears about the disproportionate impact of legalization on vulnerable groups who might feel coerced by the absence of good care alternatives (the elderly, the uninsured, minorities, the disabled, women, the poor) are not justified.[55] A Washington state ballot measure virtually identical to Oregon's Death with Dignity Act passed on November 4, 2008, by a margin of 59 percent to 41 percent. Efforts to pass similar ballot measures in Maine, Michigan, and California have failed by narrow margins in recent years.[56]

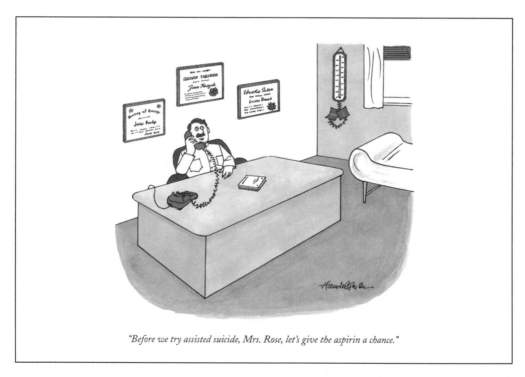

"Before we try assisted suicide, Mrs. Rose, let's give the aspirin a chance."

Although the debate on the ethics and the legality of euthanasia and assisted suicide invokes strongly held beliefs on both sides, in many respects the issue has more salience for the so-called worried well than it does for persons actually living with serious and life-threatening illness. The literature suggests that a desire for aggressive life-prolonging interventions actually increases as death draws near, and the number of persons invoking their legal right to a physician-assisted death in Oregon is small. These observations suggest that fears of loss of control and unrelieved suffering associated with hypothetical future serious illness are the primary motivators for the endorsement of legalization among healthy voters. The rational policy response to such widespread fear is to improve the quality of care for the seriously ill to the point where such concerns are no longer based in reality. This can be accomplished by investing in policies ensuring reliable access to quality palliative care for all Americans rather than by giving a very small number of sick patients access to their doctors' assistance with suicide.

RESEARCH ON CARE OF THE SERIOUSLY ILL

SUPPORT, the Study to Understand Prognoses and Preferences for Outcomes and Risks of Treatment

In the late 1980s, the Robert Wood Johnson Foundation decided to focus on how to improve the care of patients dying in hospitals. Working with a number of prominent academic researchers, the foundation invested more than $29 million in SUPPORT, a randomized multihospital trial of information-sharing for seriously ill patients and their physicians. Research nurses determined patient prognoses and asked patients about their preferences for care. This information was communicated to the treating physicians; the assumption was that information on prognosis and preferences would have an effect on care decisions near the end of life. Surprisingly, however, the intervention had no impact on care processes, patient outcomes, or costs.

Although SUPPORT was a dramatic failure, it did yield important data on the experiences of patients and their families with the medical care system (Table 1). The SUPPORT investigators were among the first to examine the impact of a serious illness on family members, identifying adverse financial, medical, and social consequences that affected the majority. The study demonstrated that high levels of pain were common across all diagnostic categories, even among people who were actively dying and those who had been hospitalized for more than a week. It found that the odds of dying in a hospital had little to do with patient preferences or with physician recognition of prognosis but rather were largely determined by the availability of hospital beds in the community. The publication of the major paper from SUPPORT was covered by all the major media and was a key factor in creation of the "burning platform"—public and professional recognition of a serious quality problem in the care of Americans with advanced illness.

TABLE 1. Key Findings from SUPPORT

Pain	Families of 50% of conscious patients reported moderate to severe pain at least half the time during the last three days of life.[57] 40 to 60% of patients reported moderate to severe pain after 8 to 12 days in the hospital.[58]
Families	Serious illness in a family member required high levels of caregiving from family members in 34%; led to job loss or other major life change in 20%; resulted in loss of all or most of family savings in 31%; and resulted in loss of major source of income in 29%.[59]
Prognosis	Prognosis is variable and uncertain even close to the time of death.[60]
Preferences	Doctor, nurse, and surrogate knowledge of patient wishes is only slightly better than chance. Patients and doctors rarely discuss patient preferences.[61]
Advance directives	Advance directives had no measurable impact on care actually received.[62]
Communication	53% of doctors did not know their patients' preferences about CPR.[63]
Intensity of hospital care	38% of those who died spent at least ten days in an ICU.[64]
Location of death	Location of death is primarily determined by hospital bed availability, not by patient, family, or doctor preferences.[65]
Age and health care spending	Compared with that of similar, younger patients, the care of seriously ill older adults involves fewer procedures and lower costs.[66]

Summarizing the findings from SUPPORT, Joanne Lynn, one of the principal investigators, wrote:

> The problem was not just that physicians were not asking patients their views. In addition, patients were not seeking to talk with physicians. . . . No one involved talks much—not physicians, families, or patients. Decisions are made very late in the course of the illness—a practice that risks some harm and precludes planning but protects most patients from having to consider the issues at all and spares families from confronting mortality until doing so is unavoidable. Surely we can do better. . . . It may well be that change requires a much more fundamental restructuring of service supply, incentives, and rewards.[67]

The Institute of Medicine Reports

In 1997, two years after the release of the SUPPORT findings, the Institute of Medicine (IOM) published *Approaching Death: Improving Care at the End of Life,* the culmination of a yearlong study.[68] Preparation for the report included public meetings, forty-seven testimonials from stakeholder groups, review of the literature, and consultation with a broad range of experts. The report called for radical restructuring of the health care system to include fundamental changes in care delivery, policy, financing, education, research priorities, and public and community engagement. In particular, the report recommended:

- A new subspecialty of palliative medicine
- Reform of burdensome constraints on the prescription of opioid analgesics
- Substantial investment in palliative care research by the National Institutes of Health (NIH) and other research establishments
- Revision of textbooks and other curricular materials to include core content on palliative care
- Mandatory health professional education in palliative care across disciplines and levels of training

With support from private sector philanthropy, many of these recommendations were implemented in whole or in part in subsequent years. The IOM subsequently released two additional reports—*Improving Palliative Care for Cancer*[69] and *When Children Die: Improving Palliative and End-of-Life Care for Children and Their Families.*[70]

Variation and Its Implications: The Dartmouth Atlas

Using Medicare claims data and small-area analyses, researchers at the Dartmouth Medical School have identified wide variation in the provision of effective care (for example, underuse of beta blockers after heart attacks) and utilization of health care resources during chronic illness, due primarily to the number of physicians and hospital beds in different regions.[71] More specialists and more hospital beds in a given community encourage more specialist visits and more and longer hospital admissions for patients living in that community. The extra spending on doctors' visits, specialist consultations, procedures, tests, and hospital stays in the high-utilization regions do not appear to buy either a longer or a better life. If anything, the data suggest that the higher the utilization of health care, the *higher* the mortality rate—due, perhaps, to the greater risk of medical errors, poor coordination and poor communication, and other potential harms.[72] Additionally, family members of seriously ill patients living in high-intensity hospital service areas report lower satisfaction with the health care system and lower quality of emotional support, shared decision making, information about what to expect, and respectful treatment.[73] Similarly, physicians practicing in high-intensity service regions report more difficulty arranging elective admissions, obtaining specialty referrals, maintaining good doctor-patient relations, and delivering high-quality care.[74]

If more high-technology medicine applied to care of the seriously ill neither improves care, prolongs lives, nor increases satisfaction of patients, families and their physicians, why are we spending so much money on it, and how do we reorganize the system to facilitate access to truly effective medical care? This question underscores the need to develop different approaches to the care of the seriously and chronically ill, approaches that can lead to changes in deeply entrenched and highly patterned physician practice styles, starting with the place where this care variation leads to the highest costs and the greatest potential harms—the hospital. As demonstrated by SUPPORT, successful interventions to change physician behavior are notoriously elusive; hence the need for system- and bedside-level interventions to try to change the physician's usual path of decision making for seriously ill hospitalized patients.

PRIVATE SECTOR PHILANTHROPY AS CATALYST OF SOCIAL CHANGE

Despite the widespread belief that government is the main driver of innovation and quality assurance in health care, the American health care system has little to no centralized organizing authority and is instead influenced by multiple stakeholders, including industry manufacturers of devices and pharmaceuticals, payers, and providers. Unlike other developed nations with centralized national health care plans, the United States has a health care marketplace that comprises an amalgam of for-profit industries and special interest groups (such as commercial insurers, pharmaceutical and device manufacturers, and for-profit hospitals, nursing homes, and hospices), not-for-profit care settings, public payers (Medicare, Medicaid), employer-based insurance (of diminishing affordability and availability) for those under sixty-five, and a rising crisis in access to quality health care for insured and uninsured alike. Although major public policy advances during the last century led to Medicare coverage for all older adults and disabled persons, as well as the Medicare hospice benefit and the Medicare Part D prescription drug coverage plan, to date government has been unable to impose incentives and constraints on overuse and lack of primary care coordination, leading to fragmented, poor-quality care for the seriously ill. Private sector philanthropy, specifically major foundations committed to improving health and health care, stepped into the breach with the substantial and sustained investments necessary to build and integrate a new field of medicine into the mainstream of health care in the United States.

These philanthropic initiatives evolved in a context of the growing interest in patients' rights, advance care planning, the hospice movement, the "right to die" movement, and Jack Kevorkian's challenge to mainstream medicine. In the early 1980s, the W. K. Kellogg Foundation, along with the Arthur Vining Davis Foundation, funded the creation of protocols for end-of-life care, pain management, and nursing services. The standards they set regarding care for the dying were recognized by the U.S. government through the creation of the Medicare hospice benefit. As a result of these early foundation-funded efforts, millions of dollars in federal support now flow to the care of over one-third of dying Americans who are served by the more than four thousand hospice programs nationwide.

The other major early investor in this effort was the Robert Wood Johnson Foundation; its commitment was precipitated in part by the difficult personal experiences of several board members. Since the late 1980s, the Robert Wood Johnson Foundation has invested more than $180 million in end-of-life and palliative care—an investment that helped to create a new and now thriving academic and clinical field in health care.[75]

In 1994, George Soros, the Open Society Institute founder and chairman, in response to his personal experiences with the deaths of his parents, convened a national group of experts and launched the Project on Death in America. This nine-year, $45 million investment in "understanding and transforming the culture and experience of dying and bereavement" in the United States supported career development for academic leaders, professional and public education, the arts, research, clinical care, and public policy in end-of-life and palliative care.[76]

In combination, the Open Society Institute and the Robert Wood Johnson Foundation programs led to:

- Career development support for leaders in medicine, nursing, and social work

- Development and dissemination of medical and nursing curricula in palliative care

- Technical assistance for palliative care capacity building in American hospitals

- Development of new models and settings to enhance access to palliative care

- Regulatory and policy changes supportive of access to quality palliative care through The Joint Commission

- Investment in consensus efforts to define quality palliative care through the National Consensus Project for Quality Palliative Care and the National Quality Forum

- Grassroots coalition building in communities across the United States

- Public outreach through media, including the Bill Moyers four-part PBS series *On Our Own Terms: Moyers on Dying*

These initiatives collectively marshaled the resources and built the momentum necessary to launch and begin to sustain a new field. Both entities ceased or greatly reduced their funding in the field (the Open Society Institute in 2003 and the Robert Wood Johnson Foundation in 2006). The work of these and other philanthropic foundations is summarized in the table that forms the appendix to this chapter ("Major Foundation Investments in Building Palliative Care").

THE GROWTH OF PALLIATIVE CARE

The goal of palliative care is to prevent and relieve suffering and to support the best possible quality of life for patients and their families, regardless of the stage of the disease or the need for other therapies. Palliative care is both a philosophy of care and an organized, highly structured system for delivering care. Palliative care expands traditional disease-model medical treatments to include the goals of enhancing quality of life for patient and family, optimizing function, helping with decision making, and providing opportunities for personal growth. As such, it can be delivered concurrently with life-prolonging care or as the main focus of care.

National Consensus Project for Quality Palliative Care and National Quality Forum.[77]

Many social forces are shaping the emergence of the palliative care movement in the United States. These forces, combined with a strategic infusion of hundreds of millions of private sector philanthropic dollars over the last twenty years, have crystallized palliative care as a solution to many problems facing people with chronic conditions and serious illnesses—a solution that did not require a revolution in health care financing. The major factors contributing to the recent rapid growth in the field include:

- The unprecedented increase in numbers and needs of the elderly

- Recognition of the growing numbers of family caregivers and their unmet needs

- The transformation of demands on the health care system from acute care of infections and heart attacks to long-term management of chronic diseases

- Large numbers of baby boomers in leadership roles learning about the failures of the health care system during care for their parents

- The unsustainable rise in per capita and total health care spending due to expensive new technologies and drugs and more people receiving them

- The influence of the right-to-die movement and the attention of the public to high-profile cases such as Karen Ann Quinlan and Terri Schiavo.

- The recurring debate on the pros and cons of legalized physician-assisted dying, precipitated in part by Jack Kevorkian and his activities.

- Broad media coverage (for example, the film *Sicko,* the Bill Moyers PBS series *On Our Own Terms*) of bad experiences with the health care system

- The ascendancy of subspecialty medicine and the associated fragmentation in care, coupled with the collapse of primary care in the United States.

The health care sector has seen fifty years of stunning growth through rapid development of and profit from life-prolonging technologies. As these technologies (drugs, procedures, devices, imaging) are routinely applied to chronically ill people with advanced disease—mostly elderly populations, for whom these treatments have increasingly marginal benefit—the nation's ability to provide access to them will be challenged.

> *The relief of suffering and the cure of disease must be seen as twin obligations of a medical profession that is truly dedicated to the care of the sick. Physicians' failure to understand the nature of suffering can result in medical intervention that (though technically adequate) not only fails to relieve suffering but becomes a source of suffering itself.*
>
> Eric J. Cassell, M.D., 1982[78]

Palliative Care: A Key Part of the Solution

Palliative care has emerged as both a response and a possible solution. The predominant delivery model of palliative care in the United States is the hospital consultation service involving a team of professionals (typically physicians, nurses, and social workers, with additional contributions from massage therapists, chaplains, psychologists, psychiatrists, rehabilitation experts, and others as needed) who provide recommendations and support to primary and specialist physicians caring for seriously ill patients in the hospital. Palliative care teams, which vary in composition based on the stage of the program and the size and needs of the institution, focus on assessing and treating symptoms such as pain, fatigue, and depression; communicating with patient, family, and colleagues inside and out of the hospital in order to gain a full understanding of the medical situation and ascertain the patient's and family's preferences and needs; developing and communicating a plan of care consistent with the patient's and family's needs and preferences; and assuring the necessary coordination, communication, and follow-up to optimize continuity and quality of care throughout the course of the illness.

In the last ten years, much progress has been made:

- Through the National Consensus Project for Quality Palliative Care, leaders in the field established a consensus process and defined guidelines for quality palliative care in 2004.[79] Building on these guidelines, the National Quality Forum (the nation's public-private entity for determining the quality of health care) has developed a preferred practice framework for the field.[80] Quality guidelines call for extending palliative care upstream from the dying phase, requiring hospice and palliative care programs to form seamless continuums of care between hospital and community (home and nursing home) settings.

- The Joint Commission, the country's major accrediting body for health care organizations, now requires assessment and treatment of pain as a condition of accreditation, and the Joint Commission is considering release of a new voluntary certificate program for hospital palliative care programs in 2009–2010.[81]

- Palliative care is increasingly understood as appropriate, independent of prognosis, to be offered to patients with complex or advanced illness in light of patient (and family) needs, whether they will live for years or days.

- As of 2006, the American Board of Medical Specialties has recognized palliative medicine as a subspecialty of medicine, with an unprecedented ten primary parent boards.

- More than sixteen thousand nurses have received nursing certification in palliative care.[82]

- Physician, nursing, and social work education, from undergraduate to midcareer professional levels, has been strengthened in the last ten years, primarily through private sector initiatives supported by both national and regional foundations.

- More than 30 percent of American hospitals report having a palliative care program; and of the larger hospitals that serve the majority of patients (those with more than 250 beds), three-quarters reported an active program in 2006.

- The number of patients served by hospice has increased by 162 percent since 1996—to 1.4 million in 2007—and more than 38 percent of all patients in the United States are served by a hospice program before their death.[83]

- The topic of serious illness and even death and dying is more commonplace in the media and popular entertainment (for example, *Away from Her;* HBO's *Six Feet Under; My Life Without Me; Big Fish; The Savages; Wit; The Year of Magical Thinking; The Diving Bell and the Butterfly*).

- Medical schools and residency training programs now require some training in aspects of palliative care as a condition of accreditation.

Medical, Nursing, and Social Work Education

The remarkable growth in the number of palliative care programs over the last five to ten years has not been matched by growth in the number of trained clinicians to lead and staff these programs. The mismatch between the nature of the patients served by medical professionals (chronically and in hospitals, seriously ill), their needs (expert symptom management, available and responsive communication about goals of care and how to achieve them, practical and psychosocial support for family caregivers, well-coordinated and communicated care across settings), and the inadequacy of training in the content areas necessary to meet their needs is striking.

PALLIATIVE CARE: 2008[84]

- Board-certified physicians: 2,883
- Board-certified nurses:
    - RN: 11,268
    - Nurse practitioners: 394
- Postgraduate palliative medicine fellowship programs: 65
- Postgraduate advanced practice nursing programs in palliative care: 10
- Peer-reviewed journals: *Journal of Palliative Medicine; Journal of Pain and Symptom Management; American Journal of Hospice & Palliative Medicine; Journal of Psychosocial Oncology; Death Studies*
- Textbooks (English language): More than 20
- Hospital palliative care programs: 1,299 (2006 data)
- Hospices: More than 4,700
- Patients served by hospice: 1.4 million, 38 percent of all deaths (2007 data)

Survey research and reports from patients and their families indicate that physicians, nurses, and social workers—who deliver the vast majority of direct care to chronically and seriously ill patients—are poorly trained to provide effective and timely palliative care to patients with serious and complex illness. The poor quality of pain and symptom management, doctor-patient communication, and coordination and continuity of care can be traced at least in part to the inadequacy of curricular content in these areas in both undergraduate and graduate medical, nursing, and social work education. It is not reasonable to expect physicians, nurses, or social workers to be expert in knowledge, attitudes, and skills that they were not taught during many years of undergraduate and postgraduate education. Despite little exposure during training, physicians recognize the importance of palliative care to quality health care. In an international poll conducted by the *British Medical Journal* in 2008, when physicians were asked which of five public health priorities would make the "greatest difference" to health care, palliative care came in a strong first with 38 percent of the vote, ahead of combating drug-resistant infections in poor nations (22 percent), improving care (17 percent) and pain management (12 percent) in the elderly, reducing excess drinking in young women (8 percent), and reducing adverse drug reactions in the elderly (3 percent).[85]

A number of strategies have been employed to improve medical and nursing education in palliative care, including the pursuit of subspecialty status for palliative medicine and nursing; advocacy for changes in undergraduate and graduate medical, nursing, and social work education accreditation standards; and numerous philanthropically funded efforts to train midcareer physicians and nurses.

Palliative Medicine Specialty Status In an effort to gain the credibility afforded to other specialties in medicine—status that is necessary to have influence on training curricula, allocation of research dollars, and improved access to quality care for patients and families—palliative care advocates have pursued formal specialty status as a key strategy. Britain was the first country to make palliative medicine a subspecialty, in 1987, followed by Australia, Hong Kong, New Zealand, Poland, Romania, Singapore, and Taiwan. In 2006, the American Board of Medical Specialties, which confers specialty and subspecialty status, approved subspecialty status for palliative medicine in the United States. The first official ABMS-certified board examination for physicians was given in 2008. It remains to be seen how physicians practicing in ten different medical fields will be served by a single examination.

Nursing Subspecialty Certification In an effort to standardize and assure the quality of palliative care delivery by nursing professionals, nurses have also developed formal accreditation requirements and certification examinations for nurse practitioners, registered nurses, certified nursing assistants, and licensed practical nurses. In 2007, the American Board of Nursing Specialties approved accreditation for a master's-level hospice and palliative care certification program that allows certified nurses to bill insurers for their services. Similarly, the National Board for Certification of Hospice and Palliative Nurses successfully fulfilled National Commission for Certifying Agencies' accreditation requirements for licensed practical nurses and nursing assistants in hospice and palliative care.

Medical School Education   Surveys of medical school deans by the Liaison Committee on Medical Education (the undergraduate medical education accrediting body) and of graduating medical students by the Association of American Medical Colleges in the 1990s showed that palliative and end-of-life care was covered only minimally in the coursework and the clinical clerkships of medical schools, and almost none of it was required.[86]

Infusing new content areas into an overcrowded and ever-expanding medical and nursing school curriculum has required strategy and persistence, and it remains a work in progress. In 2000, influenced by the 1997 Institute of Medicine report *Approaching Death,* the Liaison Committee on Medical Education added a requirement for training in end-of-life care and doctor-patient communication. Subsequent surveys suggest that 87 percent of medical schools are providing some curriculum on these topics, but the range of hours required is broad, and the content and impact of the teaching are unknown.[87] A 2006 survey conducted by the Association of American Medical Colleges comparing changes in American medical students' perceptions of their training in palliative care between 1998 and 2006 demonstrated a significant improvement in the proportion reporting that their exposure was at least adequate for care at the end of life (from 71 percent to 80 percent), pain management (from 34 percent to 55 percent), and palliative care (from 60 percent to 75 percent).[88] Although it is not possible to know the extent to which medical students' opinions translate into improved practice, this change in their perceptions is a positive sign.

A recent systematic review of palliative care training in medical schools found that clinical exposure to palliative care and hospice patients, as opposed to lecture-based classroom teaching, was particularly effective in improving student knowledge and attitudes.[89] No data are available to assess the number of American medical schools providing mandatory clinical rotations in palliative medicine. Barriers to requiring palliative care clinical rotations in the medical school curriculum include entrenched local politics and habits influencing medical school course content and priorities; lack of palliative care content in medical school certifying examinations and competency evaluations in clinical training rotations; inadequate numbers of palliative medicine faculty to teach quality care for this patient population; and lack of palliative care program staff capacity to provide bedside teaching. Experts in medical education have called for mandatory required coursework in palliative care, increasing the number of palliative care faculty as role models and teachers, and the establishment of academic medical school departments to lead and strengthen these advances.[90]

Paying for the faculty necessary to provide palliative care teaching for physicians in training has been a challenge. With few exceptions, philanthropy has been the sole investor in developing academic faculty leaders at medical schools and teaching hospitals, and most of this foundation support has concluded. New funding focused on financial incentives (such as loan forgiveness for physicians and nurses who pursue graduate training in palliative care) to build the palliative care workforce is needed. A report of the Center to Advance Palliative Care and the International Longevity Center called for the federal government to provide funding for core palliative medicine faculty at each of the 129 medical schools in the country—an investment of approximately $10.5 million a year over twenty years.[91] These faculty members, in turn, will be charged with educating and training the next generation of physicians, expanding the workforce pipeline, and conducting the research necessary to create a more robust evidence base to guide palliative care clinicians. To date, the necessary legislation has not been passed.

BASIC PRINCIPLES FOR ENHANCING UNDERGRADUATE MEDICAL EDUCATION IN PALLIATIVE CARE

1. The care of dying persons and their families is a core professional task of physicians. Medical schools have a responsibility to prepare students to provide skilled, compassionate end-of-life care. Additional resources will be required to implement these changes.

2. The following key content areas related to end-of-life care must be appropriately addressed in undergraduate medical education. *Note*: This list will differ according to the setting and, to some extent, the patient population (for example, children versus adults):

   a. Medical education should encourage students to develop positive feelings about dying patients and their families and about the role of the physician in terminal care.

   b. Enhanced teaching about death, dying, and bereavement should occur throughout the span of medical education.

   c. Educational content and process should be tailored to students' developmental stage.

   d. The best learning grows out of direct experiences with patients and families, particularly when students have an opportunity to follow patients longitudinally and develop a sense of intimacy and manageable personal responsibility for suffering persons.

   e. Teaching and learning about death, dying, and bereavement should emphasize humanistic attitudes.

   f. Teaching should address communication skills.

   g. Students need to see physicians offering excellent medical care to dying people and their families, and finding meaning in their work.

   h. Medical education should foster respect for patients' personal values and an appreciation of cultural and spiritual diversity in approaching death and dying.

   i. The teaching process itself should mirror the values to which physicians aspire in working with patients.

Continued

Continued

    j. A comprehensive, integrated understanding of and approach to death, dying, and bereavement is enhanced when students are exposed to the perspectives of multiple disciplines working together.

    k. Faculty should be taught how to teach about end-of-life care, including how to be mentors and to model ideal behaviors and skills.

    l. Student competence in managing prototypical clinical settings related to death, dying, and bereavement should be evaluated.

    m. Educational programs should be evaluated using state-of-the-art methods.

Source: Billings and Block, 1997[92]

Graduate Medical Education Postgraduate medical education—internship, residency, and subspecialty fellowship training—is widely acknowledged to have the greatest impact on the development of medical professionals. These are the years when new physicians are charged with direct (albeit supervised) responsibility for the care of patients in teaching hospitals and associated community settings. The hours are typically arduous, and exposure to chronically and very seriously ill and dying patients in acute care hospital settings constitutes a major part of the training experience. These are patient populations with extreme burdens of disease with multiple coexisting illnesses, a high prevalence of symptom distress, and overburdened and exhausted family caregivers. Developing skill in symptom assessment and management, doctor-patient-family communication, and transitions of care for patients and families are obvious priorities for residency training.

Little research has been conducted on the adequacy and impact of graduate medical education in palliative care. Annual surveys of residency training program directors conducted by the American Medical Association indicate that 60 percent of training programs report a "structured curriculum in end-of-life care." However, no information was sought on the content, the time committed, or the effectiveness of these curricula. A survey of residency programs in family medicine, internal medicine, pediatrics, and geriatrics published in 1995 found that 26 percent of all residency programs in the United States offered a standard course in end-of-life care, almost 15 percent of programs offered no formal training in care of terminally ill patients, only 8 percent required a hospice rotation, and 9 percent offered an elective.[94]

More recent surveys of medical residents found that they perceived their training as adequate to manage pain and symptoms in 72 percent, telling patients they are dying in 62 percent, describing what to expect with the dying process in 38 percent, and responding to a patient's request for aid in dying in 32 percent.[95] No direct observational data are available to validate whether residents' perceptions of the "adequacy" of exposure to these topic areas correlates with the knowledge, skills, and attitudes they will need once in practice. In a 2005 survey of residents reporting how they were

FACULTY URGENTLY NEEDED

In 1997, the Institute of Medicine called for fundamental changes in the content and quality of health professional education through the development of "a cadre of palliative care experts whose numbers and talents are sufficient to: a) provide expert consultation and role models for colleagues, students, and other members of the health professions; b) supply leadership for scientifically based and practically useful undergraduate, graduate, and continuing medical education; and c) organize and conduct biomedical, clinical, behavioral, and health services research." To achieve the IOM's goals, a policy report from the Center to Advance Palliative Care and the International Longevity Center–USA recommends five years of academic career development support for at least three faculty members at each medical and osteopathic school in the United States. These Palliative Care Academic Career Awards would be modeled after the successful Geriatric Academic Career Awards currently administered by the Health Resources and Services Administration (HRSA), which have funded several hundred new geriatric faculty members since their inception in 1999. No action has been taken on the IOM's recommendation.[93]

taught palliative care, few reported having received useful feedback from a resident (8 percent) or an attending physician (7 percent) about their ability to discuss advance care planning. An even smaller number reported that bedside work and attending rounds (4–5 percent) were frequent settings for learning about palliative care. Despite residents' self-evaluation as adequately competent for such discussions, by their own report they fail to engage in recommended behaviors for such discussions.[96]

Exposure to palliative medicine teaching at both undergraduate and graduate levels has improved in the last ten years, presumably as a consequence of increased programmatic support from private sector philanthropy, academic leadership by palliative medicine physician faculty, growing integration of community hospice programs with medical education and the gradual adoption of curricular standards and competencies for medical trainees. As of 2006, more than 80 percent of the member hospitals of the Council of Teaching Hospitals and Health Systems reported a clinical palliative care program.[97] The future challenge is to assure that these programs have the capacity and the opportunity to incorporate mandatory clinical rotations for both medical students and residents into their existing clinical responsibilities.

Nursing Education   Other than family members, nurses provide the great majority of care to patients living with chronic and advanced illness. Nurses witness and remain present for patients when physicians and other professionals have left the bedside. Through their presence and their ability to be with patients who are suffering, nurses are in a unique position to reduce the isolation and loneliness that accompany serious illness.

> *Nurses recognize that witnessing suffering is a part of their daily work, yet they seek to understand each person who is suffering as a unique individual. Nurses respond to suffering primarily through identifying its sources and offering presence. As witnesses to suffering, they serve as compassionate voices and recognize the human response to illness in the confusing and often depersonalized healthcare environment.*
>
> Betty Ferrell and Nessa Coyle, 2008[98]

Expertise in symptom assessment and treatment, communication about the primary concerns of patients and families, and assuring well-coordinated and well-communicated care are core competencies for nursing professionals. Unfortunately, an extensive literature on nursing education documents that, as is true of physicians, nurses receive inadequate education in palliative care, at both undergraduate and postgraduate levels.[99] In an effort to improve nursing education, private sector philanthropy has supported work to assess and strengthen textbook and certifying examination content as well as curricular resources and faculty preparation. The End-of-Life Nursing Education Consortium (ELNEC), administered by the American Association of Colleges of Nursing, has developed and widely disseminated palliative care curricular resources for undergraduate, graduate, faculty, and various specialty audiences, including geriatrics, pediatrics, critical care, and oncology.[100] Nursing certification examinations for advance practice nurses, registered nurses, licensed practical nurses, and certified nursing assistants are offered by the National Board for Certification of Hospice and Palliative Care Nurses and more than ten postgraduate master's-level palliative nurse practitioner programs are now available in the United States.

Social Work Education Social workers are central to counseling, case management, and advocacy services for persons with serious illness and their family caregivers. With their focus on the psychosocial aspects of illness, they work not only with patients but also with families and others in making decisions about treatment options, marshaling resources, and helping families cope with the serious illness and death of a relative. The demands on social workers have changed over time. A major reason is the rising pressure to shift seriously ill and dying patients out of hospitals "quicker and sicker" and into less resource-intense settings such as nursing homes and hospices. This pressure to discharge requires social workers to coordinate a broadening array of services and providers and to navigate an ever more complex and changing set of insurance eligibility and payment rules and regulations.

As is true of physicians and nurses, social work students receive little training in palliative care.[101] Several post–master's degree programs on palliative care for social workers have been developed, a critical resource for training the faculty members needed to teach this content in social work training programs. Competencies to guide the development of curricular content, credentialing criteria, and new initiatives promoting palliative care curricular content requirements are under way through the Social Work in Hospice and Palliative Care Network.[102] In 2008, the National Association of Social Workers and the National Hospice and Palliative Care

Organization partnered to develop the first palliative care credentialing process for social workers.

Palliative Care Content in Textbooks   One reason that practicing physicians, nurses, and social workers completed their training with so little expertise in core palliative care skills had been the nearly complete absence of these topics from their major textbooks. Several studies analyzed palliative care content in general medical, subspecialty, and nursing textbooks and found little to no content on how to care for patients in the late stages of the major chronic and serious illnesses, other than vague recommendations to provide "supportive care."[103] A physician or a nurse consulting these texts could be forgiven for assuming that the management of symptoms, planning for a peaceful death, and supporting families and seriously ill patients in the community is somebody else's job. Many textbook publishers, to their credit, responded quickly and have added to existing chapters or added new chapters in forthcoming editions of their books.

Activities of Professional Organizations

Standard-setting and accrediting organizations such as the Joint Commission have made major contributions to focusing the attention of institutions on assessment and relief of pain, communication and coordination of care, and support for families. In an important step, the Joint Commission is considering the launch in 2009–2010 of a voluntary certificate program in palliative care, built on the National Consensus Project for Quality Palliative Care's and the National Quality Forum's *National Framework and Preferred Practices for Palliative and Hospice Care.* A certification process signals legitimacy and critical mass for hospital palliative care services and is both evidence of and stimulus for the increased importance of palliative care programs in American hospitals.[104]

Palliative Care in Hospitals

Based on data from the 2008 American Hospital Association annual survey of hospitals, some 31 percent, or 1,299 of 4,136 responding hospitals, answered "yes" to a question asking whether their institution had "an organized program providing specialized medical care, drugs, or therapies for the management of acute or chronic pain and/or the control of symptoms administered by specially trained physicians and other clinicians; and supportive care services, such as counseling on advanced directives, spiritual care, and social services, to patients with advanced disease and their families." Such programs have increased in number by 106 percent since 2000. The percentage of hospitals reporting a palliative care program varies dramatically by hospital type and geographic region—the larger the hospital, the more likely it is to provide palliative care. Similarly, faith-based hospitals, teaching hospitals, and nonprofit hospitals are significantly more likely to report the presence of a palliative care program, while smaller hospitals, safety net and sole community provider hospitals, for-profit hospitals, and hospitals located in the South of the United States are significantly less likely to report a program.[105] The Veterans Health Administration has made a strong commitment to assuring access to quality palliative care for veterans across the nation, including hospital palliative care services, home-based hospice care, and development of coordinated delivery systems across care settings.

Regions with greater access to hospital palliative care services are associated with lower rates of in-hospital death and intensive care unit use.[106] A 2008 state-by-state report card comparing access to palliative care across the United States is available at www.capc.org/reportcard.

The statistics point to the rising availability of palliative care services at larger hospitals, where the majority of seriously ill Americans receive their care, and the strong presence of programs in teaching hospitals, where medical students, residents, and fellows receive their training (Table 2). The survey does not tell us anything about the quality of these services or about the likelihood that a patient in need actually accesses palliative care. Similarly, the presence of a palliative care program in a teaching hospital represents an opportunity for training but is no guarantee that students and residents are actually exposed to the program. Finally, the striking absence

TABLE 2. **2006 American Hospital Association Annual Hospital Survey: Hospitals Reporting a Palliative Care Program**

	Palliative Care Programs	Hospitals	%
Hospital size			
1–74 adult beds	455	2,523	18
75–149 adult beds	339	847	40
150–249 adult beds	291	488	60
250+ adult beds	214	278	77
Hospital features			
Joint Commission–accredited	1118	2938	38
Residency training, ACGME-approved	503	832	60
Council of Teaching Hospital member	226	288	78
Catholic Church–operated	310	537	58
American Cancer Society–approved cancer program	698	1203	58
For-profit, investor-owned	57	610	9
Nonprofit, nongovernment	1015	2460	41
Federal government, including VA	60	94	64

Source: Goldsmith B, Dietrich J, Du Q, et al. Variability in access to hospital palliative care in the United States. *J Pal Med.* 2008;11(8):1094–1102. Reprinted with permission.

of palliative care programs in the for-profit and public hospital sector represents a major opportunity for improvement in both quality and efficiency of services in those settings.

Palliative Care in Nursing Homes

The demographics of nursing homes are changing with the aging of our country. Residents are staying longer—often for several years—and the number of people dying in nursing homes is also increasing dramatically (currently 22 percent of all deaths in the United States occur in nursing homes, projected to rise to 50 percent by 2020). These trends point to the importance of well-integrated and culturally sensitive palliative care services in nursing homes. Nursing home leaders have called for improvements in advance care planning and pain and symptom management, and better coordination of transitions between hospitals and nursing homes.[107] There are no national survey data on the presence of skilled and trained palliative care professionals or programs in nursing homes, and little on the satisfaction of patients and families with such care. Teno and colleagues reported low satisfaction with pain management, emotional support, and doctor-patient-family communication among families of Medicare patients who died in four settings (hospital, home care, hospice, nursing home), with nursing homes ranking at or near the bottom.[108] Similarly, Bernabei and colleagues reported high levels of untreated pain among nursing home residents with cancer.[109] The financial stress, perceived and real regulatory barriers, staff turnover, and predominance of for-profits in the nursing home industry all pose significant barriers to wider application of palliative care principles and practices. Recent trends in the growth of assisted-living facilities and other less regulated alternatives to nursing home care point to the need for more research on access to quality palliative care across the long-term-care industry. Neither the public nor the private sector has invested adequately in research to identify and test new models to assure access to quality palliative care for this highly vulnerable population.

A report on palliative care practices in a selected group of progressive American nursing homes revealed the emergence of four dominant models:[110]

- Outside palliative care consultants (physicians or advance practice nurses) called in on an as-needed basis

- Hospice staff providing nonhospice palliative care services

- "Training up" of nursing home staff on core palliative care competencies, including symptom assessment and management

- Improved access to the Medicare hospice benefit for residents meeting the six-month prognosis criterion

These models enable development of tools to help other nursing homes develop similar services. Technical assistance and quality guidelines for these models, as well as health professional training to help frontline nursing home providers meet the palliative care needs of their patients, are required. The opportunity and the obligation to ensure that quality of life and quality of dying are reliable components of nursing home and other long-term care settings in the future remain unmet. Palliative care training and programmatic supports are among the key solutions to this challenge.

Palliative Care Research

Despite its remarkable growth, the field of palliative care rests on an evidence base wholly inadequate to guide quality of care. Three Institute of Medicine reports, two National Institutes of Health state-of-the-science conferences, and the report of the research committee of the American Academy of Hospice and Palliative Medicine have all called for major investments in palliative care research, specifically in the areas of pain and symptom management, communication skills, care coordination, and models of care delivery.[111]

A recent analysis of sources of funding for palliative care found that fewer than 5 percent of palliative care investigators (identified from PubMed keyword searches between 2003 and 2005) received any NIH funding. More than half of published palliative care research reported only private sector philanthropic support, while less than a third reported NIH support; the remaining palliative care research was conducted with no reported extramural funding of any kind.[112] Compounding this concern, and despite the fact that the leading causes of death and advanced chronic illness in the United States are cancer, dementia, and diseases of heart, brain, lung, and kidney, less than 1 percent of all grants funded by the major NIH institutes were for research on palliative care aspects of these common disease states.[113]

Reasons advanced to account for the inadequacy of federal funding for palliative care research include the disease-specific focus of most NIH institutes and the associated lack of an NIH institute focused on palliative medicine; the fact that those NIH study sections composed of scientists charged with peer review and scoring of grant proposals include at most one to two palliative medicine researchers; and the associated fact that, unlike our neighbors in Canada, no NIH study section focuses specifically on the science of palliative medicine and no dollars are dedicated to palliative medicine research. Recommendations aimed at redressing this situation include federal funding for palliative care research; the designation of one or more palliative medicine study review sections; and the development of mechanisms similar to those already well established at the NIH such as investigator-initiated research, center grants, and career development awards in palliative medicine.[114]

Continued support from the private sector is also crucial for pilot studies and career development support necessary to prepare young and established investigators alike to compete for federal funding. In an effort to catalyze these goals, the Kornfeld Foundation in New York City established the National Palliative Care Research Center (NPCRC) in 2005, with additional support from the Brookdale, Ho-Chiang, and Olive Branch Foundations, and the American Cancer Society, the American Academy of

Hospice and Palliative Medicine, and the National Institute on Aging. In the first year, the request for proposals yielded 101 applications for career development awards and pilot and exploratory projects.

THE NATIONAL PALLIATIVE CARE RESEARCH CENTER

The mission of the National Palliative Care Research Center is to improve care for patients with serious illness and to help with the needs of their families by promoting palliative care research. In partnership with the Center to Advance Palliative Care, the center will rapidly translate research findings into clinical practice.

Specifically, the NPCRC provides a mechanism to

- Establish priorities for palliative care research.
- Develop a new generation of researchers in palliative care.
- Coordinate and support studies focused on improving care for patients and families living with serious illness.

In a parallel effort to catalyze palliative care research for cancer patients, the American Cancer Society has recently invested over $1.5 million in palliative care research, established an expert group of palliative care grant reviewers, and received more than 136 applications in response to its first call for proposals. Although a substantial proportion of these proposals scored in the fundable range, because of a lack of funds only 5 percent were awarded. This experience demonstrates a widespread demand for funding for palliative care research, the availability of qualified investigators to conduct it, and the need for a major federal funding commitment.

THE FAMILY CAREGIVER

In American society, family caregiving has become the linchpin of the long-term-care system. The reasons include the growth in numbers of persons surviving into old age with serious chronic conditions and the trend toward deinstitutionalization—maintaining dependent persons as much as possible in their communities rather than nursing homes, and discharging them from hospitals as quickly as possible, preferably to their homes. Complicating matters, families are no longer clustered in the same community; women often work full time, and the current payment system does not cover long-term care unless one is poor enough to qualify for Medicaid or is terminally ill and eligible for hospice.

It is no exaggeration to say that patients living with chronic and complex illness are abandoned by the health care system unless they require hospital care for an acute illness, a brief period of skilled nursing care after a hospital stay, or are terminally ill and eligible for hospice, all of which are covered by Medicare and most commercial insurers. All other patients—that is, the vast majority with multiple chronic conditions or a serious illness—are left to coordinate and oversee their own care, find their own transportation to their doctor's office, locate a doctor from the shrinking pool of primary care providers, assure communication between all their specialists, check to be sure there are no risks from taking drugs prescribed by multiple providers, find a doctor who accepts Medicare or Medicaid, and, when these responsibilities become overwhelming, call 911 for a trip to the emergency room.

The interim report of the Citizens' Health Care Working Group (an entity mandated by Congress, with members appointed by the Comptroller General of the United States) reported, after six hearings, thirty-one community meetings in thirty states and the District of Columbia, review of all major public opinion polls focused on health that were conducted between 2002 and 2006, some ten thousand responses to Web polls, and review of five thousand individual commentaries:

> A picture has been sketched for us of a health care system that is unintelligible to most people. They see a rigid system with a set of ingrained operating procedures that long ago became disconnected from the mission of providing people with humane, respectful, and technically excellent health care.[115]

In the absence of an effective health care delivery system, the responsibility for nearly all aspects of a loved one's care needs falls to families.

Who Are the Caregivers?[116]

More than forty-four million adults (21 percent of the adult population) provide unpaid care to other adults who are sick or disabled. Spending an average of twenty-one hours a week providing the care, they are by far the largest source of long-term-care services in the country. About a third of these caregivers are elderly themselves.[117] The estimated cost equivalent of this uncompensated care (at an estimated hourly rate of $8 an hour) is $257 billion a year—more than three-quarters of the total dollars ($336 billion) spent in 2005 on Medicare.[118] Perhaps not surprisingly, nearly nine out of ten seriously ill patients say they need help with the sorts of things not covered by health insurance, such as transportation to the doctor's office and help with homemaking (buying groceries, cooking, cleaning) (see Figure 8).[119]

The typical caregiver is a woman in her midforties who works full time and spends at least twenty hours a week providing care to her mother. Roughly 60 percent of caregivers are women, and women are more likely to provide the most demanding kinds of care, such as helping with bathing, dressing, and toileting for the most physically dependent patients. About a third of caregivers (40 percent of women and 26 percent of men) report emotional strain, a major predictor of morbidity and mortality among caregivers.

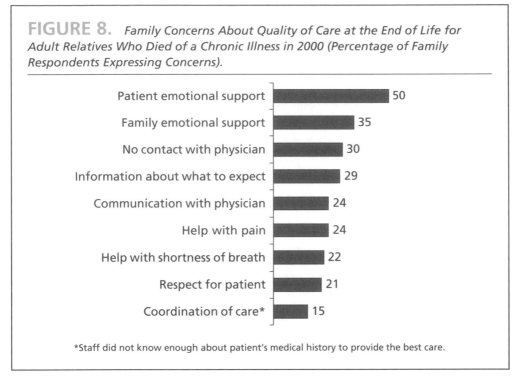

FIGURE 8. *Family Concerns About Quality of Care at the End of Life for Adult Relatives Who Died of a Chronic Illness in 2000 (Percentage of Family Respondents Expressing Concerns).*

Patient emotional support	50
Family emotional support	35
No contact with physician	30
Information about what to expect	29
Communication with physician	24
Help with pain	24
Help with shortness of breath	22
Respect for patient	21
Coordination of care*	15

*Staff did not know enough about patient's medical history to provide the best care.

Data Source: The Commonwealth Fund; Study of Care at the Last Place of Care (Teno, J. M. et al. 2004. *JAMA* 291:88-93). Reprinted with permission.
Source: McCarthy and Leatherman, Performance Snapshots, 2006. www.cmwf.org/snapshots.

The Loneliness of the Long-Term Caregiver

In addition to holding a full-time job, I manage all my husband's care and daily activities. Being a caregiver requires grit and persistence. It took me 10 days of increasingly insistent phone calls to get my managed-care company to replace my husband's dangerously unstable hospital bed. When the new bed finally arrived—without notice, in the evening, when there was no aide available to move him—it turned out to be the cheapest model, unsuitable for my husband's condition. In these all-too-frequent situations, I feel that I am challenging Goliath with a tiny pebble. More often than not, Goliath just puts me on hold.

Carol Levine, 1999[120]

Impact of Caregiving on Caregivers

Although the majority of family caregivers report low emotional stress, physical strain, and financial hardship, those taking on high burdens of physical care, who report poor health themselves, and who feel they had no choice in taking on the caregiver role are more likely to report significant emotional strain. Emotional strain in caregivers is

FIGURE 9. *Family Caregivers and the SUPPORT Study.*

Patient needed large amount of family caregiving:	34%
Lost most family savings:	31%
Lost major source of income:	29%
Major life change in family:	20%
Other family illness from stress:	12%
At least one of the above:	**55%**

Source: *JAMA* 1995; 272:1839. Reprinted with permission.

associated with a 63 percent increase in risk of death (see Figure 9),[121] and the Nurses Health Study (a large longitudinal study of more than fifty thousand nurses) found an 80 percent increase in risk of heart attack or cardiac death among nurses caring nine or more hours a week for a disabled or seriously ill spouse.[122]

What Do Caregivers Need?

Caregiver advocacy organizations call for fundamental changes in federal policies addressing family caregiver concerns, including:

- Protection of caregivers from the health and financial consequences of their role
- Building infrastructure for accessible and safe respite care
- Development of family-friendly workplace policies such as flextime, working at home, and job sharing
- Education and training to prepare caregivers for their role
- Access to a reliable and coordinated "medical home" or primary care provider
- Reliable availability of a trained and supervised direct-care workforce
- Coverage for regular professional assessment and reassessment of the long-term care situation at home.[123]

The capacity to give one's attention to a sufferer is a very rare and difficult thing; it is almost a miracle; it is a miracle.

Simone Weil, *Waiting for God*, 2000

PAYING FOR PALLIATIVE CARE

The United States spends more than $2 trillion a year on health care, at a per capita spending rate far higher than that of any other developed nation. Despite continued growth in spending, the United States ranks low on a number of quality benchmarks, including access, quality, equity, and efficiency.[124] At least in part, this paradox can be traced to a fee-for-service payment system that rewards unnecessary subspecialty care as well as excessive and inefficient medical service. Despite the evidence that primary care leads both to better quality and lower costs,[125] the perverse payment incentives and very high levels of medical student indebtedness upon graduation have led to growth in the number of well-reimbursed "proceduralists" (subspecialist physicians who focus on specific procedures) and a shrinking number of poorly reimbursed primary care and generalist physicians.[126]

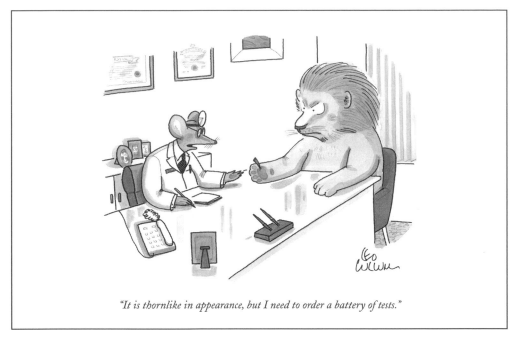

"It is thornlike in appearance, but I need to order a battery of tests."

Palliative care specialists are not proceduralists. Their expertise involves:

- Comprehensive patient and family assessment (for example, levels of pain and other symptoms, and equipment and care needs in the home)

- Provision of treatment designed to meet those needs (for example, pain medications or ordering a hospital bed and visiting nurse services)

- Discussion with colleagues, family members, and the patient about the patient's condition, the treatment options, and their concordance with the patient's goals

- Establishment of a feasible care plan

- Assurance that the plan is coordinated and carried out in the setting that best meets the needs of the patient and family

The current fee-for-service payment system does not compensate physicians and other health care professionals adequately for these kinds of cognitive services, even though they are of higher quality and lower cost than fragmented subspecialty care.[127] In many ways, it fails to pay for cognitive services at all. For example, the current Medicare payment system will not compensate physicians for the conduct of goals-of-care meetings with family members of seriously ill patients, whether in the hospital, in the office, or at home. Nor will Medicare reimburse the necessary collaborative process of decision making or the services of the interdisciplinary team required to deliver quality palliative care. If a clinician (a physician or a nurse practitioner) is not appropriately recognized and compensated for the intensive and repeated coordination and communication required, it should come as no surprise that the necessary communication and coordination seldom occurs.[128]

> *The average Medicare beneficiary sees an average of six unique physicians, and those with five or more chronic conditions see fourteen different physicians.*
> Gallup Serious Chronic Illness Survey, 2002

Emotionally demanding and skilled discussions about prognosis, treatment alternatives and their pros and cons, and gaining an in-depth understanding of the patient's wishes and values are time-consuming but crucial to the development of a rational and patient-centered plan of care. Failure to conduct such meetings results in a default to multiple fee-for-service specialists, each focused on a specific organ system or disease state, with no single professional synthesizing the inputs and taking responsibility for care of the whole patient. Not only is such care expensive, it is all too often of either marginal or no benefit to the patient.

Although palliative care providers do bill Medicare and other payers for the care they provide, the reimbursement for time-intensive but nonprocedural services fails to cover the salaries of these professionals. As a result, the recent growth in hospital palliative care services has been financed not by fee-for-service reimbursement to hospitals and providers but rather by hospital operating budgets. Hospitals have chosen to absorb the costs of palliative care services because they are persuaded by the business case for palliative care—namely, that hospitals will save money by delivering high-quality palliative care to their sickest and most vulnerable patients, helping them to avoid long hospital and ICU stays and costly interventions of marginal or no benefit.[129] In other words, hospitals have underwritten the costs of palliative care programs for cost-avoidance reasons. This is a frail reed on which to base support for a field so critical to quality care of the growing population of chronically and seriously ill patients.

EXPLAINING THE RAPID GROWTH OF PALLIATIVE CARE: QUALITY AND COST

In the chaotic context that is today's health care system, the growth of and demand for palliative care is nothing short of stunning. Many factors—including substantial private sector philanthropic investment, the perception of the public and health professionals that modern medicine is failing to meet the most fundamental needs of the most seriously ill, and the persistent search among idealistic professionals for ways of putting the needs of patients and their families first—have contributed to this phenomenon. First among these factors, however, is the positive impact of palliative care services on both the quality and the costs of care provided to seriously ill individuals and their families.

Palliative Care Is Quality Care

> *The secret of the care of the patient is in caring for the patient.*
> Francis Peabody, 1925[130]

The National Quality Forum, a national not-for-profit membership organization created to develop and implement a national strategy for health care quality measurement and improvement, defines quality as health care that meets six goals:

- Patient-centered (based on the patient's wishes and goals)
- Beneficial (likely to help the patient)
- Safe (not likely to harm the patient)
- Timely (delivered when it is appropriate, not too early and not too late)
- Equitable (available and applied to all who could benefit)
- Efficient (not wasteful of health resources and patient's time and effort)[131]

The health care quality movement recognizes that high-quality care depends a great deal more on effective systems than on individual behavior. It seeks to develop standards, best practices, and guidelines and to strengthen public reporting so that high-quality care will be routinely available to patients and their families. The evidence makes clear that palliative care delivers high-quality care in terms of benefit to patients, patient-centered focus, safety, and efficiency—but it is not yet timely or equitable.

- It is patient-centered because the palliative care plan is based on the goals and wishes of patients and families.
- It is beneficial; multiple studies have demonstrated reduced symptoms and improved satisfaction among patients (and their families) receiving palliative care as compared with similar patients who are not.
- It is safe; that is, it is not associated with earlier death.
- It is efficient, as demonstrated by reductions in health care utilization and resulting cost savings.

Palliative Care Is Patient-Centered and Beneficial

Recent studies confirm that survivors of patients who died in American hospitals, nursing homes, or at home without hospice have significant concerns about quality of care, with hospitals, nursing homes, and home health agencies all ranking substantially worse than hospice (see Figure 10).[132]

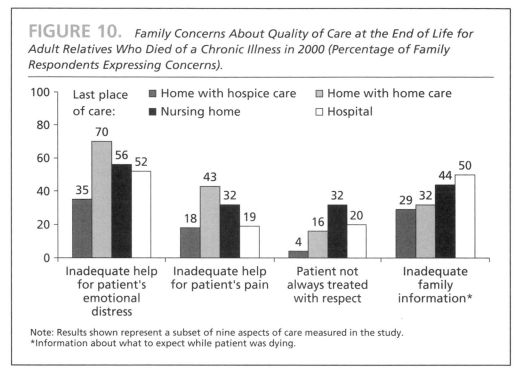

FIGURE 10. *Family Concerns About Quality of Care at the End of Life for Adult Relatives Who Died of a Chronic Illness in 2000 (Percentage of Family Respondents Expressing Concerns).*

Note: Results shown represent a subset of nine aspects of care measured in the study.
*Information about what to expect while patient was dying.

Data Source: The Commonwealth Fund; Study of Care at the Last Place of Care (Teno, J. M. et al. 2004. *JAMA* 291:88-93). Reprinted with permission.
Source: McCarthy and Leatherman, Performance Snapshots, 2006. www.cmwf.org/snapshots.

Multiple studies have demonstrated the benefits of palliative care in reducing pain and symptom burden and improving patient and family satisfaction with care.[133] For example, a recent study conducted among more than five hundred family survivors of seriously ill veterans demonstrated a marked superiority of palliative care over usual care in terms of emotional and spiritual support, adequacy of information and communication, care at time of death, access to services in the community, support for well-being and sense of dignity, receipt of care in a setting concordant with patient preferences, and relief of pain and symptoms of post-traumatic stress disorder.[134] Another randomized controlled trial of a brochure plus communications and listening intervention for families of dying ICU patients demonstrated significantly less anxiety, depression, and post-traumatic stress symptoms, for the intervention families as assessed ninety days after the death of their loved one.[135]

Palliative Care Is Efficient

In addition to the evidence of its positive impact on quality, palliative care has been shown to reduce hospital costs. Most hospitals in the United States are reimbursed by Medicare through diagnosis-related groups (DRGs), by which they receive a single lump-sum payment per hospital stay, regardless of what the stay actually costs the hospital. For example, the DRG payment for pneumonia with complications is the same whether the patient is discharged after five days or twenty-five days, and whether the actual total costs of the stay were $3,500 or $35,000. This payment method gives hospitals a clear financial incentive to invest in programs that can safely reduce both length of hospital stay as well as the costs of each day spent in the hospital.

Palliative care lowers costs for hospitals by reducing both the number of days spent in the hospital and the intensive care unit[136] and the use of costly diagnostic and therapeutic interventions of marginal or no benefit to patients, such as imaging studies, pharmaceuticals, and subspecialty consultations.[137] Studies have shown no difference in mortality or other adverse events associated with hospital palliative care, and, at least in the hospice setting, palliative care appears to be associated with both better survival and lower costs.[138]

Palliative care professionals are able to reduce hospitalizations and costly interventions primarily through enhanced communication with patients and their families. They are able to have open discussions about the realities of the illness and its likely course, and the treatment alternatives and their benefits and risks. Palliative care professionals are skilled at eliciting the primary concerns and goals of patients and their families, an understanding that leads to the development of care plans that will optimize the chances of patients' achieving their goals. This process often results in a different set of decisions by patients and families—decisions that help them use their time optimally and that typically (but not always) involve lower-intensity and lower-cost settings (such as going home with hospice or moving out of an intensive care unit that is no longer benefiting the patient). Recognition of the so-called cost-avoidance impact of palliative care programs in hospitals has been a major influence on their rapid spread. Palliative care is an exemplar of the growing recognition that lower cost and higher quality actually go hand in hand. There remain, however, some concerns about the way palliative care is currently delivered in the United States.

Palliative Care Is Not Timely

Though data are lacking, palliative care does not appear to be timely. The data that do exist suggest that about 30 percent of hospice patients are not referred until their last week of life, and 10 percent in their last twenty-four hours of life—too late to have much impact on the experience of their illness.[139] Similarly, though most data are from single-institution studies, a large proportion of palliative care referrals in acute care hospitals occur late in the hospital stay, well after opportunities to assess goals and make care plans accordingly have been missed.[140]

Palliative Care Is Not Equitable

As in virtually all other aspects of America's health care system, palliative care is not equitably accessible, both in terms of geographic location and patient race and ethnicity. Hospice statistics suggest that African American, Hispanic, and Asian minorities are less likely to receive hospice care than whites.[141] Furthermore, there is considerable geographic variation in access to both hospice and palliative care in the United States (see Figure 11).[142]

FIGURE 11. *State-by-State Variation in Hospice Use: Percent Using Hospice during Last Six Months of Life, Fee-for-Service Medicare Beneficiaries with Severe Chronic Illnesses Who Died During 2000–2003.*

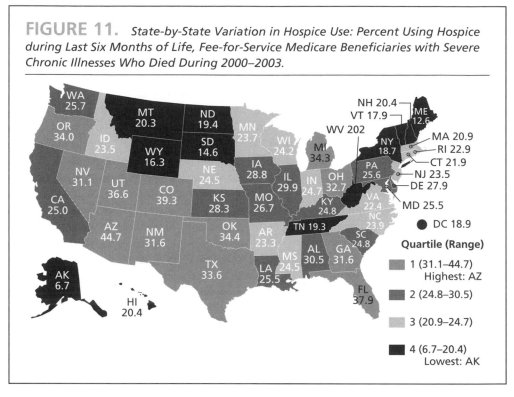

Note: Rates were adjusted for differences in age, sex, race, and prevalence of twelve chronic illnesses. Excludes Medicare beneficiaries enrolled in managed care plans.
Source: Data: Dartmouth Atlas Project 2006. Adapted and reprinted with permission.

THE WAY FORWARD

Building a Continuum of Palliative Care

One could be forgiven for thinking that seriously ill people spend most of their illness in hospitals, since that is the setting where nonhospice palliative care is most frequently provided. Although about 75 percent of Americans actually die in either a hospital or a nursing home, the vast majority of all serious illnesses are lived through at home, and the burden of care is assumed primarily by family members, with minimal support from the insurance system (unless the patient is eligible and ready for hospice care). If a patient is eligible and ready for hospice (that is, willing to give up insurance payment for life-prolonging or curative therapies and certified by two doctors as likely to be dead within six months), comprehensive interdisciplinary palliative care paid for through the Medicare hospice benefit is largely delivered at home. However, for the patient who is ineligible or unwilling to enter a hospice program, in most communities it is all but impossible to obtain palliative care services at home, in a doctor's office, or in a nursing home.

Although patients and families trying to manage complex and chronic illness clearly need and benefit from care that is carefully transitioned and well coordinated, the current fee-for-service payment system rewards procedures, hospitalization, and multiple specialist visits. Further, these perverse payment incentives, while rewarding fragmented care in the most expensive settings, simultaneously deny adequate payment for so-called cognitive (non-procedure-based) services involving coordination, communication, and oversight of the patient as a whole person. Because of this lack of appropriate payment incentives, no clear business case for supporting a continuum of palliative care has emerged outside of hospital settings.

Despite the current fragmented and counterproductive reimbursement system, models to provide palliative care across settings have been successfully developed in some communities, primarily through the efforts of strong community hospice program leaders. These hospice leaders have expanded their services to deliver both hospice and nonhospice palliative care across a range of care settings within their communities.

The efforts are exemplified by the work of two well-established and large community hospice programs: the Hospice and Palliative Care Center of the Bluegrass,[143] in Lexington, Kentucky, and the Midwest Hospice and Palliative Care Center,[144] in Evanston, Illinois. Leaders of these community hospice programs recognized that substantial numbers of patients in hospitals and nursing homes and at home were in need of palliative care but were not receiving it because they were ineligible for, or unwilling to access, hospice care. Over time, both programs developed nonhospice hospital palliative care consultation services, hospital inpatient palliative care units, office- and home-based palliative care practices, and palliative care consultation teams for nursing homes. Thus, no matter what the stage of illness, the diagnosis, the prognosis, or the insurance coverage, patients served by these programs can obtain palliative care where they are and when they need it. This diversification of service lines builds continuity into the system; eventually, the illnesses of most patients progress to a point where they are both eligible for and willing to receive hospice care. The transition from usual care to hospice care is less abrupt and easier for patients and their families when they have gained familiarity with the benefits of nonhospice palliative care.

The leaders of these two programs were able to develop these innovations by focusing on the needs of patients first, working out the payment mechanisms later, and relying on economies of scale and enhanced income (for example, from more and longer hospice stays) in some areas to compensate for losses in others.[145] Their programs are a model for what can be accomplished with appropriate leadership and strong community and philanthropic support. However, palliative care will be not be reliably available across the country in all care settings until the financial incentives rewarding hospitalization, specialty care, and high-technology drugs and devices are shifted to a system rewarding coordination, communication, and patient-centered services at home and in the community (see Figure 12).

Policies to Improve Access to Palliative Care within the Current Payment System

In the absence of fundamental change in the way that health care is organized and compensated, incremental efforts to improve quality are necessary. Achieving the goal of assuring access to high-quality palliative care for all Americans who need it—regardless of geography, diagnosis, prognosis, care setting, stage of illness, family situation, or social class—will require more than the innovative programs described above.

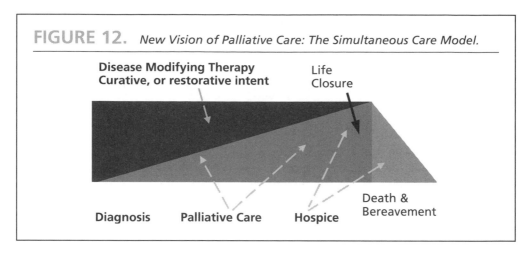

FIGURE 12. *New Vision of Palliative Care: The Simultaneous Care Model.*

Source: National Hospice Work Group; Adapted from work of the Canadian Palliative Care Association and Frank Ferris, MD. Reprinted with permission.

It will require:

- *A public knowledgeable about what palliative care is and when they should demand it*

- *Health care professionals with the knowledge, skill, and attitudes necessary to provide palliative care*

- *Hospitals, nursing homes, office practices, home care agencies, and others equipped with the resources necessary to deliver palliative care services*

These requirements have policy implications, as illustrated in Table 3.

TABLE 3. **Policy Recommendations to Improve Access to Quality Palliative Care**

Goals	Policy Recommendations
Patients and families will know what palliative care is and when to demand it.	Federal and private sector investment in a major social marketing campaign
Medical professionals have the knowledge and skills to provide quality palliative care.	Legislation will assure that NIH funding for palliative care will at least quadruple from its current level to approximately 2 percent of the total NIH grants budget. All major NIH Institutes will fund palliative care research. To assure peer review, study sections of grant reviewers responsible for evaluating palliative care research will include at least three palliative care scientists, and one or more palliative care specific study sections will be formed.

	Regulatory and accrediting bodies responsible for undergraduate and postgraduate medical, nursing, and other health professional education will mandate adequate and required curricular content and time commitment to palliative care skills and knowledge.
	Both the federal and private sector will support junior faculty palliative care career development awards similar to the Geriatric Academic Career Award.
	Reimbursement will be commensurate with complexity for cognitive and prolonged professional services through establishment of palliative care professional current procedural terminology (CPT) billing codes.
	Lift the government cap on hospital graduate medical education (GME) training slots to assure salary support for ACGME-accredited palliative medicine fellowship training programs. Develop additional private sector support for palliative medicine fellowship training.
Hospitals and other care settings are equipped to deliver and support palliative care services.	Change regulatory and accreditation requirements so that health care institutions must deliver quality palliative care as a condition of accreditation.
	Medicare and other payers create payment incentives for hospital and provider delivery of palliative care to appropriate patient populations.
	Public and private investment in development and testing of clinical models for effective efficient delivery of palliative care in nursing home, office practice, home care, and long term-acute care settings.

In summary, government and regulatory policy is required to bring the palliative care innovation to scale. Success will be achieved when all patients with advanced illness and their families can reliably access high-quality palliative care no matter where they live, what illness(es) they have, what their stage of disease, and where they need care. Policy solutions range from the quick and easy (career development awards for palliative medicine and nursing faculty; lifting the cap on GME dollars for palliative medicine fellowships accredited by the Accreditation Council for Graduate Medical Education; increasing NIH allocations for palliative care research) to more complex long-term efforts (such as payment reform, accreditation requirements, and curricular change).

BACK TO BASICS: WHAT ARE THE ENDS OF MEDICINE? WHAT ARE THE ENDS OF A SOCIETY?

We are all in this together. Consider the kind of health care system we would design for our future selves if we had the choice and could not know what family we'd be born into. It would include health care available to everyone regardless of social class or income, with priority for surviving childbirth and childhood, treatment of curable and remediable illness, assurance of relief for those who suffer, and practical support for family caregivers and community resources. Even if our societal resources are infinite, all of us will still die. All of us are profoundly interdependent and interrelated. All of us need our families to help care for us when our turn comes, and all of us rely on societal infrastructure and resources to help us when we are in need, protect our families from financial ruin imposed by illness, and assure us an equal shot at a long and healthy life.

Palliative care has emerged in American health care on the platform of these truths. It cuts through our cherished myths of personal immortality and the false god of the technology imperative. It recognizes that serious illness and the suffering that accompanies it is a universal human condition, affecting every one of us. It is designed to address the fact that serious illnesses in modern America are almost always chronic—we live for a very long time with what will eventually kill us. It recognizes that families are the mainstay of the ill and that families need information, guidance, and support to help them fulfill their responsibilities. It strives to redress the fragmentation and discontinuities of the health care system, recognizing that the patient and the family still need care when they leave the hospital or the doctor's office. Palliative care wins trust because it begins and ends with what patients and families say they want and need: relief from pain and other symptom distress; kind and respectful treatment; information necessary to retain control over decisions; help for families; and an opportunity to strengthen relationships with others, seeking meaning through human connection "as deep calls to deep in the roar of waters" (Psalms 42:7).

APPENDIX

Major Foundation Investments in Building Palliative Care[146]

Research	SUPPORT, which clearly demonstrated poor quality care in terms of pain, communication, family burden, health care utilization	Robert Wood Johnson Foundation
	Research on spirituality during serious illness and near the end of life	Fetzer Institute; Nathan Cummings Foundation
	Grief Research: Report on Gaps, Needs, and Actions	Open Society Institute
	Improving pain management through research, training, technical assistance	Mayday Fund
	Establishment of the National Palliative Care Research Center	Initial funding by Emily Davie and Joseph F. Kornfeld Foundation; subsequent funding by Olive Branch Fund, Brookdale and Ho Chiang Foundations, American Cancer Society, American Academy of Hospice and Palliative Medicine, and National Institute on Aging
Leadership Development	Faculty Scholars Program of the Project on Death in America: 87 grantees at more than 60 medical and nursing schools, building the academic and clinical field	Open Society Institute
	Social Work Leadership Development Awards	Open Society Institute
	Palliative Medicine Leadership Forum: Annual retreat to strengthen and build academic physician leaders	Robert Wood Johnson Foundation
	Faculty Development in the Veterans Health Administration	Robert Wood Johnson Foundation

Physician Education	2,000 EPEC (Education in Palliative and End-of-Life Care) graduates, and millions trained by these graduates	Robert Wood Johnson Foundation
	Improving Residency Training in End-of-Life, Medical College of Wisconsin	Robert Wood Johnson Foundation
	Promoting "caring attitudes" among health professionals; improving communication and self-care skills in physicians in training	Arthur Vining Davis Foundation
	Harvard Medical School's Program in Palliative Care Education and Practice: Intensive two-week midcareer training; more than 400 graduates as of December 2008	Robert Wood Johnson, Good Samaritan, Jane and the late Charles Weingarten, and Green Family Foundations; Open Society Institute
	The Initiative for Pediatric Palliative Care	Open Society Institute; Aetna, Schwartz, Nathan Cummings, and Argosy Foundations
	End of Life/Palliative Education Resource Center (EPERC): Provides curricular materials on the Web	Robert Wood Johnson Foundation
	Stanford University Medical School Faculty Development Program, 10/1/98–9/30/02	Department of Health and Human Services; Department of Veterans Affairs; John A. Hartford, Robert Wood Johnson, and Josiah Macy Foundations
	Palliative medicine fellowship training	Emily Davie and Joseph S. Kornfeld Foundation; Open Society Institute
Nursing Education	As of December 2007, 4,200 graduates who have educated more than 125,000 nurses using train-the-trainer model via End of Life Nursing Education Consortium (ELNEC)	Robert Wood Johnson Foundation, Aetna Archstone, Oncology Nursing and California HealthCare Foundations, Open Society Institute, and the National Cancer Institute.
	Nursing Leadership Consortium on End of Life Care	Open Society Institute

	End-of-life educational materials for nursing school faculty and practicing nurses, University of Washington School of Nursing	Robert Wood Johnson Foundation
	Strengthening Nursing Education in Pain Management and End-of-Life Care, City of Hope National Medical Center	Robert Wood Johnson Foundation
Exploring New Care Models	Promoting Excellence in End-of-Life Care: 22 demonstration projects delivering palliative care to special populations (e.g., children, mentally ill, the poor, Native Americans), medical conditions (Alzheimer's, HIV/AIDS), and challenging settings (prisons, rural areas, nursing homes, cancer centers)	Robert Wood Johnson Foundation
Capacity Building	Center to Advance Palliative Care: Disseminates technical assistance and tools in support of hospital palliative care programs, 1999–present	Robert Wood Johnson, John A. Hartford, Aetna, JEHT, Milbank Rehabilitation, Brookdale, Donaghue, Fan Fox and Leslie R. Samuels, Ho Chiang, and Archstone Foundations; Department of Veterans Affairs, 1999–present
	Investment in palliative care program capacity building in New York City hospitals	Open Society Institute; United Hospital Fund; Greenwall, Fan Fox and Leslie R. Samuels and JM Foundations
	Investment in palliative care program capacity building in California	Archstone and California HealthCare Foundations
	United Hospital Fund of New York City: Hospital Palliative Care Initiative and Community-Oriented Palliative Care Initiative in New York City	Open Society Institute; United Hospital Fund; United Way of New York City

	Initiative to Improve Palliative Care for African-Americans: Developed research education policy agenda and built coalitions to improve access	U.S. Cancer Pain Relief Committee; Open Society Institute; Dade Community Foundation; Foundation for End-of-Life Care
	Duke Institute on Care at the End of Life: Develops professional and public educational materials, coalitions, and outreach through faith and cultural communities	Open Society Institute; Robert Wood Johnson Foundation
	Palliative Care in Prisons and Jails: Development of National Guidelines (*Guiding Responsive Action in Corrections at End-of-Life*)	Robert Wood Johnson Foundation
Quality Guidelines and Practice Standards	Joint Commission on Accreditation of Healthcare Organizations (JCAHO): Issued standards for hospice participation, 1981	W. K. Kellogg and Arthur Vining Davis Foundations
	National Consensus Project Guidelines for Quality Palliative Care	Robert Wood Johnson, Arthur Vining Davis, California HealthCare, Charitable Leadership, and Milbank Rehabilitation Foundations; Mayday Fund
	Development of the National Quality Forum's national framework for palliative and hospice care quality measurement and reporting	Robert Wood Johnson Foundation
Textbook Project	Reviews of palliative care content in major medical, nursing, and social work textbooks, demonstrating near complete absence of palliative care content, resulted in addition of content to many major texts	Robert Wood Johnson Foundation; Open Society Institute

Public Outreach	Public education and community organizing about end of life care (the Last Acts campaign), including a four-part PBS program, *On Our Own Terms: Moyers on Dying*, seen by more than 20 million people; the Writers Project, which developed scripts and story lines on care of the dying for popular television; technical support from the Media Resource Center for the film *Wit*; and American RadioWorks' *The Hospice Experiment*	Robert Wood Johnson, Nathan Cummings, Kohlberg, John D. and Catherine T. MacArthur, and JL Foundations; Open Society Institute; Laurance S. Rockefeller Fund; Mutual of America Life Insurance Company
	Community grief and bereavement initiative: Model interfaith, schools, prison, and community programs in support of bereavement	Open Society Institute
	American Pain Foundation: To improve consumer access to information about pain and its management	Open Society Institute; Anderson Family Living Trust; Disabled American Veterans Charitable Service Trust; Gess Donor Fund; Kamish Living Trust; Nathan Bruckenthal Memorial Trust; Reflex Sympathetic Dystrophy Hope Group; California Community; Emmert Hobbs, Herb Block, Mary R. and Joseph R. Payden, Medtronic, Milbank Rehabilitation, and William and Joanne Moeller Foundations
	Grief at School Program: Trained school-based professionals to identify and help grieving children.	Open Society Institute
Professional Journals	Supported a series of articles on palliative care topics in major medical and nursing journals	Robert Wood Johnson Foundation

Accreditation and Regulation	Supported addition of pain as a fifth vital sign as Joint Commission accreditation requirement for hospitals and nursing homes	Robert Wood Johnson Foundation
Medical Licensure Examinations	Supported the National Board of Medical Examiners to assess and add palliative care questions to the U.S. Medical Licensing Examination	Robert Wood Johnson Foundation
Health Policy	Community-State Partnerships to Improve End-of-Life Care: Developed community coalitions in 21 states	Robert Wood Johnson Foundation
	Systematic analysis of drug regulations and their impact on pain management via the Pain & Policy Studies Group	Open Society Institute
	Pioneer Programs in Palliative Care: 9 case studies	Milbank Memorial Fund; Robert Wood Johnson Foundation
	Palliative Academic Career Awards: Policy report calls for federal funding of career development awards for junior faculty in palliative medicine	Open Society Institute; Greenwall Foundation
	Protecting Americans from religious restrictions at end of life; promoting policy to strengthen advance care planning	Nathan Cummings Foundation
	Americans for Better Care of the Dying: Social, policy, and professional reform	Open Society Institute
Organized Medicine	Cosponsored three Institute of Medicine reports calling for fundamental change in financing, structure, education, and research for the seriously ill: *Approaching Death: Improving Care at the End of Life* (1997), *Improving Palliative Care for Cancer* (2001), and *When Children Die: Improving Palliative and End-of-Life Care for Children and their Families* (2003)	Open Society Institute; Robert Wood Johnson, Greenwall, Culpeper, Archstone, and James Irvine Foundations; Milbank Memorial Fund; Commonwealth Fund

	Support for palliative care professional membership organizations (American Academy of Hospice and Palliative Medicine, Hospice and Palliative Nursing Association) and for Social Work Summit on Palliative and End-of-Life Care	Open Society Institute
	Support for National Hospice and Palliative Care Organization	Open Society Institute; Robert Wood Johnson Foundation
	Support for standards for training, practice, and certification by the American Board of Hospice and Palliative Medicine; led to establishment of American Board of Medical Specialties–approved subspecialty for palliative medicine	Open Society Institute; Robert Wood Johnson Foundation
Spirituality and Palliative Care	George Washington Institute for Spirituality and Health	Templeton Foundation
Building Private Sector Investment	Grantmakers Concerned with Care at the End of Life	Robert Wood Johnson and Nathan Cummings Foundations; Open Society Institute; Commonwealth Fund
	Collaborative to Advance Funding in Palliative Care	Open Society Institute; Robert Wood Johnson, Emily Davie and Joseph S. Kornfeld, Fan Fox and Leslie R. Samuels, and Altman Foundations along with 15 other participant foundations
Arts and Humanities	Engaged artists in diverse media on topics of serious illness and death	Open Society Institute

NOTES

1. U.S. lags behind other countries in life expectancy. *International Herald Tribune.* August 11, 2007.

2. Ford ES, Ajani UA, Critchley JA, et al. Explaining the decrease in U.S. deaths from coronary disease, 1980–2000. *N Engl J Med.* 2007; 356:2388–98; Crimmins EM, Saito Y. Trends in healthy life expectancy in the United States, 1970–1990: gender, racial, and educational differences. *Soc Sci Med.* 2001; 52:1629–1641; Mor V. The compression of morbidity hypothesis: a review of research and prospects for the future. *J Am Geriatr Soc.* 2005: 53(9s): S308–S309.

3. US Census Bureau. *US Census Bureau survey of income and program participation.* June-Sept, 2002.

4. McNeil J. Americans with disabilities: 1997. *Current Population Reports, P70–73, US Census Bureau.* Washington DC: US Government Printing Office; 2000.

5. Poisal JA, Truffer C, Smith C, et al. Health spending projections through 2016: modest changes obscure Part D's impacts. *Health Affairs.* February 12, 2007:W242–253.

6. Schoen C. In chronic condition: experience of patient with complex care need in 8 countries. *Health Affairs* web exclusive. November 13, 2008:W1–16.

7. Schoen C, Collins SR, Kriss JL, Doty, MM. How Many Are Underinsured? Trends Among U.S. Adults, 2003 and 2007. *Health Affairs* web exclusive. June 10, 2008: W298–w309.

8. Callahan D. Conservatives, liberals, and medical progress. *The New Atlantis.* 2005; 10:3–16.

9. Employee Benefit Research Institute. *2006 Health Confidence Survey: dissatisfaction with health care system doubles since 1998.* Nov. 2006;27(11). Available at: http://www.ebri.org/publications/notes/index.cfm?fa=notesDisp&content_id=3758. Accessed April 26, 2009.

10. The Commonwealth Fund. *Commonwealth Fund survey of public views of the healthcare system, 2006.* Available at: http://www.commonwealthfund.org/surveys/surveys_show.htm?doc_id=394593. Accessed April 26, 2009.

11. Teno JM, Clarridge BR, Casey V, et al. Family perspectives on end-of-life care at the last place of care. *JAMA.* 2004; 291:88–93; Audet AJ, Doty MM, Shamasdin J, et al. *Physician's view of quality care: findings from the Commonwealth Fund National Survey of Physicians and Quality Care.* The Commonwealth Fund, May 2005.

12. Ariès P. *The Hour of our Death.* New York: Oxford University Press; 1991.

13. Tolstoy L. *The Death of Ivan Ilych and Other Stories.* New York: Barnes and Nobles Classics; 2004,127.

14. Gorer G. *Death, Grief and Mourning in Contemporary Britain.* London: Cresset Press; 1965.

15. Schweitzer A. *On the Edge of the Primeval Forest.* London: Home Farm Books; 2006.

16. Dickinson E. *The Selected Poems of Emily Dickinson.* New York, The Modern Library; 2000, 14.

17. Oral History Project of the John C. Liebeskind History of Pain Collection of the UCLA Louise M. Darling Biomedical Library, manuscript collection no. 127.16.

18. Melzack R, Wall P. Pain mechanisms: a new theory. *Science.* 1965; 150:171–79.

19. Mitchell SW. *Injuries of Nerves and Their Consequences.* Philadelphia: J.B. Lippincott; 1872.

20. Livingston WK. *Pain Mechanisms.* New York: Plenum Press; 1943.

21. Bonica JJ. *The Management of Pain.* In: Lea and Febiger, 2nd ed. Philadelphia: Lippincott Williams & Wilkins; 1990.

22. Schmitt P. Rehabilitation of chronic pain: a multi-disciplinary approach. *J Rehabil.* 1985; 51:72.

23. Hardt J, Jacobsen C, Goldberg J, et al. Prevalence of chronic pain in a representative sample in the United States. *Pain Medicine.* 2008; 9:803–12.

24. American Pain Foundation. *Pain Fact & Figures.* Available at: http://www.painfoundation.org/page.asp?file=Newsroom/PainFacts.htm. Accessed April 26, 2009.

25. American Pain Foundation, 2008.

26. Desbiens NA, Wu AW. Pain and suffering in seriously ill hospitalized patients. *J Am Geriatr Soc.* 2000; 48: S183–186.

27. Von Roenn JH, Cleeland CS, Gonni R, et al. Physician attitudes and practice in cancer pain management. A survey from the Eastern Cooperative Oncology Group. *Ann Intern Med.* 1993; 119(2):121–6.

28. Nguyen M, Ugarte C, Fuller I, Portenoy RK. Access to care for chronic pain: racial and ethnic differences. *J Pain.* 2005; 6:301–14.

29. Breuer B, Pappagallo M, Tai JY, et al. U.S. Board certified pain physician practices: uniformity and census data of their locations. *J Pain.* 2006; 8:244–50.

30. Clay, MC. *The Medieval Hospitals of England.* Whitefish, MT: Kessinger Publishing; 2006, 236.

31. Abel EK. The hospice movement: institutionalizing innovation. *Int J. Health Serv.* 1986; 16(1):71–85; Stoddard S. *The Hospice Movement.* New York: Vintage; 1992; Ryndes T, et al. The development of palliative medicine in the USA, in *Textbook of Palliative Medicine,* Bruera E, et al., editors. London; Hodder Arnold; 2006:29–35.

32. Saunders, C. 1958 Available at: http://www.bmj.com/cgi/content/full/331/7509/DC1

33. Saunders C. *Living with Dying: a Guide to Palliative Care.* New York: Oxford University Press; 1995.

34. Wald FS. Towards development of a nursing practice theory. In Folta JR, Dock ES. *A Social Framework for Patient Care.* San Francisco: Wiley; 1966, 309.

35. Kübler-Ross E. *On Death and Dying.* New York: Scribner; 1965.

36. Biewen, J. *The Hospice Experiment.* American Radio Works; June 2004. Available at: http://americanradioworks.publicradio.org/features/hospice/. Accessed April 26, 2009.

37. Taylor DH, Ostermann J, Van Houtven CH, et al. What length of hospice use maximizes reduction in medical expenditures near death in the US Medicare program? *Soc Sci Med.* 2007; 65:1466–78.

38. http://www.nhpco.org/files/pblic/Statistics_Research/NHPCO_facts-and-figures_2008.pdf

39. Connor SR, Elwert F, Spence C, Christakis NA. Geographic variation in hospice use in the United States in 2002. *J Pain Symptom Manage.* 2007; 34:277–85.

40. Sack K. In Hospice Care, Longer Lives Mean Money Lost. *New York Times*; November 27, 2007:1.

41. Morrison RS, Meier DE. Palliative care. *N Engl J Med.* 2004; 350:2582–2590.

42. Caplan A, McCartney JJ, Sisti D, editors. *The Case of Terri Schiavo: Ethics at the End of Life.* Amherst NY: Prometheus Books; 2006.

43. Hammes BJ, Rooney BL. Death and end of life planning in one Midwestern community. *Arch Intern Med.* 1998; 158:383–90; Hickman SE, Hammes BJ, Moss AH, Tolle SW. Hope for the future: achieving the original intent of advance directives. *Hastings Ctr Rep.* 2005; November-December: S26.

44. Jackson EA, Yarzebeski, JL, Goldberg, RJ, et al. DNR orders in patients hospitalized with acute MI. *Arch Int Med* 2004; 164:776–83; Zweig SC et al. Effect of DNR orders on hospitalization of NH residents evaluation for LRI. *J Amer Geri Soc.* 2003; 52:51–8.

45. Burt RA. The end of autonomy. *Hastings Ctr Rep.* 2005; 35:S9–13.

46. http://ohsu.edu/ethics/polst/.

47. Hickman SE, Tolle SW, Brummel-Smith K, et al. Use of the physician orders for life sustaining treatment program in Oregon nursing facilities: beyond resuscitation status. *J Amer Geriatr Soc.* 2004; 52:1424–9.

48. McCormack RA. *The Living Will Handbook.* Winter Park: Hastings House; 1991, 18.

49. Quill TE, Cassel CK, Meier DE. Care of the hopelessly ill. Proposed clinical criteria for physician-assisted suicide. *N Engl J Med.* 1992; 327(19):1380–4; Miller FG, Quill TE, Brody H, Fletcher JC, Gostin LO, Meier DE. Regulating physician-assisted death. *N Engl J Med.* 1994; 331(2):119–23.

50. Gallup A, Newport F. *The Gallup Poll.* New York: Rowman and Littlefield; 2006, 179.

51. Cassel CK, Meier DE. Morals and moralism in the debate over euthanasia and assisted suicide. *N Engl J Med.* 1990; 323(11):750–752.

52. Whatever its legality or illegality, the practice is not unknown. A national representative survey of American physicians conducted in 1996 found that since entering practice, 18.3 percent of the physicians reported having received a request from a patient for assistance with suicide and 11.1 percent had received a request for a lethal injection (a practice that is illegal in all states.). Sixteen percent of the physicians receiving such requests reported that they had written at least one prescription to be used to hasten death, and 4.7 percent said that they had administered at least one lethal injection.

53. Charatan F. US Supreme Court upholds Oregon's Death with Dignity Act. *Br Med J.* 2006; 332:195.

54. Oregon Department of Human Services. *Summary of Oregon's Death with Dignity Act.* Available at: http://egov.oregon.gov/DHS/ph/pas/docs/year9.pdf. Accessed on December 10, 2008.

55. Battin MP, van der Heide A, Ganzini L, et al. Legal physician-assisted dying in Oregon and the Netherlands: evidence concerning the impact on patients in "vulnerable" groups. *J Med Ethics.* 2007; 33(10):591–7.

56. http://seattletimes.nwsource.com/html/nationaworld/2008352350_assistesuicdie05.m.html.

57. SUPPORT. A controlled trial to improve care for seriously ill hospitalized patients. The study to understand prognoses and preferences for outcomes and risks of treatments (SUPPORT). *JAMA.* 1995; 274:1591–8.

58. Desbiens NA, Wu AW. Pain and suffering in seriously ill hospitalized patients. *J Am Geriatr Soc.* 2000; 48(5 suppl):S183–S186.

59. Covinsky KE. Is economic hardship on families of the seriously ill associated with patient and surrogate care preferences? *Arch Int Med.* 1996; 156:1737–41; Covinsky KE, Goldman L, Cook EF, et al. Impact of serious illness on patient's families. *JAMA.* 1994; 272:1839–44.

60. Fox E, Landrum-McNiff K, Zhong ZS, et al. Evaluation of prognostic criteria for determining hospice eligibility in patients with heart, lung, or liver disease. *JAMA.* 1999; 282:1638–45.

61. Covinsky KE, Fuller JD, Yaffe K, et al. Communication and decision-making in seriously ill patients: findings of the SUPPORT project. *J Am Geriatr Soc.* 2000; 48: S187–93.

62. Covinsky KE, Fuller JD, Yaffe K, et al.; Teno JM, Lynn J, Connors AF Jr, et al. The illusion of end-of-life resource savings with advanced directives. *J Am Geriatr Soc.* 1997; 45:513–18.

63. SUPPORT, 1995.

64. SUPPORT, 1995.

65. Lynn J, Arkes HR, Stephens M, et al. Rethinking fundamental assumptions: SUPPORT's implications for future reform. *J Am Geriatr Soc.* 2000; 48: S214–221.

66. Hamel MB, Phillips RS, Teno JM, et al. Seriously ill hospitalized older adults: do we spend less on older patients? *J Am Geriatr Soc.* 1996; 44:1043–8.

67. Joanne Lynn. Unexpected Returns. *The Robert Wood Johnson Foundation Anthology 1997.* San Francisco: Jossey-Bass; 1997.

68. Institute of Medicine. *Approaching Death: Improving Care at the End of Life.* Washington, DC: National Academies Press; 1997.

69. Institute of Medicine. *Improving Palliative Care for Cancer.* Washington, DC: National Academies Press; 2001.

70. Institute of Medicine. *When Children Die: Improving Palliative and End of life Care for Children and Their Families.* Washington, DC: National Academies Press; 2002.

71. Fisher ES, Wennberg DE, Stukel TA, et al. The implications of regional variations in Medicare spending. Part 1: the content, quality, and accessibility of care. *Ann Intern Med.* 2003; 138(4):273–87. Fisher ES, Wennberg DE, Stukel TA, et al. The implications of regional variations in Medicare spending. Part 2: health outcomes and satisfaction with care. *Ann Intern Med.* 2003; 138(4):288–98. Fisher ES, Welch HG. Avoiding the unintended consequence of growth in medical care: how might more be worse? *JAMA.,* 1999; 281(5):446–453.

72. Dartmouth Atlas Project. The Care of Patients with Severe Chronic Illness: An Online Report on the Medicare Program by the Dartmouth Atlas Project. *The Dartmouth Atlas of Health Care 2006.* Center to the Evaluative Clinical Sciences Dartmouth Medical School. Available at: www.dartmouthatlas.org/atlases/2006_Chronic_Care_Atlas.pdf. Accessed April 26, 2009.

73. Teno JM, Mor V, Ward N, et al. Bereaved family members perceptions of quality of end-of-life care in US regions with high and low usage of intensive care unit care. *J Am Geriatr Soc.* 2005; 53:1905–11.

74. Sirovich BE, Gottleib DJ, Welsch HD, et al. Regional variations in health care intensity and physician perceptions of quality of care. *Annals Intern Med.* 2006; 144:641–649.

75. Bronner E. The Foundation's End of Life Programs: Changing the American Way of Death. *To Improve Health and Health Care, Volume VI: The Robert Wood Johnson Foundation Anthology.* San Francisco: Jossey-Bass; 2003.

76. McGlinchey L, editor. *Transforming the Culture of Dying: The Project on Death in America, October 1994— December, 2003.* New York: Open Society Institute; 2004.

77. National Consensus Project for Quality Palliative Care; National Quality Forum.

78. Cassel E. The nature of suffering and the goals of medicine, *N Engl J Med.* 1982; 306:639–645.

79. National Consensus Project for Quality Palliative Care. Clinical Practice Guidelines (2004). Available at: http://www.nationalconsensusproject.org/Guidelines_Download.asp. Accessed April 26, 2009.

80. National Quality Forum. *A National Framework and Preferred Practices for Palliative and Hospice Care*; December 2006. Available at: http://www.qualityforum.org/publications/reports/palliative.asp. Accessed April 26, 2009.

81. The Joint Commission. Services Certification. Available at: http://www.jointcommission.org/CertificationPrograms/HCS/. Accessed April 26, 2009.

82. National Board of Certification of Hospice & Palliative Care Nurses. Available at: http://www.nbchpn.org/DisplayPage.aspx?Title=Why%20Certification. Accessed April 26, 2009.

83. National Hospice and Palliative Care Organization. Available at: http://www.nhpco.org/files/public/Statistics_Research/NHPCO_facts-and-figures_2008. Accessed April 26, 2009.

84. Sources: American Board of Hospice and Palliative Medicine. Available at: www.abhpm.org. Accessed April 26, 2009; National Board of Certified Hospice and Palliative Care Nurses. Available at: http://www.nbchpn.org/Certificants_Map.aspx?Cert=CHPN. Accessed April 26, 2009; American Academy of Hospice and Palliative Medicine. Available at: http://www.aahpm.org/fellowship/directory.html. Accessed April 26, 2009; Hospice and Palliative Care Nurses Association. Available at: http://www.hpna.org/DisplayPage.aspx?Title=Degree%20Programs. Accessed April 26, 2009; Center to Advance Palliative Care. Available at: http://www.capc.org/research-and-references-for-palliative-care/journals. Accessed April 26, 2009; National Hospice and Palliative Care Organization. Available at: http://www.nhpco.org/files/public/Statistics_Research/NHPCO_facts-and-figures_2008.pdf. Accessed April 26, 2009.

85. http://resources.bmj.com/bmj/interactive/polls, April 2008. Accessed April 26, 2009.

86. Baransky B, Jonas HS, Etzel SI. Educational programs in U.S. medical schools. 1990–1999. *J Amer Med Assoc.* 1999; 282:840–6; Billings JA, Block S. Palliative care in undergraduate medical education. *J Amer Med Assoc.* 1997; 278(9):733–738.

87. Barzansky B, Etzel SI. Educational programs in US medical schools, 2002–2003. *J Amer Med Assoc.* 2003; 290:1190–6; Dickinson GE. Teaching end-of-life issues in US medical schools: 1975 to 2005. *Am J Hosp Palliat Care.* 2006; 23:197–204.

88. Sulmasy DP, Cimino JE, He MK, et al. U.S. medical students' perceptions of the adequacy of their schools' curricular attention to care at the end of life: 1998–2006. *J Palliative Med.* 2008; 11:707–716.

89. Bickel-Swenson D. End of life training in U.S. medical schools: a systematic literature review. *J Palliat Med.* 2007; 10:229–235.

90. Hammel JF, Sullivan AM, Block SD, et al. End of life and palliative care education for final year medical students: a comparison of Britain and the United States. *J Palliat Med.* 2007; 10:1356.

91. International Longevity Center-USA. *Palliative Care Academic Career Awards: A Public Private Partnership to Improve Care for the Most Vulnerable.* Policy Report. Available at: www.ilcusa.org/media/pdfs/palliativecare.pdf. Accessed April 26, 2009.

92. Billings JA, Block S. Palliative care in undergraduate medical education—status report and future directions. *JAMA.* 1997;278; 278:733–738.

93. Institute of Medicine, 1997.

94. Hill TP. Treating the dying patient: the challenge for medical education. *Arch Intern Med* 1995; 155:1265–1269.

95. Weissman DE, Ambuel B, Norton AJ, et al. A survey of competencies and concerns in end-of-life care for physician trainees. *J Pain Symptom Manage.* 1998; 15(2):82–90; Buss MK, Alexander GC, Switzer GE, et al. Assessing competence of residents to discuss end-of-life issues. *J Palliat Med.* 2005; 8(2):363–371.

96. Buss MK, Alexander GC, Switzer GE, et al. Assessing competence of residents to discuss end of life issues. *J Palliat Med.* 2005; 8:363–71.

97. Goldsmith B, Dietrich J, Du Q, et al. Variability in access to hospital palliative care in the United States. *J Palliat Med.* 2008; 11(8):1094–1102.

98. Ferrell B, Coyle N, The nature of suffering and the goals of nursing. *Oncol Nursing Forum.* 2008;35:241; 35:241–247.

99. Ferrell BR, Virani R, Grant M, et al. Evaluation of the end of life nursing education consortium undergraduate faculty training program. *J Palliative Med.* 2005; 8(1):107–114. Paice JA, Ferrell BR, Virani R, Grant M, Malloy P, Rhome A. Graduate nursing education regarding end of life care. *Nurs Outlook.* 2006; 54(1):46–52.

100. Ferrell BR. Evaluation of the end of life nursing education consortium project in the USA. *Intl J Pal Nursing.* 2006; 12:269–276; Ferrell BR, Virani R, Grant M, et al. *J Palliat Med.* 2005; 8(1):107–114; Ferrell BR, Grant M, Virani R. Strengthening nursing education to improve end of life care. *Nurs Outlook.* 1999; 47:252–256.

101. Stein GL, Sherman PA. Promoting effective social work policy in end-of-life and palliative care. *J Palliat Med.* 2005; 8(6):1271–1281; Christ GH, Blacker S. Series introduction: the profession of social work in end-of-life and palliative care. *J Palliat Med.* 2005; 8(2):415–417; Sheldon FM. Dimensions of the role of the social worker in palliative care. *Pal Med.* 2000; 14:491–498; Christ GH, Sormanti M. Advancing social work practice in end of life care. *Soc Work in Health Care.* 1999; 30:81.

102. Brandsen CK. Social work and end-of-life care: reviewing the past and moving forward. *J Soc Work End Life Palliat Care.* 2005; 1:45–70; Gwyther LP, Altilio T, Blacker S, et al. Social work competencies in palliative and end-of-life care. *J Soc Work End Life Palliat Care.* 2005; 1(1):87–120; http://swhpn.org/lhp/.

103. Carron AT, Lynn J, Keaney P. End of life care in medical textbooks. *Ann Intern Med.* 1999; 130:82–86. Rabow MW, Hardie GE, Fair JM, et al. End of life care content in nursing textbooks. *Onc Nurs Forum.* 1999; 26:869–76. Ferrell B, Virani R, Grant M. Analysis of end of life content in nursing textbooks. *Onc Nurs Forum.* 1999; 26:869–76

104. The Joint Commission. Health Care Staffing Service Certification. Available at: http://www .jointcommission.org/CertificationPrograms/HealthCareStaffingServices/. Accessed April 26, 2009.

105. Goldsmith B, Dietrich J, Du Q, et al. Variability in access to hospital palliative care in the United States. *J Pal Med.* 2008; 11(8):1094–1102.

106. Goldsmith B, Dietrich J, Du Q, et al., 2008.

107. http://www.nhqualitycampaign.org/star_index.aspx?controls=goals. Accessed February 23, 2009.

108. Teno JM, Clarridge BR, Casey V, et al. 2004

109. Bernabei R, Gambassi G, Lapane K, et al. Management of pain in elderly patients with cancer. *J Amer Med Assoc.* 1998; 279:1877–1882.

110. http://www.capc.org/support-from-capc/capc_publications/nursing_home_report.pdf.

111. www.npcrc.org/about/about_show.htm?doc_id=374985. Accessed on February 23, 2009.

112. Gelfman LP, Morrison RS. Research funding for palliative medicine. *J Palliat Med.* 2008; 11:36–43.

113. Gelfman LP, Morrison RS, 2008.

114. Gelfman LP, Morrison RS, 2008.

115. Citizen's Health Care Working Group. *Health Care that Works for All Americans, Final Recommendations*; June 1; 2006:1. Available at: www.citizenshealthcare.gov. Accessed April 26, 2009.

116. National Alliance for Caregiving and AARP. *Caregiving in the U.S.* April 2004. Available at: http://www.caregiving.org/data/04finalreport.pdf. Accessed April 26, 2009.

117. Emanuel EJ, Fairclough DL, Slutsman J, et al. Assistance from family members, friends, paid care givers, and volunteers in the care of terminally ill patients. *N Engl Jour Med.* 1999; 341:956–963.

118. Medicare Payment Advisory Commission. Report to the Congress: Medicare Payment Policy. March, 2007. Available at: http://www.medpac.gov/chapters/Mar07_Ch01.pdf. Accessed April 26, 2009; Medicare Payment Advisory Commission. *Report to the Congress: Healthcare Spending and the Medicare Program.* June, 2007. Available at: http://www.medpac.gov/chapters/Jun07DataBookSec1.pdf. Accessed April 26, 2009.

119. Emanuel EJ, Fairclough DL, Slutsman J, et al. Understanding economic and other burdens of terminal illness: the experience of patients and their caregivers. *Ann Intern Med.* 2000; 132:451.

120. Levine C. The loneliness of the long-term caregiver. *N Engl J Med.* 1999;340:1587; 340:1587–1590.

121. Schulz R, Beach SR. Caregiving as a risk factor for mortality: the caregiver health effects study. *JAMA.* 1999; 282:2215–2219.

122. Lee S, Colditz GA, Berkman LF. Care giving and risk of coronary heart disease in U.S. women: a prospective study. *Am J Prev Med.* 2003; 24(2):113–119.

123. National Alliance for Care Giving. Family Care Giving and Public Policy: Principles for Change. December 1, 2003. Available at: http://www.caregiving.org/data/principles04.pdf. Accessed April 26, 2009.

124. Schoen C., et al. U.S. Health system performance: a national scorecard. *Health Affairs* Web exclusive. Sept. 20, 2006: w457–w475; The Commonwealth Fund Commission on a High Performance Health System Bending the Curve: Options for Achieving Savings and Improving Value in U.S. Health Spending, December 2007. Available at; http://www.commonwealthfund.org/publications/publications_show .htm?doc_id=620087. Accessed on December 10, 2008; Davis K, Schoen C, Schoenbaum SC, et al. *Mirror, Mirror on the Wall: An International Update on the Comparative Performance of American Health Care.* The Commonwealth Fund. May 2007. Available at: http://www.commonwealthfund.org/usr_doc/1027_Davis_ mirror_mirror_international_update_final.pdf. Accessed April 26, 2009.

125. Starfield B, Shi L, Macinko J. Contribution of primary care to health systems and health. *Milbank Q.* 2005; 83:457–502.

126. Steinwald BA. Crisis in the Primary Care Workforce. Primary Care Professionals: Recent Supply Trends, Projections, and Valuation of Services. *Testimony before the US Senate Committee on Heath, Education, Labor, and Pensions.* US Government Accounting Office, GAO-08–472T. February, 2008. Available at: http://www.gao.gov/new.items/d08472t.pdf. Accessed April 26, 2009.

127. Smith TJ, Coyne P, Cassel C, et al. A high volume specialist palliative care unit and team may reduce in-hospital end of life care cost. *J Pall Med.* 2003: 6:5; http://www.capc.org/research-and-references-for-palliative-care/add-resources-websites/

128. Harrington SE, Smith TJ. The role of chemotherapy at the end of life: "When is enough, enough?'' *JAMA.* 2008; 299:2667–78.

129. Morrison RS; Penrod JD, Cassel B, et al. Cost savings associated with United States hospital palliative care consultation programs. *Arch Int Med* 2008. 168; 16:1783–1790.

130. Peabody FW. The care of the patient. *JAMA.* 1927; 88:877–882.

131. National Quality Forum, www.qualityforum.org; Institute for Healthcare Improvement www.ihi.org.

132. Teno JM, Clarridge BR, Casey V, et al., 2004.

133. www.capc.org/research-and-references-for-palliative-care/citations; Jordhoy MS, Fayers P, Saltnes T, et al. A palliative-care intervention and death at home: a cluster randomized trial. *Lancet.* 2000; 356(92330): 888–93; Higginson, JPSM 2002 and 2003; Teno JM, 2004; Finlay IG, Higginson IJ, Goodwin DM, et al. Palliative care in hospital, hospice, at home: results from a systematic review. *Ann Oncol.* 2002; 13:257–64. http://www.hsrd.research.va.gov/research/abstracts.cfm?Project_ID=2141694967&UnderReview=no. Accessed on February 23, 2009.

134. Casarett D, Pickard A, Bailey FA. Do palliative consultations improve patient outcomes? *J Am Geriatr Soc.* 2008; 56:593–99.

135. Lautrette A, Darmon M, Megarbane B, et al. A communication strategy and brochure for relatives of patients dying in the ICU. *N Engl J Med.* 2007; 365: 469–478.; Lilly CM, Daly BJ. The healing power of listening in the ICU. *N Engl J Med.* 2007; 365:513–515.

136. Ciemins EL, Blum L, Nunley M, et al. The economic and clinical impact of an inpatient palliative care consultation service. *J Palliat Med.* 2007; 10:1347–55.

137. Morrison RS; Penrod JD, Cassel B, et al., 2008; Smith TJ, Coyne P, Cassel C, et al., 2003.

138. Taylor DH, Ostermann J, Van Houtven CH, et al. What length of hospice use maximizes reduction in medical expenditures in the US Medicare program? *Soc Sci Med.* 2007; 65:1466–78; Connor SR, Pyenson B, Fitch K, et al. Comparing hospice and nonhospice patient survival among patients who die within a three-year window. *J Pain Sympt Manage.* 2007; 33:238–246.

139. Teno JM, Shue JE, Casarett D et al. Timing of referral to hospice and quality of care: length of stay and bereaved family members perception of the timing of hospice referral. *J Pain Sympt Manage.* 2007; 34:120–125.

140. Manfredi PL, Morrison RS, Morris J, Goldhirsch SL, et al. *J Pain Symptom Manage.* 2000; 20(3):166–73; Back AL, Li YF, Sales AE. *J Palliat Med.* 2005; 8(1):26–35; Penrod JD, Deb P, Luhrs C, et al. *J Palliat Med.* 2006 Aug; 9(4):855–60. Erratum in: *J Palliat Med.* 2006 Dec; 9(6):1509; Morrison RS, Penrod JD, Cassel JB, et al. Palliative Care Leadership Centers' Outcomes Group. *Arch Intern Med.* 2008 Sep 8; 168(16):1783–90.

141. Cohen LL. Racial/ethnic disparities in hospice care: a systematic review. *J Palliat Med.* 2008; 11:63–768.

142. Goldsmith B, Dietrich J, Du Q, et al., 2008.

143. Hospice of the Bluegrass. Available at: http://www.hospicebg.com/programsservices.html. Accessed April 26, 2009.

144. Midwest Palliative & Hospice Care Center. Available at: www.midwestpalliativeandhospicecarecenter.org. Accessed April 26, 2009.

145. Meier DE, Beresford L. Hospitals and hospices partner to extend the continuum of palliative care. *J Palliat Med.* 2007; 10:1231–35; Center to Advance Palliative Care. *Navigating palliative care: positioning hospice for the 21st Century.* Available at: http://www.capc.org/palliative-care-across-the-continuum/hospital-hospice/. Accessed April 26, 2009.

146. The number and diversity of foundation and philanthropic investments in the field of palliative care is remarkable. This list was culled from websites, publications, and personal communications with program leaders and funders and is not intended to be a complete chronicle. Apologies to funders who should have been but are not included in this list.

CARE OF THE SERIOUSLY ILL: WHY IS IT AN IMPORTANT ISSUE?

Marilyn J. Field and Christine K. Cassel, editors, for the Committee on Care at the End of Life, Institute of Medicine, "Approaching Death: Improving Care at the End of Life"

Council on Ethical and Judicial Affairs, American Medical Association, "Decisions Near the End of Life"

APPROACHING DEATH: IMPROVING CARE AT THE END OF LIFE

MARILYN J. FIELD AND CHRISTINE K. CASSEL, EDITORS
For the Committee on Care at the End of Life, Institute of Medicine

EDITORS' INTRODUCTION

This highly influential IOM report, edited by Marilyn J. Field and Christine K. Cassel, called for fundamental change in health professionals' education, research priorities, and the structure of the health care system. It served as a blueprint for the investment of hundreds of millions of dollars in private sector philanthropy. Many of the report's key recommendations have been accomplished, but others, equally important to assuring access to quality care during advanced illness, remain unfinished or are works in progress.

■ ■ ■

SUMMARY

Dying is at once a fact of life and a profound mystery. Death comes to all, yet each person experiences it in ways that are only partly accessible to the physician or family member, the philosopher or researcher. In principle, humane care for those approaching death is a social obligation as well as a personal offering from those directly involved. In reality, both society and individuals often fall short of what is reasonably—if not simply—achievable. As a result, people have come both to fear a technologically overtreated and protracted death and to dread the prospect of abandonment and untreated physical and emotional distress.

A humane care system is one that people can trust to serve them well as they die, even if their needs and beliefs call for a departure from typical practices. It honors and protects those who are dying, conveys by word and action that dignity resides in people—not physical attributes—and helps people to preserve their integrity while coping with unavoidable physical insults and losses. Such reliably excellent and respectful care at the end of life is an attainable goal, but realizing it will require many changes in attitudes, policies, and actions. System changes—not just changes in individual beliefs and actions—are necessary.

A number of developments suggest that the time is right for action at all levels to improve care at the end of life and to assure people that they will be neither abandoned nor maltreated as they approach death. This Institute of Medicine report is intended to support such action by strengthening popular and professional understanding of what constitutes good care at the end of life and by encouraging a wider societal commitment to caring well for people as they die. More specifically, it is intended to stimulate health professionals and managers, researchers, policy makers, funders of health care, and the public at large to develop more constructive perspectives on dying and death and to improve the practices and policies under their control. To these ends, this report stresses several themes.

- Too many dying people suffer from pain and other distress that clinicians could prevent or relieve with existing knowledge and therapies.

- Significant organizational, economic, legal, and educational impediments to good care can be identified and, in varying degrees, remedied.

- Important gaps in scientific knowledge about the end of life need serious attention from biomedical, social science, and health services researchers.

- Strengthening accountability for the quality of care at the end of life will require better data and tools for evaluating the outcomes important to patients and families.

CONTEXT AND TRENDS

In the United States, death at home in the care of family has been widely superseded by a technological, professional, and institutional process of treatment for the dying. That process—its benefits notwithstanding—often isolates the final stage of life from the rest of living. Likewise, the mobility of Americans quite literally puts distance between many younger and older family members. Many adults, even in middle age, have not lived with or cared for someone who was dying.

Because Americans, on average, live much longer now than they did at the end of the nineteenth century, a much larger proportion of the population dies at an advanced age. More than 70 percent of those who die each year are age sixty-five or over, and those who die in old age tend to die of different causes than those who die young. For both younger and older people, the major causes of death and the typical experience of dying differ from one hundred years ago. The dying process today tends to be more extended, in part because medical treatments can manage pneumonia, infections, kidney failure, and other immediate causes of death that come in the wake of cancer and other "slow killers."

The field of palliative care is one response to the changing profile of death in the twentieth century. It focuses on the prevention and relief of suffering through the meticulous management of symptoms from the early through the final stages of an illness; it attends closely to the emotional, spiritual, and practical needs of patients and those close to them. Other community, professional, and governmental responses include the development of hospice programs, bereavement support groups, and policies and programs that encourage communication about people's goals and preferences as they approach death.

The twenty-first century will bring new realities as well as continuing problems and opportunities in care at the end of life. It will undoubtedly deliver improvements in what medical science can do to prevent and relieve distress for those approaching death, but demographic, economic, and other trends will strain systems that already find it difficult to deliver what clinical knowledge currently allows—and what compassion should grant.

The next century will see the final demographic consequences of the post–World War II baby boom. The oldest members of the baby boom generation will reach age sixty-five in the year 2011, and the youngest members will do so nearly twenty years later. The elderly will constitute a larger proportion of the population than today, and the absolute numbers of dying patients will be substantially higher. Although health care and social service providers have a long lead time compared with the educators and communities who had to scramble to provide schooling for the baby boom generation, the difficulties that policy makers are already having with Social Security and Medicare do not bode well for the nation's ability to cope with the social, medical, economic, and other effects of an aging population.

Contrary to some popular thinking, however, the increase in overall personal health care spending is not explained by disproportionate growth in costs for end-of-life care. The small percentage of people who die each year do account for a significant proportion of health care expenditures, but the share of spending accounted for by this group does not appear to have changed much since the 1970s. Overall, increased health care spending is primarily accounted for by population growth, general inflation in the economy, and additional medical care inflation. One reason for the attention to the cost of care at the end of life is that such care is, in considerable measure, funded through Medicare, Medicaid, veterans, and other public programs.

Pressures to control public and private health care costs will continue and, indeed, will likely intensify with consequent restructuring of how health care is organized, delivered, and financed. More older people with advanced disease will be served by different kinds of managed care organizations. If effective quality monitoring and improvement methods are in place, the strengths and limitations of these varied arrangements will become clearer as their experience with end-of-life care grows. Possible problem areas include contracting, payment, and review mechanisms that limit access to clinicians and care teams experienced in palliative care; patient scheduling norms that limit time for careful patient-clinician communication; and marketing strategies that may discourage enrollment by seriously ill people.

CONCEPTS AND PRINCIPLES

Notions of "good" and "bad" deaths are threaded throughout discussions about dying and death. These concepts are not fixed in meaning but rather are shaped by people's experiences, spiritual beliefs, and culture and by changes in social mores, technology, and options for dying. Reflecting its members' personal and professional experiences and philosophical perspectives, the study committee that developed this report proposed that people should be able to expect and achieve a decent or good death—*one that is free from avoidable distress and suffering for patients, families, and caregivers; in general accord with patients' and families' wishes; and reasonably consistent with clinical, cultural, and ethical standards.* A bad death is characterized by needless suffering, disregard for patient or family wishes or values, and a sense among participants or observers that norms of decency have been offended.

The committee that prepared this report was guided by a set of working principles that reflect a combination of value judgments and empirical assumptions. Only the first of the following principles applies exclusively to care at the end of life.

Care for those approaching death is an integral and important part of health care. Everyone dies, and those at this stage of life deserve attention that is as thorough, active, and conscientious as that granted to those for whom cure or longer life is a realistic goal.

Care for those approaching death should involve and respect both patients and those close to them.
Particularly for patients with a grim prognosis, clinicians need to consider patients in the context of their families and close relationships and to be sensitive to their culture, values, resources, and other characteristics.

Good care at the end of life depends on strong interpersonal skills, clinical knowledge, and technical proficiency, and it is informed by scientific evidence, values, and personal and professional experience.
Clinical excellence is important because the frail condition of dying patients leaves little margin to rectify errors.

Changing individual behavior is difficult, but changing an organization or a culture is potentially a greater challenge—and often is a precondition for individual change.
Deficiencies in care often reflect flaws in how the health care system functions, which means that correcting problems will require change at the system level.

The health care community has special responsibility for educating itself and others about the identification, management, and discussion of the last phase of fatal medical problems.
Although health care professionals may not have a central presence in the lives of some people who are dying, many others draw heavily on physicians, nurses, social workers, and others for care—and caring. Thus, health care professionals are inescapably responsible for educating themselves and helping to educate the broader community about good care for dying patients and their families.

More and better research is needed to increase our understanding of the clinical, cultural, organizational, and other practices or perspectives that can improve care for those approaching death.
The committee began—and concluded—its deliberations with the view that the knowledge base for good end-of-life care has enormous gaps and is neglected in the design and funding of biomedical, clinical, psychosocial, and health services research.

CARING AT THE END OF LIFE: DIMENSIONS AND DEFICIENCIES

Care for most dying patients involves several basic elements: (1) understanding the physical, psychological, spiritual, and practical dimensions of caregiving; (2) identifying and communicating diagnosis and prognosis; (3) establishing goals and plans; and (4) fitting palliative and other care to these goals. In looking at current systems and practices, the committee found much that was good, including clinical, organizational, and ethical practices of palliative medicine that are implemented through hospices, interdisciplinary care teams in varied settings, innovative educational programs, and nascent outcomes measurement and quality monitoring and improvement strategies.

Notwithstanding these positive features, the committee concluded that very serious problems remain. It identified four broad deficiencies in the current care of people with life-threatening and incurable illnesses.

First and most fundamentally, too many people suffer needlessly at the end of life, both from errors of omission (when caregivers fail to provide palliative and supportive care known to be effective) and from errors of commission (when caregivers do what is known to be ineffective or even harmful). Studies have repeatedly indicated that a significant proportion of dying patients and patients with advanced disease experience serious pain, despite the availability of effective pharmacological and other options for relieving most pain. Other symptoms are less well studied, but the information available to the committee suggested a similar pattern of inadequate care. In perverse counterpoint to the problem of undertreatment, the aggressive use of ineffectual and intrusive interventions may prolong and even dishonor the period of dying. Some of this care is knowingly accepted; some is provided counter to patients' wishes; much is probably provided and accepted with little knowledge or consideration of its probable benefits and burdens.

Second, legal, organizational, and economic obstacles conspire to obstruct reliably excellent care at the end of life. Outdated and scientifically flawed drug-prescribing laws, regulations, and interpretations by state medical boards continue to frustrate and intimidate physicians who wish to relieve their patients' pain. Addiction to opioids appropriately prescribed to relieve pain and other symptoms is virtually nonexistent, whereas underuse of these medications is a well-documented problem. Fragmented organizational structures often complicate coordination and continuity of care and impede the further development and application of palliative care strategies in patient care, professional education, and research. Medicare hospice benefits have made palliative services more available to a small segment of dying patients, but many more have illnesses that do not readily fit the traditional hospice model or government benefit requirements. Traditional financing mechanisms—including arrangements based on discounted fees—still provide incentives for the overuse of procedural services and the underprovision or poor coordination of the assessment, evaluation, management, and supportive services so important for people with serious chronic or progressive medical problems.

Third, the education and training of physicians and other health care professionals fail to provide them the attitudes, knowledge, and skills required to care well for the dying patient. Many deficiencies in practice stem from fundamental prior failures in professional education. Undergraduate, graduate, and continuing education do not sufficiently prepare health professionals to recognize the final phases of illnesses, understand and manage their own emotional reactions to death and dying, construct effective strategies for care, and communicate sensitively with patients and those close to them.

Fourth, current knowledge and understanding are insufficient to guide and support the consistent practice of evidence-based medicine at the end of life. Biomedical and clinical research have focused almost exclusively on the development of knowledge that contributes to the prevention, detection, or cure of disease and to the prolongation of life. Research on the end stages of diseases and the physiological bases of symptoms and symptom relief has had negligible support. Epidemiological and health services research has likewise not provided a strong base for understanding the degree to which people suffer symptoms (except, perhaps, cancer pain), experience death alone rather than in the company of those who care, comprehend diagnostic and prognostic information, and achieve a dying that is reasonably consistent with their preferences, palliative care principles, and community norms. Methods development is important to define and measure outcomes other than death (including patient and family perceptions) and to monitor and improve the quality of care for those approaching death.

More generally, this committee concluded that people in this country have not yet discovered how to talk realistically but comfortably about the end of life, nor have they learned how to value the period of dying as it is now experienced by most people. Except for the occasional newspaper feature or television documentary, the reality of dying as most often experienced in the United States has been largely shunned by the news, information, and entertainment media as distasteful or uninteresting. One result is an unhelpful combination of fear, misinformation, and oversimplification that contributes to a public perception of misery as inescapable, pain as unavoidable, and public spending as misdirected for people approaching death.

RECOMMENDATIONS AND FUTURE DIRECTIONS

Seven recommendations address different decision makers and different deficiencies in care at the end of life. Each applies generally to people approaching death, including those for whom death is imminent and those with serious, eventually fatal illnesses who may live for some time. Each is intended to contribute to the achievement of a compassionate care system that dying people and those close to them can rely on for respectful and effective care.

Recommendation 1: **People with advanced, potentially fatal illnesses and those close to them should be able to expect and receive reliable, skillful, and supportive care.**

Educating people about care at the end of life is a critical responsibility of physicians, hospitals, hospices, support groups, public programs, and media. Most patients and families need information not only about diagnosis and prognosis but also about what support and what outcomes they should reasonably be able to expect. They should, for example, not be allowed to believe that pain is inevitable or that supportive care is incompatible with continuing efforts to diagnose and treat. They should learn—before their last few days of life—that supportive services are available from hospices and elsewhere in the community and that those involved in their care will help arrange such services. Patient and family expectations and understanding will be aided by advance care planning that considers needs and goals, identifies appropriate surrogate decision makers, and avoids narrow preoccupation with written directives. To these ends, health care organizations and other relevant parties should adopt policies regarding information, education, and assistance related to end-of-life decisions and services. For those who seek to build public understanding of dying as a part of life and to generate public demand for better supportive services, one model can be found in the perspectives, spirit, and strategies that have guided efforts to promote effective prenatal care and develop mother- and family-oriented arrangements for childbirth.

Recommendation 2: **Physicians, nurses, social workers, and other health professionals must commit themselves to improving care for dying patients and to using existing knowledge effectively to prevent and relieve pain and other symptoms.**

Patients often depend on health care professionals to manage the varying physical and psychological symptoms that accompany advanced illness. To meet their obligations to their patients, practitioners must hold themselves responsible for using existing knowledge and available interventions to assess, prevent, and relieve physical and emotional distress. When they identify organizational and other impediments to good practice, practitioners have the responsibility as individuals and members of larger groups to advocate for system change.

Recommendation 3: **Because many problems in care stem from system problems, policy makers, consumer groups, and purchasers of health care should work with health care practitioners, organizations, and researchers to:**

a. **strengthen methods for measuring the quality of life and other outcomes of care for dying patients and those close to them;**

b. **develop better tools and strategies for improving the quality of care and holding health care organizations accountable for care at the end of life;**

c. **revise mechanisms for financing care so that they encourage rather than impede good end-of-life care and sustain rather than frustrate coordinated systems of excellent care; and**

d. **reform drug prescription laws, burdensome regulations, and state medical board policies and practices that impede effective use of opioids to relieve pain and suffering.**

Although individuals must act to improve care at the end of life, systems of care must be changed to support such action. Better information systems and tools for measuring outcomes and evaluating care are critical to the creation of effective and accountable systems of care and to the effective functioning of both internal and external systems of quality monitoring and improvement. Policy makers and purchasers need to consider both the long-recognized deficiencies of traditional fee-for-service arrangements and the less thoroughly understood limitations of alternatives, including various kinds of capitated and per-case payment methods. Particularly in need of attention are payment mechanisms that fail to reward excellent care and that create incentives for under- or overtreatment of those approaching death.

State medical societies, licensing boards, legislative committees, and other groups should cooperate to review drug prescribing laws, regulations, board practices, and physician attitudes and practices to identify problem areas and then devise revisions in unduly burdensome statutes and regulations. Such regulatory change is not enough. It must be accompanied by education to increase knowledge and correct misperceptions about the appropriate medical use of opioids and about the biological mechanisms of opioid dependence, addiction, and pain management.

The committee identified characteristics of community care systems that would more effectively and reliably serve dying patients and their families. "Whole community" approaches to end-of-life care would include a mix of programs, settings, personnel, procedures, and practices that extend beyond health care institutions and policies to involve entire communities. The goals would be to make effective palliative care available wherever and whenever the dying patient is cared for; help dying patients and their families to plan ahead and prepare for dying and death; and establish accountability for high-quality care at the end of life. Exhibit 1.1 shows key features of a whole-community system for end-of-life care. A system with these components would reflect the understanding that there is not just one way to care for dying patients and that some flexibility is needed to respond to patients who do not comfortably fit the routines and standards that serve most patients well. Clearly, such a system represents an aspiration. The model implies cooperative effort involving public and private agencies on multiple levels—community, state, and national.

Recommendation 4: **Educators and other health professionals should initiate changes in undergraduate, graduate, and continuing education to ensure that practitioners have relevant attitudes, knowledge, and skills to care well for dying patients.**

Dying is too important a part of life to be left to one or two required (but poorly attended) lectures, to be considered only in ethical and not clinical terms, or to be set aside on the grounds that medical educators are already swamped with competing demands for time and resources. Every health professional who deals directly with patients and families needs a basic grounding in competent and compassionate care for seriously ill and dying patients. For clinicians and others to be held truly accountable for their care of the dying, educators must be held accountable for what they teach and what they implicitly and explicitly honor as exemplary practice. Textbooks and other materials likewise need revision to reflect the reality that people die and that dying patients are not people for whom "nothing can be done." Exhibit 1.2 outlines the fundamental elements of professional preparation for skillful, compassionate, and respectful care at the end of life.

EXHIBIT 1.1.   A Whole-Community Model for Care at the End of Life

Programs and settings of care suited to the needs and circumstances of different kinds of dying patients

- Home hospice programs
- Other palliative care arrangements for patients that do not fit the home care model
    - Day programs in hospitals and nursing homes, similar to those developed by geriatricians
    - "Step down" arrangements, including nursing homes that permit a less intensive and less expensive level of inpatient care when appropriate
    - Specialized inpatient palliative care beds for those with severe symptoms that cannot be well managed elsewhere
    - Respite programs to relieve families of patients with a long dying trajectory (for example, those with Alzheimer's disease) that imposes major physical and emotional burdens on families

Personnel, protocols, and other mechanisms that support high-quality, efficient, timely, and coordinated care

- Practical and valid assessment instruments and practice guidelines for patient evaluation and management that can be applied at both the individual and organizational level
- Protocols for evaluating patients' need for referral or transfer to other individual or organizational caregivers
- Procedures for implementing patient transitions in ways that encourage continuity of care, respect patient and family preferences and comfort, and assure the transfer of necessary patient information
- Consulting and crisis teams that extend and intensify efforts to allow patients to remain home despite difficult medical problems or crises
- Ongoing professional education programs fitted to the varying needs of all clinicians who care for dying patients
- Performance monitoring and improvement programs intended to identify and correct problems and to improve the average quality of care

Public and private policies, practices, and attitudes that help organizations and individuals

- Provider payment, coverage, and oversight policies that, at a minimum, do not restrict access to appropriate, timely palliative care and, as a goal, promote it
- Support systems provided through workplaces, religious congregations, and other institutions to ease the emotional, financial, and practical burdens experienced by dying patients and their families
- Public education programs that aim to improve general awareness, to encourage advance care planning, and to provide specific information at the time of need about resources for physical, emotional, spiritual, and practical caring at the end of life

EXHIBIT 1.2. Professional Preparation for End-of-Life Care

Scientific and clinical knowledge and skills, including

Learning the biological mechanisms of dying from major illnesses and injuries

Understanding the pathophysiology of pain and other physical and emotional symptoms

Developing appropriate expertise and skill in the pharmacology of symptom management

Acquiring appropriate knowledge and skill in nonpharmacological symptom management

Learning the proper application and limits of life-prolonging interventions

Understanding tools for assessing patient symptoms, status, quality of life, and prognosis

Interpersonal skills and attitudes, including

Listening to patients, families, and other members of the health care team

Conveying difficult news

Understanding and managing patient and family responses to illness

Providing information and guidance on prognosis and options

Sharing decision making and resolving conflicts

Recognizing and understanding one's own feelings and anxieties about dying and death

Cultivating empathy

Developing sensitivity to religious, ethnic, and other differences

Ethical and professional principles, including

Doing good and avoiding harm

Determining and respecting patient and family preferences

Being alert to personal and organizational conflicts of interests

Understanding societal/population interests and resources

Weighing competing objectives or principles

Acting as a role model of clinical proficiency, integrity, and compassion

Organizational skills, including

Developing and sustaining effective professional teamwork

Understanding relevant rules and procedures set by health plans, hospitals, and others

Learning how to protect patients from harmful rules and procedures

Assessing and managing care options, settings, and transitions

Mobilizing supportive resources (for example, palliative care consultants, community-based assistance)

Making effective use of existing financial resources and cultivating new funding sources

Recommendation 5: **Palliative care should become, if not a medical specialty, at least a defined area of expertise, education, and research.**
The objective is to create a cadre of palliative care experts whose numbers and talents are sufficient to (a) provide expert consultation and role models for colleagues, students, and other members of the health care team; (b) supply leadership for scientifically based and practically useful undergraduate, graduate, and continuing medical education; and (c) organize and conduct biomedical, clinical, behavioral, and health services research. More generally, palliative care must be redefined to include prevention as well as relief of symptoms.

Recommendation 6: **The nation's research establishment should define and implement priorities for strengthening the knowledge base for end-of-life care.**
The research establishment includes the National Institutes of Health, other federal agencies (for example, the Agency for Health Care Policy and Research, the Health Care Financing Administration, the National Center for Health Statistics), academic centers, researchers in many disciplines, pharmaceutical companies, and foundations supporting health research. One step is to take advantage of clinical trials by collecting more information on the quality of life of those who die while enrolled in experimental or treatment groups. A further step is to support more research on the physiological mechanisms and treatment of symptoms common during the end of life, including neuropsychiatric problems. Pain research appears to supply a good model for this enterprise to follow. To encourage change in the attitudes and understandings of the research establishment, the committee urges the National Institutes of Health and other public agencies to take the lead in organizing workshops, consensus conferences, and other projects that focus on what is and is not known about end-stage disease and symptom management and that propose an agenda for improvement. Demonstration projects to test new methods of financing and organizing care should be a priority for the Health Care Financing Administration. For the Agency for Health Care Policy and Research, the committee encourages support for the dissemination and replication of proven health care interventions and programs through clinical practice guidelines and other means.

Recommendation 7: **A continuing public discussion is essential to develop a better understanding of the modern experience of dying, the options available to patients and families, and the obligations of communities to those approaching death.**
Individual conversations between practitioners and patients are important but cannot by themselves provide a more supportive environment for the attitudes and actions that make it possible for most people to die free from avoidable distress and to find the peace or meaning that is significant to them. Although efforts to reduce the entertainment and news media's emphasis on violent or sensational death and unrealistic medical rescue have not been notably successful, a modicum of balance has recently been provided by thoughtful analyses, public forums, and other coverage of the clinical, emotional, and practical issues involved in end-of-life care. Regardless of how the current, highly publicized policy debate over physician-assisted

suicide is resolved, the goal of improving care for those approaching death and the barriers to achieving that goal should not be allowed to fade from public consciousness. Much of the responsibility for keeping the public discussion going will rest not with the media but with public officials, professional organizations, religious leaders, and community groups.

The committee agreed that it would not take a position on the legality or morality of physician-assisted suicide. It does, however, believe that the issue should not take precedence over those reforms to the health care system that would improve care for dying patients.

CONCLUSION

The analyses, conclusions, and recommendations presented here are offered with optimism that people, individually and together, can act to "approach" death constructively and reduce suffering at the end of life. This report identifies steps that can be taken to improve care at the end of life and to create a solid foundation for maintaining such improvements through difficult times. It also highlights the reasons for believing that professionals, policy makers, and the public are becoming more aware of what can and should be done and are ready to embrace change. These reasons range from the examples of well-known men and women facing death with grace to the more intense focus on deficiencies in care that has been stimulated by the debate over assisted suicide. In sum, the timing appears right to press for a vigorous societal commitment to improve care at the end of life. That commitment would motivate and sustain individual and collective efforts to create a humane care system that people can trust to serve them well as they die.

DECISIONS NEAR THE END OF LIFE

COUNCIL ON ETHICAL AND JUDICIAL AFFAIRS, AMERICAN MEDICAL ASSOCIATION

This article originally appeared as American Medical Association, Council on Ethical and Judicial Affairs. Decisions near the end of life. *JAMA.* 1992;267(16):2229–2233. Members of the Council on Ethical and Judicial Affairs include Richard J. McMurray, M.D., Flint, Mich., chair; Oscar W. Clarke, M.D., Gallipolis, Ohio, vice chair; John A. Barrasso, M.D., Casper, Wyo.; Dexanne B. Clohan, Arlington, Va.; Charles H. Epps Jr., M.D., Washington, D.C.; John Glasson, M.D., Durham, N.C.; Robert McQuillan, M.D., Kansas City, Mo.; Charles W. Plows, M.D., Anaheim, Calif.; Michael A. Puzak, M.D., Arlington, Va.; David Orentlicher, M.D., J.D., Chicago, Ill., secretary and staff author; Kristen A. Halkola, Chicago, Ill., associate secretary and staff author; and Anita K. Schweickart, Chicago, Ill., staff associate and principal staff author. Copyright © 1992, American Medical Association. All rights reserved. Reprinted with permission.

EDITORS' INTRODUCTION

This report from an influential committee of the American Medical Association confirmed the growing public and professional consensus that maximum possible prolongation of life is not the highest good in medicine and that a patient's wishes and the obligation to follow them act as checks on the value of life in medical decision-making. The committee rejected a distinction between withdrawing and withholding life-sustaining treatments and underscored physicians' obligation to relieve pain and suffering and promote dignity and autonomy of their dying patients.

■ ■ ■

Over the last fifty years, people have become increasingly concerned that the dying process is too often needlessly protracted by medical technology and is consequently marked by incapacitation, intolerable pain, and indignity. In one public opinion poll, 68 percent of respondents believed that "people dying of an incurable painful disease should be allowed to end their lives before the disease runs its course."[1] A number of comparable surveys indicate similar public sentiment.[2]

Since the turn of the century, there has been a dramatic shift in the places where people die. Sixty years ago, the vast majority of deaths occurred at home. Now most people die in hospitals or long-term care facilities. Approximately 75 percent of all deaths in 1987 occurred in hospitals and long-term care institutions,[3] up from 50 percent in 1949, 61 percent in 1958, and 70 percent in 1977.[4] This transition from the privacy of the home to medical institutions has increased public awareness and concern about medical decisions near the end of life. "Since deaths which occur in institutions are more subject to scrutiny and official review, decisions for death made there are more likely to enter public consciousness."[5]

The development of sophisticated life support technologies now enables medicine to intervene and forestall death for most patients. Do-not-resuscitate orders are now commonplace.[6] The Office of Technology Assessment Task Force estimated in 1988 that 3,775 to 6,575 persons were dependent on mechanical ventilation and 1,404,500 persons were receiving artificial nutritional support.[7] This growing capability to forestall death has contributed to the increased attention to medical decisions near the end of life.[5]

The council has issued opinions on withdrawing and withholding life-prolonging treatment from patients who are terminally ill or permanently unconscious[8] and has also published reports concerning do-not-resuscitate orders,[9,10] euthanasia,[11] and withdrawal of life-prolonging treatment from permanently unconscious patients.[12] This report will reexamine the council's existing positions and will expand the analysis to include physician-assisted suicide and withdrawing or withholding life-sustaining treatment for patients who are neither terminally ill nor permanently unconscious. The report will focus on competent patients in nonemergency situations. The issue of decisions near the end of life for incompetent patients is addressed in a separate report by the council.[13]

DEFINITIONS

The decisions near the end of life examined in this report are those decisions regarding actions or intentional omissions by physicians that will foreseeably result in the deaths of patients. In particular, these decisions concern the withholding or withdrawing of life-sustaining treatment, the provision of a palliative treatment that may have fatal side effects, euthanasia, and assisted suicide.

Life-sustaining treatment is any medical treatment that serves to prolong life without reversing the underlying medical condition. Life-sustaining treatment may include but is not limited to mechanical ventilation, renal dialysis, chemotherapy, antibiotics, and artificial nutrition and hydration. At one time, the term *passive euthanasia* was commonly used to describe withholding or withdrawing life-sustaining treatment. However, many experts now refrain from using the term passive euthanasia.

The provision of a palliative treatment that may have fatal side effects is also described as *double-effect euthanasia.* The intent of the treatment is to relieve pain and suffering, not to end the patient's life, but the patient's death is a foreseeable potential effect of the treatment. An example is gradually increasing the morphine dosage for a patient to relieve severe cancer pain, realizing that large enough doses of morphine may depress respiration and cause death.

Euthanasia is commonly defined as the act of bringing about the death of a hopelessly ill and suffering person in a relatively quick and painless way for reasons of mercy. In this report, the term euthanasia will signify the medical administration of a lethal agent to a patient for the purpose of relieving the patient's intolerable and incurable suffering.

Voluntary euthanasia is euthanasia that is provided to a competent person on his or her informed request. *Nonvoluntary euthanasia* is the provision of euthanasia to an incompetent person according to a surrogate's decision. *Involuntary euthanasia* is euthanasia performed without a competent person's consent. This report will not examine involuntary euthanasia further, since it clearly would never be ethically acceptable.

Euthanasia and assisted suicide differ in the degree of physician participation. Euthanasia entails a physician performing the immediate life-ending action (for example, administering a lethal injection). *Assisted suicide* occurs when a physician facilitates a patient's death by providing the necessary means and/or information to enable the patient to perform the life-ending act (for example, the physician provides sleeping pills and information about the lethal dose, while aware that the patient may commit suicide).

Discussions about life-ending acts by physicians often refer to the patient's "competence" or "decision-making capacity." The two terms are often used interchangeably. However, *competence* can also refer to a legal standard regarding a person's soundness of mind. *Decision-making capacity* signifies the ability to make a particular decision and is not considered a legal standard. "Competence" for the council's purposes will mean "decision-making capacity."

The evaluation of a person's decision-making capacity is an assessment of the person's capabilities for understanding, communicating, and reasoning. Patients should not be judged as lacking decision-making capacity based on the view that what they decide is unreasonable.[14] People are entitled to make decisions that others think are foolish as long as their choices are arrived at through a competently reasoned process and are consistent with their personal values.

ETHICAL FRAMEWORK

Determining the ethical responsibilities of physicians when patients wish to die requires a close examination of the physician's role in society. Physicians are healers of disease and injury, preservers of life, and relievers of suffering. Ethical judgments become complicated, however, when these duties conflict. The four instances in which physicians might act to hasten death or refrain from prolonging life involve conflicts between the duty to relieve suffering and the duty to preserve life.

The considerations that must be weighed in each case are (1) the principle of patient autonomy and the corresponding obligation of physicians to respect patients' choices; (2) whether what is offered by the physician is sound medical treatment; and (3) the potential consequences of a policy that permits physicians to act in a way that will foreseeably result in patients' deaths.

Patient Autonomy

The principle of patient autonomy requires that competent patients have the opportunity to choose among medically indicated treatments and to refuse any unwanted treatment. Absent countervailing obligations, physicians must respect patients' decisions. Treatment decisions often involve personal value judgments and preferences in addition to objective medical considerations. We demonstrate respect for human dignity when we acknowledge "the freedom [of individuals] to make choices in accordance with their own values."[15]

Sound Medical Treatment

The physician's obligation to respect a patient's decision does not require a physician to provide a treatment that is not medically sound. Indeed, physicians are ethically prohibited from offering or providing unsound treatments. Sound medical treatment is defined as the use of medical knowledge or means to cure or prevent a medical disorder, preserve life, or relieve distressing symptoms.

This criterion of soundness arises from the medical ethical principles of beneficence and nonmaleficence. The principle of *nonmaleficence* prohibits physicians from using their medical knowledge or skills to do harm, on balance, to their patients, while the principle of *beneficence* requires that medical knowledge and skills be used to benefit patients.

Generally, a treatment that is likely to cause the death of a patient violates the principle of nonmaleficence, and a failure to save a patient's life is contrary to beneficence. However, for these decisions near the end of life the patient does not consider his or her death to be an absolutely undesirable outcome.

Practical Considerations

Policies governing decisions near the end of life must also be evaluated in terms of their practical consequences. The ethical acceptability of a policy depends on the benefits and costs that result from the policy. In addition to the impact on individual cases (for example, patients will die according to their decision to have life supports withdrawn), there are likely to be serious societal consequences of policies regarding physicians' responsibilities to dying patients.

WITHHOLDING AND WITHDRAWING LIFE-SUSTAINING TREATMENT

The principle of patient autonomy requires that physicians respect a competent patient's decision to forgo any medical treatment. This principle is not altered when the likely result of withholding or withdrawing a treatment is the patient's death.[4] The right of competent patients to forgo life-sustaining treatment has been upheld in the courts (for example, *In re Brooks Estate,* 32 Ill2d 361, 205 NE2d 435 [1965]; *In re Osborne,* 294 A2d 372 [1972]) and is generally accepted by medical ethicists.[4]

Decisions that so profoundly affect a patient's well-being cannot be made independent of a patient's subjective preferences and values.[16] Many types of life-sustaining treatments are burdensome and invasive, so that the choice for the patient is not simply a choice between life and death.[7] When a patient is dying of cancer, for example, a decision may have to be made whether to use a regimen of chemotherapy that might prolong life for several additional months but also would likely be painful, nauseating, and debilitating. Similarly, when a patient is dying, there may be a choice between returning home to a natural death or remaining in the hospital, attached to machinery, where the patient's life might be prolonged a few more days or weeks. In both cases, individuals might weigh differently the value of additional life versus the burden of additional treatment.

The withdrawing or withholding of life-sustaining treatment is not inherently contrary to the principles of beneficence and nonmaleficence. The physician is obligated only to offer sound medical treatment and to refrain from providing treatments that are detrimental, on balance, to the patient's well-being. When a physician withholds or withdraws a treatment on the request of a patient, he or she has fulfilled the obligation to offer sound treatment to the patient. The obligation to offer treatment does not include an obligation to impose treatment on an unwilling patient. In addition, the physician is not providing a harmful treatment. Withdrawing or withholding is not a treatment, but the forgoing of a treatment.

Some commentators argue that if a physician has a strong moral objection to withdrawing or withholding life-sustaining treatment, the physician may transfer the patient to another physician who is willing to comply with the patient's wishes.[4] It is true that a physician does not have to provide a treatment, such as an abortion, that is contrary to his or her moral values. However, if a physician objects to withholding or withdrawing the treatment and forces unwanted treatment on a patient, the patient's autonomy will be inappropriately violated even if it will take only a short time for the patient to be transferred to another physician.

Withdrawing or withholding some life-sustaining treatments may seem less acceptable than others. The distinction between "ordinary" versus "extraordinary" treatments has been used to differentiate ethically obligatory versus ethically optional treatments.[17] In other words, ordinary treatments must be provided, while extraordinary treatment may be withheld or withdrawn. Varying criteria have been proposed to distinguish ordinary from extraordinary treatment. Such criteria include customariness, naturalness, complexity, expense, invasiveness, and balance of likely benefits versus burdens of the particular treatment.[17,18]

When a patient is competent, this balancing must ultimately be made by the patient. As stated earlier, the evaluation of whether life-sustaining treatment should be initiated, maintained, or forgone depends on the values and preferences of the patient. Therefore, treatments are not objectively ordinary or extraordinary. For example, artificial nutrition and hydration have frequently been cited as an objectively ordinary treatment which, therefore, must never be forgone. However, artificial nutrition and hydration can be very burdensome to patients. Artificial nutrition and hydration immobilize the patient to a large degree, can be extremely uncomfortable (restraints are sometimes used to prevent patients from removing nasogastric tubes), and can entail serious risks (for example, surgical risks from insertion of a gastrostomy tube and the risk of aspiration pneumonia with a nasogastric tube).

Aside from the ordinary-versus-extraordinary argument, the right to refuse artificial nutrition and hydration has also been contested by some because the provision of food and water has a symbolic significance as an expression of care and compassion.[19] These commentators argue that withdrawing or withholding food and water is a form of abandonment and will cause the patient to die of starvation and/or thirst. However, it is far from evident that providing nutrients through a nasogastric tube to a patient for whom it is unwanted is comparable to the typical human ways of feeding those who are hungry.[18] In addition, discomforting symptoms can be palliated so that a death that occurs after forgoing artificial nutrition and/or hydration is not marked by substantial suffering.[20,21] Such care requires constant attention to the patient's needs. Therefore, when comfort care is maintained, respecting a patient's decision to forgo artificial nutrition and hydration will not constitute an abandonment of the patient, symbolic or otherwise.

There is also no ethical distinction between withdrawing and withholding life-sustaining treatment.[4,15,17] Withdrawing life support may be emotionally more difficult than withholding life support because the physician performs an action that hastens death. When life-sustaining treatment is withheld, on the other hand, death occurs because of an omission rather than an action. However, as most bioethicists now recognize, such a distinction lacks ethical significance.[4,15,17] First, the distinction is often meaningless. For example, if a physician fails to provide a tube feeding at the scheduled time, would it be a withholding or a withdrawing of treatment? Second, ethical relevance does not lie with the distinction between acts and omissions but with other factors, such as the motivation and professional obligations of the physician. For example, refusing to initiate ventilator support, despite the patient's need and request, because the physician has been promised a share of the patient's inheritance is clearly ethically more objectionable than stopping a ventilator for a patient who has competently decided to forgo it. Third, prohibiting the withdrawal of life support would inappropriately affect a patient's decision to initiate such treatment. If treatment cannot be stopped once it is initiated, patients and physicians may be more reluctant to begin treatment when there is a possibility that the patient may later want the treatment withdrawn.[4]

While the principle of autonomy requires that physicians respect competent patients' requests to forgo life-sustaining treatments, there are potential negative consequences of such a policy. First, deaths may occur as a result of uninformed decisions, or from pain and suffering that could be relieved with measures that will not cause the patient's death. Further, subtle or overt pressures from family, physicians, or society to forgo life-sustaining treatment may render the patient's choice less than free. These pressures could revolve around beliefs that such patients' lives no longer possess social worth and are an unjustifiable drain of limited health resources.

The physician must ensure that the patient has the capacity to make medical decisions before carrying out the patient's decision to forgo (or receive) life-sustaining treatment. In particular, physicians must be aware that the patient's decision-making capacity can be diminished by a misunderstanding of the medical prognosis and options or by a treatable state of depression. It is also essential that all efforts be made to maximize the comfort and dignity of patients who are dependent on life-sustaining treatment and that patients be assured of these efforts. With such assurances, patients will be less likely to forgo life support because of suffering or anticipated suffering that could be palliated.

The potential pressures on patients to forgo life-sustaining treatments are an important concern. The council believes that the medical profession must be vigilant against such tendencies, but that the greater policy risk is of undermining patient autonomy.

PROVIDING PALLIATIVE TREATMENTS THAT MAY HAVE FATAL SIDE EFFECTS

Health care professionals have an ethical duty to provide optimal palliative care to dying patients. At present, many physicians are not informed about the appropriate doses, frequency of doses, and alternate modalities of pain control for patients with severe chronic pain.[22] In particular, inappropriate concerns about addiction too often inhibit physicians from providing adequate analgesia to dying patients. Physicians should inform the patient and the family that concentrated efforts to relieve pain will be a priority in the care of the patient, since fear of pain is "one of the most pervasive causes of anxiety among patients, families and the public."[2]

The level of analgesia necessary to relieve the patient's pain, however, may also have the effect of shortening the patient's life. The council stated in its 1988 report on euthanasia that "the administration of a drug necessary to ease the pain of a patient who is terminally ill and suffering excruciating pain may be appropriate medical treatment even though the effect of the drug may shorten life."[11] The council maintains this position and further emphasizes that a competent patient must be the one who decides whether the relief of pain and suffering is worth the danger of hastening death. The principle of respect for patient autonomy and self-determination requires that patients decide about such treatment.

The ethical distinction between providing palliative care that may have fatal side effects and providing euthanasia is subtle because in both cases the action that causes death is performed with the purpose of relieving suffering. The intent of the former is to relieve suffering despite the fatal side effects, while the intent of the latter is to cause death as a means by which relief of suffering is achieved. Most medical treatments entail some undesirable side effects. In general, the patient has a right to decide either to risk the side effects or to forgo the treatment. It does not follow from this reasoning that a patient also has a right to choose euthanasia as a medical treatment for their suffering.

An important concern is that patients who are not fully informed about their prognosis and options may make decisions that unnecessarily shorten their lives. In addition, severe pain might diminish the patient's capacity to decide whether to choose a treatment that risks death. Caution when determining decision-making capacity in this situation, therefore, must be exercised, and patients should be fully informed.

EUTHANASIA

Euthanasia is the medical administration of a lethal agent in order to relieve a patient's intolerable and untreatable suffering. Whether or not a physician may use the skills or knowledge of medicine to cause an "easy" death for a patient who requests such assistance has been debated as early as the time of Hippocrates. Recently, euthanasia has been gaining support from the public and some in the medical profession. In the Netherlands, while physician-performed euthanasia remains illegal, physicians have not been prosecuted since 1984 when they follow certain criteria.[23] These criteria include that (1) euthanasia is explicitly and repeatedly requested by the patient and there is no doubt that the patient wants to die; (2) the mental and physical suffering is severe with no prospect for relief; (3) the patient's decision is well informed, free, and enduring; (4) all options for alternate care have been exhausted or refused by the patient; and (5) the physician consults another physician.[24] The frequency of euthanasia in the Netherlands has been estimated to range from 2,000 to 20,000 persons per year.[23] Recently, the first nationwide study of the practice of euthanasia in the Netherlands estimated the incidence of euthanasia to be 1,900 persons per year.[25]

In the United States there has been growing public support for legalized euthanasia. The Hemlock Society, an organization dedicated to legalizing voluntary euthanasia and assisted suicide, has doubled its membership in the past five years to approximately 33,000.[26] Recently, an initiative in Washington State that would have legalized euthanasia for terminally ill patients was put to a vote. Although the initiative was unsuccessful, 44 percent of the voters supported the initiative.[27]

Though the principle of patient autonomy requires that competent patients be given the opportunity to choose among offered medical treatments and to forgo any treatment, it does not give patients the right to have a physician perform a treatment to which the physician has objections. Though patients have a right to refuse life-sustaining treatment, they do not have a right to receive euthanasia. There is an autonomy interest in directing one's death, but this interest is more limited in the case of euthanasia than in the case of refusing life support.

The question remains whether it is ethical for a physician to agree to perform euthanasia. To approach this question, one must look to the principles of beneficence and nonmaleficence and to the larger policy implications of condoning physician-performed euthanasia.

Can euthanasia ever constitute sound medical treatment? Any treatment designed to cause death is generally considered detrimental to the patient's well-being, and therefore unsound. However, proponents of euthanasia argue that euthanasia is a sound treatment of last resort for the relief of intolerable pain and suffering. From the perspective of competent patients who request euthanasia in the face of such suffering, death may be preferable, on balance, to continued life.

On the other hand, most pain and suffering can be alleviated. The technology of pain management has advanced to the point where most pain is now controllable. The success of the hospice movement illustrates the extent to which aggressive pain control and close attention to patient comfort and dignity can ease the transition to death.[22]

There may be cases, however, where a patient's pain and suffering are not reduced to a tolerable level and the patient requests a physician to help him or her die.[2,22] If a patient's pain and suffering are unrelievable and intolerable, using medical expertise to aid an easy death on the request of the patient might seem to be the humane and beneficent treatment for the patient.

However, there are serious risks associated with a policy allowing physician-performed euthanasia. There is a long-standing prohibition against physicians killing their patients, based on a commitment that medicine is a profession dedicated to healing, and that its tools should not be used to cause patients' deaths. Weakening this prohibition against euthanasia, even in the most compelling situations, has troubling implications.[28,29] Though the magnitude of such risks is impossible to predict accurately, the medical profession and society as a whole must not consider these risks lightly. Two noted ethicists have expressed the role of this prohibition:

> The prohibition of killing is an attempt to promote a solid basis for trust in the role of caring for patients and protecting them from harm. This prohibition is both instrumentally and symbolically important, and its removal would weaken a set of practices and restraints that we cannot easily replace.[17]

If euthanasia by physicians were to be condoned, the fact that physicians could offer death as a medical treatment might undermine public trust in medicine's dedication to preserving the life and health of patients.[30] Some patients may fear the prospect of involuntary or nonvoluntary euthanasia if their lives are no longer deemed valuable as judged by physicians, their family, or society.[30] Other patients who trust their physicians' judgments may not feel free to resist the suggestion that euthanasia may be appropriate for them.[30-32]

Another risk is that physicians and other health care providers may be more reluctant to invest their energy and time serving patients whom they believe would benefit more from a quick and easy death. Caring for dying patients is taxing on physicians, who must face issues of their own mortality in the process, and who often perceive such care as a reminder of their failure to cure these patients.[4,15] In addition, the increasing pressure to reduce health care costs may serve as another motivation to favor euthanasia over longer-term comfort care.

Allowing physicians to perform euthanasia for a limited group of patients who may truly benefit from it will present difficult line-drawing problems for medicine and society. In specific cases it may be hard to distinguish which cases fit the criteria established for euthanasia. For example, if the existence of unbearable pain and suffering was a criterion for euthanasia, the definition of unbearable pain and suffering could be subject to different interpretations.

Furthermore, determining whether a patient will benefit from euthanasia requires an intimate understanding of the patient's concerns, values, and pressures that may be prompting the euthanasia request. In the Netherlands, physicians who provide euthanasia generally have a lifelong relationship with the patient and the patient's family, which enables the physician to have access to this vital information.[33] In the United States, however, physicians rarely have the depth of knowledge about their patients that would be necessary for an appropriate evaluation of the patient's request for euthanasia.

More broadly, the line-drawing necessary for the establishment of criteria for euthanasia is also problematic. If competent patients can receive euthanasia, can family members request euthanasia for an incompetent patient? Would it be acceptable for physicians to perform euthanasia on any competent individuals who request it? Furthermore, since it will be physicians and the state who ultimately answer these questions, value judgments about patients' lives will be made by a person or entity other than the patients.

Since it is unclear at this time where these lines should be drawn, the proposition of allowing euthanasia is particularly troublesome. A potential exists for a gradual distortion of the role of medicine into something that starkly contrasts with the current vision of a profession dedicated to healing and comforting.

Furthermore, in the United States there is currently little data regarding the number of euthanasia requests, the concerns behind the requests, the types and degree of intolerable and unrelievable suffering, or the number of requests that have been granted by health care providers. Before euthanasia can ever be considered a legitimate medical treatment in this country, the needs behind the demand for physician-provided euthanasia must be examined more thoroughly and addressed more effectively. A thorough examination would require a more open discussion of euthanasia and the needs of patients who are making requests. The existence of patients who find their situations so unbearable that they request help from their physicians to die must be acknowledged, and the concerns of these patients must be a primary focus of medicine. Rather than condoning physician-provided euthanasia, medicine must first respond by striving to identify and address the concerns and needs of dying patients.

PHYSICIAN-ASSISTED SUICIDE

Physician-assisted suicide has only recently become the focus of public attention. In June 1990, Dr Jack Kevorkian assisted the death of a person with the use of a "suicide machine," which he invented. This case has been criticized by many for the irresponsible way in which it was carried out by the physician.[26] Kevorkian has since used his suicide machine to assist the suicides of two more persons. Last March, an article was published in the *New England Journal of Medicine* by a physician who described his role in assisting his patient's suicide.[34] The care and compassion evidenced by the physician and the reasoned decision-making process of the patient marked this account as truly compelling. Besides these very public cases of physician-assisted suicide, there is reason to believe that it has been occurring for some time.[2]

There is an ethically relevant distinction between euthanasia and assisted suicide that makes assisted suicide an ethically more attractive option. Physician-assisted suicide affords a patient a more autonomous way of ending his or her life than does euthanasia. Since patients must perform the life-ending act themselves, they would have the added protection of being able to change their minds and stop their suicides up until the last moment.

However, the ethical objections to physician-assisted suicide are similar to those of euthanasia, since both are essentially interventions intended to cause death. Physician-assisted suicide, like euthanasia, is contrary to the prohibition against using the tools of medicine to cause a patient's death. Physician-assisted suicide also has many of the same societal risks as euthanasia, including the potential for coercive financial and societal pressures on patients to choose suicide. Further, determining the criteria for assisting a patient's suicide and determining whether a particular patient meets the criteria is as problematic as deciding who may receive euthanasia.

While in highly sympathetic cases physician-assisted suicide may seem to constitute beneficent care, due to the potential for grave harm the medical profession cannot condone physician-assisted suicide at this time. The medical profession instead must strive to identify the concerns behind patients' requests for assisted suicide and make concerted efforts at finding ways to address these concerns short of assisting suicide, including providing more aggressive comfort care.

CONCLUSIONS

■ The principle of patient autonomy requires that physicians must respect the decision to forgo life-sustaining treatment of a patient who possesses decision-making capacity. Life-sustaining treatment is any medical treatment that serves to prolong life without reversing the underlying medical condition. Life-sustaining treatment may include but is not limited to mechanical ventilation, renal dialysis, chemotherapy, antibiotics, and artificial nutrition and hydration.

- There is no ethical distinction between withdrawing and withholding life-sustaining treatment.

- Physicians have an obligation to relieve pain and suffering and to promote the dignity and autonomy of dying patients in their care. This includes providing effective palliative treatment even though it may foreseeably hasten death. More research must be pursued examining the degree to which palliative care reduces the requests for euthanasia or assisted suicide.

- Physicians must not perform euthanasia or participate in assisted suicide. A more careful examination of the issue is necessary. Support, comfort, respect for patient autonomy, good communication, and adequate pain control may decrease dramatically the demand for euthanasia and assisted suicide. In certain carefully defined circumstances, it would be humane to recognize that death is certain and suffering is great. However, the societal risks of involving physicians in medical interventions to cause patients' deaths is too great in this culture to condone euthanasia or physician-assisted suicide at this time.

REFERENCES

1. Associated Press/Media General. *Poll No. 4*. Richmond, Va: Media General; February 1985.

2. Wanzer SH, Federman DD, Adelstein SJ, et al. The physician's responsibility toward hopelessly ill patients. *N Engl J Med.* 1989; 320:844–849.

3. National Center for Health Statistics. *Vital Statistics of the United States, 1987, II: Mortality, Part A*. Washington, DC: US Public Health Service; 1990.

4. *Deciding to Forego Life-Sustaining Treatment: A Report on the Ethical, Medical, and Legal Issues in Treatment Decisions*. Washington, DC: President's Commission for the Study of Ethical Problems in Medicine and Biomedical and Behavioral Research; 1987.

5. Capron AM. Legal and ethical problems in decisions for death. *Law Med Health Care.* 1986; 14:141–144.

6. Lipton HL. Do-not-resuscitate decisions in a community hospital. *JAMA.* 1986; 256:1164–1169.

7. Office of Technology Assessment Task Force. *Life-Sustaining Technologies and the Elderly*. Philadelphia, Pa: Science Information Resource Center; 1988.

8. Council on Ethical and Judicial Affairs. *Current Opinions*. Chicago, Ill: American Medical Association; 1989:13.

9. Council on Ethical and Judicial Affairs. Do-not-resuscitate orders: report B. In: *Proceedings of the House of Delegates of the AMA*; December 1987; Chicago, Ill:170–171.

10. Council on Ethical and Judicial Affairs. Guidelines for the appropriate use of do-not-resuscitate orders: report D. In: *Proceedings of the House of Delegates of the AMA*; December 1990; Chicago, Ill:180–185.

11. Council on Ethical and Judicial Affairs. Euthanasia: report C. In: *Proceedings of the House of Delegates of the AMA*; June 1988; Chicago, Ill:258–260.

12. Council on Ethical and Judicial Affairs and the Council on Scientific Affairs. Persistent vegetative state and the decision to withdraw or withhold life support: joint report. In: *Proceedings of the House of Delegates of the AMA*; June 1989; Chicago, Ill:314–318.

13. Council on Ethical and Judicial Affairs. Decisions to forgo life-sustaining treatment for incompetent patients: report D. In: *Proceedings of the House of Delegates of the AMA*; June 1991; Chicago, Ill:261–269.

14. Buchanan AE, Brock DW. *Deciding for Others: The Ethics of Surrogate Decisionmaking*. New York, NY: Cambridge University Press; 1989.

15. *Guidelines on the Termination of Life-Sustaining Treatment and the Care of the Dying: A Report by the Hastings Center*. Briarcliff, NY: Hastings Center; 1987.

16. Brock DW. Death and dying. In: Veatch RM, ed. *Medical Ethics*. Boston, Mass: Jones & Bartlett Publishing Inc; 1989.

17. Beauchamp TL, Childress JF. *Principles of Biomedical Ethics*. 3rd ed. New York, NY: Oxford University Press; 1989.

18. Lynn J, Childress JF. Must patients always be given food and water? *Hastings Cent Rep*. October 1983;17–21.

19. Ramsey P. *The Patient as Person*. New Haven, Conn: Yale University Press; 1970:113–129.

20. Schmitz P, O'Brien M. Observations on nutrition and hydration in dying patients. In: Lynn J, ed. *By No Extraordinary Means: The Choice to Forgo Life-Sustaining Food and Water*. Bloomington, Ind: Indiana University Press; 1986.

21. Billings JA. Comfort measures for the terminally ill: is dehydration painful? *J Am Geriatr Soc*. 1985; 33:808–810.

22. Rhymes J. Hospice care in America. *JAMA*. 1990; 264:369–372.

23. de Wachter MAM. Active euthanasia in the Netherlands. *JAMA*. 1989; 262:3316–3319.

24. Rigter H. Euthanasia in the Netherlands: distinguishing facts from fiction. *Hastings Cent Rep*. 1989; 19(suppl):31–32.

25. Van der Maas P, van Delden J, Pijnenborg L, Looman C. Euthanasia and other medical decisions concerning the end of life. *Lancet*. 1991; 338:669–674.

26. Gelman D, Springen K. The doctor's suicide van. *Newsweek*. June 18, 1990:46–49.

27. Merz B. Despite defeat of state's suicide initiative, issue still unsettled. *Am Med News*. November 18, 1991:29.

28. Sprung CL. Changing attitudes and practices in forgoing life-sustaining treatment. *JAMA*. 1990; 263: 2211–2215.

29. Lifton RJ. *The Nazi Doctors: Medical Killing and the Psychology of Genocide*. New York, NY: Basic Books Inc; 1986.

30. Kass LR. Neither for love nor money: why doctors must not kill. *Public Interest*. 1989; 94:25–46.

31. Orentlicher D. Physician participation in assisted suicide. *JAMA*. 1989; 262:1844–1845.

32. Kamisar Y. Some non-religious views against proposed "mercy-killing" legislation. *Minn Law Rev*. 1958; 42:969–1042.

33. Battin MP. Remarks at University of Florida Colleges of Medicine and Nursing conference: Controversies in the Care of the Dying Patient. Orlando, Fla, February 14, 1991.

34. Quill TE. Death and dignity: a case of individualized decision making. *N Engl J Med*. 1991; 324:691–694.

EFFORTS TO COPE
WITH DEATH
AND PROVIDE CARE
FOR THE DYING

COPING WITH DEATH

Elisabeth Kübler Ross, "Hope"

Eric J. Cassell, "The Nature of Suffering and the Goals of Medicine"

Betty R. Ferrell and Nessa Coyle, "The Nature of Suffering and the Goals of Nursing"

Daniel Callahan, "Death: 'The Distinguished Thing'"

Bruce Jennings, True Ryndes, Carol D'Onofrio, and Mary Ann Baily, "Access to Hospice Care: Expanding Boundaries, Overcoming Barriers"

3

HOPE

ELISABETH KÜBLER-ROSS, M.D.

EDITORS' INTRODUCTION

Elisabeth Kübler-Ross interviewed hundreds of hospitalized patients in Chicago and, through their words, brought the inner life of dying people out into the open. The international popularity of this book has persisted to this day, reflecting enormous human curiosity about our common fate and allowing recognition of the harm to patients resulting from the denial of death prevailing in U.S. hospitals.

■ ■ ■

In desperate hope I go and search for her in all the corners of my room;
I find her not.

My house is small and what once has gone from it can never be regained.

But infinite is thy mansion, my lord, and seeking her I have come to thy door.

I stand under the golden canopy of thine evening sky and I lift my eager
eyes to thy face.

I have come to the brink of eternity from which nothing can vanish—no
hope, no happiness, no vision of a face seen through tears.

Oh, dip my emptied life into that ocean, plunge it into the deepest fullness.
Let me for once feel that lost sweet touch in the allness of the universe.

Tagore, from Gitanjali, LXXXVII

We have discussed so far the different stages that people go through when they are faced with tragic news—defense mechanisms, in psychiatric terms, coping mechanisms to deal with extremely difficult situations. These means will last for different periods of time and will replace each other or exist at times side by side. The one thing that usually persists through all these stages is hope. Just as children in Barracks L 318 and L 417 in the concentration camp of Terezin maintained their hope years ago, although out of a total of about 15,000 children under fifteen years of age only around 100 came out of it alive.

The sun has made a veil of gold

So lovely that my body aches.

Above, the heavens shriek with blue,

Convinced I've smiled by some mistake.

The world's abloom and seems to smile.

I want to fly, but where, how high?

If, in barbed wire, things can bloom,

Why couldn't I? I will not die!
> Anonymous, "On a Sunny Evening," 1944

In listening to our terminally ill patients we were always impressed that even the most accepting, the most realistic patients left the possibility open for some cure, for the discovery of a new drug or the "last-minute success in a research project," as Mr. J. expressed it (his interview follows in this chapter). It is this glimpse of hope which maintains them through days, weeks, or months of suffering. It is the feeling that all this must have some meaning, will pay off eventually if they can only endure it for a little while longer. It is the hope that occasionally sneaks in, that all this is just like a nightmare and not true; that they will wake up one morning to be told that the doctors are ready to try out a new drug which seems promising, that they will use it on him and that he may be the chosen, special patient, just as the first heart transplant patent must have felt that he was chosen to play a very special role in life. It gives the terminally ill a sense of a special mission in life which helps them maintain their spirits, will enable them to endure more tests when everything becomes such a strain—in a sense it is a rationalization for their suffering at times; for others it remains a form of temporary but needed denial.

No matter what we call it, we found that all our patients maintained a little bit of it and were nourished by it in especially difficult times. They showed the greatest confidence in the doctors who allowed for such hope—realistic or not—and appreciated it when hope was offered in spite of bad news. This does not mean that doctors have to tell them a lie; it merely means that we share with them the hope that something unforeseen may happen, that they may have a remission, that they will live longer than is expected. If a patient stops expressing hope, it is usually a sign of imminent death. They may say, "Doctor, I think I have had it," or "I guess this is it," or they may put it like the patient who always believed in a miracle, who one day greeted us with the words "I think this is the miracle—I am ready now and not even afraid any more." All these patients died within twenty-four hours. While we maintained hope with them, we did not reinforce hope when they finally gave it up, not with despair but in a stage of final acceptance.

The conflicts we have seen in regard to hope arose from two main sources. The first and most painful one was the conveyance of hopelessness either on the part of the staff or family when the patient still needed hope. The second source of anguish came from the family's inability to accept a patient's final stage; they desperately clung to hope when the patient himself was ready to die and sensed the family's inability to accept this fact (as illustrated in the cases of Mrs. W. and Mr. H.).

What happens with the "pseudo–terminal syndrome" patient who has been given up by his physician and then—after being given adequate treatment—makes a comeback? Implicitly or explicitly these patients have been "written off." They may have been told that "there is nothing else we can do for you" or they may just have been sent home in unexpressed anticipation of their imminent death. When these patients are treated with all available therapy, they will be able to regard their comeback as "a miracle," "a new lease on life," or "some extra time I did not ask for," depending on previous management and communications.

The relevant message that Dr. Bell communicates is to give each patient a chance for the most effective possible treatment and not to regard each seriously ill patient as terminal, thus giving up on them. I would add that we should not "give up" on any patient, terminal or not terminal. It is the one who is beyond medical help who needs as much if not more care than the one who can look forward to another discharge. If we give up on such a patient, he may give up himself and further medical help may be forthcoming too late because he lacks the readiness and spirit to "make it once more." It is far more important to say, "To my knowledge I have done everything I can to help you. I will continue, however, to keep you as comfortable as possible." Such a patient will keep his glimpse of hope and continue to regard his physician as a friend who will stick it out to the end. He will not feel deserted or abandoned the moment the doctor regards him as beyond the possibility of a cure.

The majority of our patients made a comeback, in some way or another. Many of them had given up hope of ever relating their concerns to anyone. Many of them felt isolated and deserted; more of them felt cheated out of the opportunity of being considered in important decisions. Approximately half of our patients were discharged to go home or to a nursing home, to be readmitted later on. They all expressed their appreciation of sharing with us their concern about the seriousness of their illness and their hopes. They did not regard their discussions of death and dying as either premature or contraindicated in view of their "comeback." Many of our patients related the ease and comfort of their return home, after having settled their concerns prior to their discharge. Several of them asked to meet with their families in our presence before going home, in order to drop the façade and to enjoy the last few weeks together fully.

It might be helpful if more people would talk about death and dying as an intrinsic part of life just as they do not hesitate to mention when someone is expecting a new baby. If this were done more often, we would not have to ask ourselves if we ought to bring this topic up with a patient, or if we should wait for the last admission. Since we are not infallible and can never be sure which is the last admission, it may just be another rationalization which allows us to avoid the issue.

We have seen several patients who were depressed and morbidly uncommunicative until we spoke with them about the terminal stage of their illness. Their spirits were lightened, they began to eat again, and a few of them were discharged once more, much to the surprise of their families and the medical staff. I am convinced that we do more harm by avoiding the issue than by using time and timing to sit, listen, and share.

I mention timing because patients are no different from the rest of us in that we have our moments when we feel like talking about what burdens us and times when we wish to think about more cheerful things, no matter how real or unrealistic they are. As long as the patient knows that we will take the extra time when *he* feels like talking, when we are able to perceive his cues, we will witness that the majority of patients wish to share their concerns with another human being and react with relief and more hope to such dialogues.

If this book serves no other purpose but to sensitize family members of terminally ill patients and hospital personnel to the implicit communications of dying patients, then it has fulfilled its task. If we, as members of the helping professions, can help the patient and his family to get "in tune" to each other's needs and come to an acceptance of an unavoidable reality together, we can help to avoid much unnecessary agony and suffering on the part of the dying and even more so on the part of the family that is left behind.

The following interview with Mr. J. represents an example of the stage of anger and demonstrates—at times in a disguised way—the phenomenon of ever-present hope.

Mr. J. was a fifty-three-year-old Negro man who was hospitalized with mycosis fungoides, a malignant skin disorder which he describes in detail in the following interview. This illness necessitated his resorting to disability insurance and is characterized by states of relapses and remissions.

When I visited him the day before our seminar session, the patient felt lonely and in a talkative mood. He related very quickly in a dramatic and colorful fashion the many aspects of this unpleasant illness. He made it difficult for me to leave and held me back on several occasions. Much in contrast to that unplanned meeting, he expressed more annoyance, at times even anger, during the session behind the one-way mirror. The day before the seminar session he had initiated the discussion of death and dying, whereas during the session he said, "I don't think about dying, I think about living."

I mention this since it is relevant to our care of terminally ill patients, that they have days, hours, or minutes when they wish to talk about such matters. They may, like Mr. J. the day before, volunteer their philosophy of life and death and we may consider them ideal patients for such a teaching session. We tend to ignore the fact that the same patient may wish to talk only about the pleasant aspects of life the next day; we should respect his wishes. We did not do this during the interview, as we attempted to regain some of the meaningful material he presented the day before.

I should say that this is a danger mainly when an interview is part of a teaching program. Forcing questions and answers for the benefit of students should never occur during such an interview. The person should always come first and the patient's wishes should always be respected even if it means having a classroom of fifty students and no patient to interview.

DOCTOR: Mr. J., just for the introduction, how long have you been in the hospital?

PATIENT: This time I've been in since April the 4th of this year.

DOCTOR: How old are you?

PATIENT: I'm fifty-three years old.

DOCTOR: You have heard what we are doing in this seminar?

PATIENT: I have. Will you lead me with questions?

DOCTOR: Yes.

PATIENT: All right, you just go right ahead, whenever you are ready.

DOCTOR: I'd be curious to get a better picture of you because I know very little about you.

PATIENT: I see.

DOCTOR: You have been a healthy man, married, working, ah—

PATIENT: That's right, three children.

DOCTOR: Three children. When did you get sick?

PATIENT: Well, I went on disability in 1963. I think I first came in contact with this disease around 1948. I first started out with small rashes on my left chest, and under my right shoulder blade. And first it was no more than what anybody gets in the course of a lifetime. And I used the usual ointments, calamine lotion, Vaseline, and different things that you buy in the drug store. Didn't bother me too much. But gradually by, I'd say by 1955, the lower part of my body was involved, not to any great extent. There was a dryness, a scaliness had settled in, and I'd use a lot of greasy ointments and things like that to keep myself moist and as comfortable as possible. I still kept on working. In fact, certain periods through there I had two jobs because my daughter was going to college and I wanted to make sure that she finished. So I'd say by 1957 it had reached a point where I had started going to different doctors. I went to Dr. X for a period of about three months and he didn't make any improvement. The visits were cheap enough, but the prescriptions were about fifteen to eighteen dollars a week. When you are raising a family of three children on a workman's salary, even if you are working two jobs, you can't handle a situation like that. And I did go through the clinic and they made a casual examination which didn't satisfy me. I didn't bother to go back to them. And I just knocked around, feeling, I guess, more and more miserable all the time until in 1962 Dr. Y had me admitted to the P. Hospital. I was in there about five weeks and really nothing happened and I came out of there and finally went back to the first clinic. Finally in March of 1963 they admitted me to this hospital. I was in such bad shape by then that I went on disability.

DOCTOR: This was in '63?

PATIENT: In '63.

DOCTOR: Did you have any idea what kind of illness you had by then?

PATIENT: I knew it was mycosis fungoides and everybody else knew it.

DOCTOR: So, how long did you know the name of your illness?

PATIENT: Well, I was suspicious of it for some time, but then it was confirmed by a biopsy.

DOCTOR: A long time ago?

PATIENT: Not a long time ago, just a few months before the actual diagnosis was made. But you get one of these conditions and you read everything you can get your hands on. You listen to everything, and you learn the names of the different diseases. And from what I read, mycosis fungoides fit right into the picture and finally it was confirmed, and by then I was just about shot. My ankles had started to swell up on me, I was in a constant state of perspiration, and I was thoroughly miserable.

DOCTOR: Is that what you mean by "by then I was thoroughly shot?" That you felt so miserable? Is that what you mean?

PATIENT: Sure. I was just miserable—itching, scaling, perspiring, ankle hurting, just a completely, thoroughly, utterly miserable human being. Now, of course, these kind of times you get a little resentful. I guess you wonder, why does this happen to me. And then you come to your senses, and you say, "Well you are no better than anybody else, why not you?" That way you can sort of reconcile yourself because then everybody you see you start looking at their skin. You look if they have any blemishes, any signs of dermatitis since your whole sole interest in life is to see if they have any blemishes and who else is suffering from something similar, you know. And I guess, too, people are looking at you because you're much different-looking from them—

DOCTOR: Because this is a visible kind of illness.

PATIENT: It is a visible kind of an ailment.

DOCTOR: What does this illness mean to you? What is this mycosis fungoides to you?

PATIENT: It means to me that up to now they haven't cured anybody. They have had remissions for certain periods of time, they have had remissions for indefinite periods of time. It means to me that somewhere, someone is going to do research. There are a lot of good brains working on this condition. They might discover a cure while in the process of working on something else. And it means to me that I grit my teeth and go on from day to day and hope that some morning I'll sit up on the side of the bed and the doctor will be there and he will say, "I want to give you this shot," and it will be something like a vaccine or something, and in a few days it will clear up.

DOCTOR: Something that works!

PATIENT: I will be able to go back to work. I like my job because I did work myself into a supervisory capacity.

DOCTOR: What did you do?

PATIENT: Actually, I was active general foreman in the main post office down here. I had worked myself to the point where I was in charge of the foremen. I had seven or eight foremen who accounted to me every night. Rather than dealing with just the help, I dealt with more or less operations. I had good prospects for advancement because I knew and enjoyed my work. I didn't begrudge any time that I spent on the job. I was always helping my wife when the kids were getting up. We hoped they would be out of the way and maybe we could enjoy some of the things that we had read about and heard about.

DOCTOR: Like what?

PATIENT: Traveling a little, I mean we never had a vacation. Our first child was a premature baby and it was touch and go for a long time. She was sixty-one days old before she came home. I still have a sack of receipts from the hospital at home now. I paid her bill out at two dollars a week and in those days I was only making about seventeen dollars a week. I used to get off the train and rush two bottles of my wife's breast milk to the hospital, pick up two empty bottles, come back to the station, and go on to my job in the city. I would then work all day and bring those two empty bottles home at night. And she had enough milk for, I guess, for all the premature kids in the nursery over there. We kept them pretty well supplied and this meant to me that we got over the hump with everything. I would soon be in a salary bracket where you don't have to pinch every nickel. It just meant for me that we would maybe sometime look forward to a planned vacation instead of, well, we can't go anywhere, this kid has to have some dental work or something like that. That's all it meant to me. It meant a few good years of more or less relaxed living.

DOCTOR: After a long, hard life of trouble.

PATIENT: Well, most people put in a longer and harder struggle than I do. I never considered it much of a struggle. I worked in that foundry and we did piece work. I could work like a demon. I had fellows that came to my house and told my wife that I worked too hard. Well, she jumped all over me about that, and I would tell her it was a matter of jealousy when you work around men with muscle, they don't want you to have more muscle than they have and I definitely did, because wherever I went to work, I worked. And whenever there was any advancement, I made it, whatever advancement there was to be made. In fact, they called me into the office over where I was working and they told me when we make a colored foreman, you will be it. I was elated for a moment but when I went out—they said *when*—that could be anywhere from now to the year two thousand. So it deflated me to an extent that I had to work under those conditions. But still nothing was hard for me in those days. I had plenty of strength, I had my youth, and I just believed I could do anything.

DOCTOR: Tell me, Mr. J., now that you are not that young anymore, and maybe you can't do all those things anymore, how do you take it? Presumably there is no doctor who stands there with an injection, a medical cure.

PATIENT: That's right. You learn how to take these things. You first get that realization that maybe you won't ever get well.

DOCTOR: What does that do to you?

PATIENT: It shakes you up, you try not to think about things like that.

DOCTOR: Do you ever think about it?

PATIENT: Sure, there are a lot of nights I don't sleep very well. I think about a million things during the night. But you don't dwell on those things. I had a good life as a child and my mother is still living. She comes out here quite often to see me. I can always run back over my mind and go over some incident that happened. We used to take the jalopy and travel within our area. We did quite a bit of traveling in those days when they had very few paved roads and the other roads were muddy. You'd get somewhere, stuck on a muddy road up to the hubcaps, and you might have to push or pull or something like that. And so I guess I had a pretty nice childhood, my parents were very nice. There was no harshness or ill temper in our house. It made for a pleasant life. I think in terms of those things and I realize I'm pretty well blessed because there has been a rare man put in this world who has nothing but misery. I look around and find that I have had what I call a few bonus days.

DOCTOR: You have had a fulfilled life is really what you are saying. But does it make dying any easier?

PATIENT: I don't think about dying. I think about living. I think, you know, I used to tell the kids, they were coming up, I would tell them, now, do your best under all circumstances, and I said lots of times you are still gonna lose. I said, now, you remember in this life you have to be lucky. That was an expression I used. And I always considered myself lucky. I look back and I think of all the boys who came along with me and are in jail and various prisons and places like that. And I had as good a chance as they had but I didn't make it. I always pulled away when they were about to get started into something that wasn't right. I had a lot of fights on account of that, they think you are afraid. But it is better to be leery of those things, and fight for what you believe in, than it is to kick in and say, well, I'll go along. Because invariably sooner or later you are involved in something that can start you off on a life that you can't reverse. Oh, they say you can pull yourself up by your boot straps and all that, but you get yourself some kind of a record and the first thing that happens in your neighborhood, and I don't care how old you get to be, they pick you up and want to know where were you such and such a night. I was fortunate enough to steer clear of all of that. So when I look it all over I have to say that I've been lucky and I project that a little further. I still have a little luck left. I mean, I have had some rough luck, you might call it, so sooner or later this thing has to even out and that's going to be the day that I walk out of here and people won't even recognize me.

DOCTOR: Is this what kept you from ever getting desperate?

PATIENT: Nothing keeps you from ever getting desperate. I don't care how well adjusted you are, you will get desperate. But I will say this has kept me from the breaking point. You get desperate. You get to a place where you can't sleep and after a while you are fighting it. The harder you fight it, the harder it is on you, because it can actually get to be a physical battle. You will break out into a sweat just as though you are exerting yourself physically but it's all mental.

DOCTOR: How do you fight it? Does religion help you? Or certain people help you?

PATIENT: I don't call myself a particularly religious man.

DOCTOR: What gives you the strength to do this for twenty years? It's just about twenty years, isn't it?

PATIENT: Well, yes, I guess your sources of strength come from so many different angles, it would be pretty hard to say. My mother has a deep abiding faith. Any effort that I give this thing less than my full effort, I would feel that I am letting her down. So I say with the help of my mother. My wife has a deep abiding faith, so it is also with the help of my wife. My sisters, it always seems to be the females in the family who have the deeper religion, and they are the ones who are, I guess, the most sincere in their prayers. To me, the average person praying is begging for something. Always had too much pride to actually beg. I think maybe that's why I can't put all the full feeling into what I say here. I can't give vent to all my feelings along those lines, I guess.

DOCTOR: What did you have as a religious background, Catholic or Protestant . . . ?

PATIENT: I'm a Catholic now, I was converted Catholic. One of my parents was Baptist and one was Methodist. They made it fine.

DOCTOR: How did you become a Catholic?

PATIENT: It seemed to fit into my idea of what a religion should be.

DOCTOR: When did you make that change?

PATIENT: When the kids were small. They went to Catholic schools. In the early '50s, I figure.

DOCTOR: Was this in any way connected with your illness?

PATIENT: No, because at the time the skin didn't bother me too much and I just thought that as soon as I get a chance to settle down and go to a doctor this will be cleared up, you know?

DOCTOR: Ah—

PATIENT: But it never happened like that.

DOCTOR: Is your wife Catholic?

PATIENT: Yes, she is. She was converted at the time I was.

DOCTOR: Yesterday you told me something. I don't know if you want to bring it up again. I think it would be helpful. When I asked you how you take all this, you gave me the whole scale of possibilities of how a man can become—ending it all and thinking about suicide, and why this is not possible for you. You mentioned also a fatalistic approach, can you repeat that again?

PATIENT: Well, I said that I had a doctor once who told me, "I couldn't, I don't know how you take it. I'd kill myself."

DOCTOR: That was a doctor who said that?

PATIENT: Yes. So then I said, killing myself is out because I'm too yellow to kill myself. That eliminates one possibility that I don't have to think about. I finally rid my mind of encumbrances as I go on, so that I have less and less and less to think about. So I eliminated the idea of killing myself by the process of eliminating death. Then I reached the conclusion that, well, you're here now. Now you can either turn your face to the wall and you can cry. Or you can try to get whatever little fun and pleasure out of life you can, considering your condition. And certain things happen. You may watch a good TV program or listen to interesting conversation and after a few minutes you are not aware of the itching and the uncomfortable feeling. All these little things I call bonuses and I figure that if I can have enough bonuses together, one of these days everything will be a bonus and it will stretch out to infinity and every day will be a good day. So I don't worry too much. When I have my miserable feelings I just more or less distract myself or try to sleep. Because, after all, sleep is the best medicine that has ever been invented. Sometimes I don't even sleep, and I just lie there quietly. You learn how to take these things, what else can you do? You jump up and scream and holler and you can beat your head against the wall, but when you do all that you're still itching, you're still miserable.

DOCTOR: It's the itching that seems to be the worst part of your illness. Do you have any pain?

PATIENT: So far the itching has been the worst, but right along the bottom of my feet it is so sore that it's like torture to put any weight on them. So I'd say up to now the itching, and the dryness and the scaliness, has been my biggest problem. I have a personal warfare on these scales. It gets to be a funny thing. You get your bed full of scales and you make a brush like that, and ordinarily any kind of debris just sails right off. The scales jump up and down in one place like they have claws and it gets to be a frantic effort.

DOCTOR: To get rid of them?

PATIENT: To get rid of them, because they will fight you to a standstill. You'll be exhausted and you'll look and they are still there. So I even thought about a small vacuum cleaner, to keep myself clean. Staying clean gets to be an obsession with you because by the time you take a bath and put all this goo on you, you don't feel clean anyway. So right away you feel like you need another bath. You could spend your life going in and out of the bath.

DOCTOR: Who is most helpful in this trouble? As long as you are in the hospital, Mr. J.?

PATIENT: Who is the most helpful? I'd say you couldn't meet anybody around here, everybody, they anticipate my needs and help. They do a lot of things I don't even think about. One of the girls noticed that my fingers were sore and I was having trouble lighting a cigarette. I heard her tell the rest of the girls, "When you come through here, you check with him and see if he wants a cigarette." Why, you can't beat that.

DOCTOR: They really care.

PATIENT: You know, it's a wonderful feeling, but everywhere I have been and all through my life, people have liked me. I am profoundly thankful for that. I am humbly thankful. I have never gone out of my way, I don't think, to be a do-gooder. But I can find any number of people in this city who could point out times on various jobs that I helped them out. I don't even know why, it was just a part of me to put a person mentally at ease. I would go to the effort to help this person adjust himself. And I can find so many people and they tell other people how I helped them. But by the same token everybody I have ever known has helped me. I don't believe I have an enemy in the world. I don't believe I know a person in the world who wishes me any kind of harm. My roommate from college was here a couple of years ago. We talked about the days we were in school together. We remembered the dormitory when at any hour of the day someone would make a suggestion, let's go down and turn out so-and-so's room. And they would come down and throw you out bodily, out of your own room. Good clean horseplay, rough, but good fun. And he was telling his son how we used to stand them off and stack them up like cord wood. We were both strong, we were both the tough type. And we would actually stack them up in that hall, they never turned our room out. We had one roommate in there with us and he was on the track team and he ran the hundred-yard dash. Before five guys came in the door he could get out of that door and down that hall, was about seventy yards long. Nobody would have had him once he got started. So way late he would come back, we would have order restored and the room cleaned up and everything, and we'd all go to bed.

DOCTOR: Is this one of the bonuses you think about?

PATIENT: I look back on it and I think of the foolish things we did. Some guys came up one night and the room was cold. We wondered who could stand the most cold and naturally each one of us knew we could stand the most cold. So we decided to raise the window. No heat coming up or anything and it was seventeen below zero outside. I remember I had one of those woolen skullcaps on and two pair of pajamas and a robe and two pair of socks. I guess everybody else did the same thing. But when we awakened in the morning, everything, every glass, and everything else in that room, was frozen solid. And any wall you touched you were just liable to stick to it, it was just frozen solid. It took us four days to thaw out that bedroom and warm it up. I mean, that's the kind of foolish thing you would do, you know. And sometimes somebody looks at me and sees a smile across my face, and thinks the guy is nuts, he is finally cracking. But it's just some incident that I think about that I get a kick out of. Now yesterday, you asked me what is the main thing that the doctors and nurses could do to help a patient. It depends a lot on the patient. It depends a lot on how sick the patient is. If you are really sick, you don't want to be bothered at all. You would just like to lay there and you don't want anybody fumbling over you or taking your blood pressure or your temperature. I mean, it seems that every time you relax someone has to do something with you. I think the doctors and the nurses should disturb you as little as possible. Because the minute you feel better, you are going to raise your head and be interested in things. And that's the time for them to come in and start gradually cheering you up and coaxing you.

DOCTOR: But Mr. J., when the very sick people are left alone, aren't they more miserable and more scared?

PATIENT: I don't think so. It's not a matter of leaving them alone, I don't mean to isolate these people or anything like that. I mean you are there in the room and you are resting nicely and there's someone plumping your pillows, you don't want your pillows plumped. Your head is resting nicely. They all mean well, so you go along with them. Then someone else comes along, and "Do you want a glass of water?" Why, really, if you wanted a glass of water you could ask for it, but they will pour you a glass of water. They are doing this out of sheer kindness of heart, trying to make you more comfortable. Whereas under certain conditions if everybody would just ignore you—just for the time being, you feel much better.

DOCTOR: Would you like to be left alone now, too?

PATIENT: Not, not too much, last week I had—

DOCTOR: I mean now, now during this interview. Is this making you tired, too?

PATIENT: Oh, I say tired, I mean I've got nothing to do but go down there and rest anyway. But, ah, I don't see much point in this thing too much longer because after a while you get repetitious.

DOCTOR: You had some concern about that yesterday.

PATIENT: Yes, well, I had reason to be concerned because a week ago, had you seen me, you would not have even considered me for an interview because I was speaking in half sentences, I was speaking in half thoughts. I would not have known my name. But, ah, I've come a long way since then.

CHAPLAIN: How do you feel about what has happened in this past week? Is this another stroke of your bonus?

PATIENT: Well, I look forward to having it happen like this, this thing travels in cycles, you know, like a big wheel. It goes around and with the new medicine they tried on me, I look for some extenuation of these different feelings. I either expect to feel real well or feel real bad at first. I went through the bad spell and now I will have a good spell and I will feel pretty good because it happens like that. Even if I don't take any kind of medicine, if I just let things go.

DOCTOR: So you are entering your good cycle now, right?

PATIENT: I think so.

DOCTOR: I think we will take you back to your room now.

PATIENT: Appreciate it.

DOCTOR: Thank you, Mr. J., for coming.

PATIENT: You are quite welcome.

Mr. J., whose twenty years of illness and suffering had made him somewhat of a philosopher, shows many signs of disguised anger. What he is really saying in this interview is "I have been so good, why me?" He describes how tough and strong he was in his younger years, how he endured cold and hardship; how he cared for his children and family, how hard he worked and never allowed the bad guys to tempt him. After all this struggle, his children are grown up and he hoped for a few good years to travel, to take a vacation, to enjoy the fruits of his labor. He knows on some level that these hopes are in vain. It takes all his energy now to stay sane, to fight the itching, the discomfort, the pain, which he so adequately describes.

He looks back at this fight, and eliminates step by step considerations which pass his mind. Suicide is "out," an enjoyable retirement is out of the question as well. His field of possibilities shrinks as the illness progresses. His expectations and requirements become smaller and he has finally accepted the fact that he has to live from one remission to the next. When he feels very bad he wants to be left alone to withdraw and attempt to sleep. When he feels better he will let people know that he is ready to communicate again and becomes more sociable. "You have got to be lucky" means that he maintains the hope that there will be another remission. He also maintains the hope that some cure may be found, some new drug developed in time to relieve him of the suffering.

He maintained this hope to the very last day.

THE NATURE OF SUFFERING
AND THE GOALS
OF MEDICINE

ERIC J. CASSELL, M.D.

EDITORS' INTRODUCTION

Proving the adage that everything worth saying has already been said and said better, Eric J. Cassell argued twenty-six years ago against the Cartesian dualism of either cure *or* comfort, and instead makes the case for a simultaneous care model, integrating appropriate life-prolonging treatments with care focused on relief of suffering. In this seminal article, he distinguishes suffering from physical symptoms and underscores the need for the medical profession to recognize the assault on identity and self-concept imposed by serious illness.

■ ■ ■

The obligation of physicians to relieve human suffering stretches back into antiquity. Despite this fact, little attention is explicitly given to the problem of suffering in medical education, research, or practice. I will begin by focusing on a modern paradox: Even in the best settings and with the best physicians, it is not uncommon for suffering to occur not only during the course of a disease but also as a result of its treatment. To understand this paradox and its resolution requires an understanding of what suffering is and how it relates to medical care.

Consider this case: A thirty-five-year-old sculptor with metastatic disease of the breast was treated by competent physicians employing advanced knowledge and technology and acting out of kindness and true concern. At every stage, the treatment as well as the disease was a source of suffering to her. She was uncertain and frightened about her future, but she could get little information from her physicians, and what she was told was not always the truth. She had been unaware, for example, that the irradiated breast would be so disfigured. After an oophorectomy and a regimen of medications, she became hirsute, obese, and devoid of libido. With tumor in the supraclavicular fossa, she lost strength in the hand that she had used in sculpturing, and she became profoundly depressed. She had a pathologic fracture of the femur, and treatment was delayed while her physicians openly disagreed about pinning her hip.

Each time her disease responded to therapy and her hope was rekindled, a new manifestation would appear. Thus, when a new course of chemotherapy was started, she was torn between a desire to live and the fear that allowing hope to emerge again would merely expose her to misery if the treatment failed. The nausea and vomiting from the chemotherapy were distressing, but no more so than the anticipation of hair loss. She feared the future. Each tomorrow was seen as heralding increased sickness, pain, or disability, never as the beginning of better times. She felt isolated because she was no longer like other people and could not do what other people did. She feared that her friends would stop visiting her. She was sure that she would die.

This young woman had severe pain and other physical symptoms that caused her suffering. But she also suffered from some threats that were social and from others that were personal and private. She suffered from the effects of the disease and its treatment on her appearance and abilities. She also suffered unremittingly from her perception of the future.

What can this case tell us about the ends of medicine and the relief of suffering? Three facts stand out: The first is that this woman's suffering was not confined to her physical symptoms. The second is that she suffered not only from her disease but also from its treatment. The third is that one could not anticipate what she would describe as a source of suffering; like other patients, she had to be asked. Some features of her condition she would call painful, upsetting, uncomfortable, and distressing, but not a source of suffering. In these characteristics her case was ordinary.

In discussing the matter of suffering with laypersons, I learned that they were shocked to discover that the problem of suffering was not directly addressed in medical education. My colleagues of a contemplative nature were surprised at how little they knew of the problem and how little thought they had given it, whereas medical students tended to be unsure of the relevance of the issue to their work.

The relief of suffering, it would appear, is considered one of the primary ends of medicine by patients and laypersons, but not by the medical profession. As in the care of the dying, patients and their friends and families do not make a distinction between physical and nonphysical sources of suffering in the same way that doctors do.[1]

A search of the medical and social science literature did not help me in understanding what suffering is; the word "suffering" was most often coupled with the word "pain," as in "pain and suffering." (The databases used were *Psychological Abstracts,* the *Citation Index,* and the *Index Medicus.*)

This phenomenon reflects a historically constrained and currently inadequate view of the ends of medicine. Medicine's traditional concern primarily for the body and for physical disease is well known, as are the widespread effects of the mind-body dichotomy on medical theory and practice. I believe that this dichotomy itself is a source of the paradoxical situation in which doctors cause suffering in their care of the sick. Today, as ideas about the separation of mind and body are called into question, physicians are concerning themselves with new aspects of the human condition. The profession of medicine is being pushed and pulled into new areas, both by its technology and by the demands of its patients. Attempting to understand what suffering is and how physicians might truly be devoted to its relief will require that medicine and its critics overcome the dichotomy between mind and body and the associated dichotomies between subjective and objective and between person and object.

In the remainder of this paper I am going to make three points. The first is that suffering is experienced by persons. In the separation between mind and body, the concept of the person, or personhood, has been associated with that of mind, spirit, and the subjective. However, as I will show, a person is not merely mind, merely spiritual, or only subjectively knowable. Personhood has many facets, and it is ignorance of them that actively contributes to patients' suffering. The understanding of the place of the person in human illness requires a rejection of the historical dualism of mind and body.

The second point derives from my interpretation of clinical observations: Suffering occurs when an impending destruction of the person is perceived; it continues until the threat of disintegration has passed or until the integrity of the person can be restored in some other manner. It follows, then, that although suffering often occurs in the presence of acute pain, shortness of breath, or other bodily symptoms, suffering extends beyond the physical. Most generally, suffering can be defined as the state of severe distress associated with events that threaten the intactness of the person.

The third point is that suffering can occur in relation to any aspect of the person, whether it is in the realm of social roles, group identification, the relation with self, body, or family, or the relation with a transpersonal, transcendent source of meaning. Below is a simplified description or "topology" of the constituents of personhood.

"PERSON" IS NOT "MIND"

The split between mind and body that has so deeply influenced our approach to medical care was proposed by Descartes to resolve certain philosophical issues. Moreover, Cartesian dualism made it possible for science to escape the control of the church by assigning the noncorporeal, spiritual realm to the church, leaving the physical world as the domain of science. In that religious age, "person," synonymous with "mind," was necessarily off limits to science.

Changes in the meaning of concepts like that of personhood occur with changes in society, while the word for the concept remains the same. This fact tends to obscure the depth of the transformations that have occurred between the seventeenth century and today. People simply *are* "persons" in this time, as in past times, and they have difficulty imagining that the term described something quite different in an earlier period when the concept was more constrained.

If the mind-body dichotomy results in assigning the body to medicine, and the person is not in that category, then the only remaining place for the person is in the category of mind. Where the mind is problematic (not identifiable in objective terms), its very reality diminishes for science, and so, too, does that of the person. Therefore, so long as the mind-body dichotomy is accepted, suffering is either subjective and thus not truly "real"—not within medicine's domain—or identified exclusively with bodily pain. Not only is such an identification misleading and distorting, for it depersonalizes the sick patient, but it is itself a source of suffering. It is not possible to treat sickness as something that happens solely to the body without thereby risking damage to the person. An anachronistic division of the human condition into what is medical (having to do with the body) and what is nonmedical (the remainder) has given medicine too narrow a notion of its calling. Because of this division, physicians may, in concentrating on the cure of bodily disease, do things that cause the patient as a person to suffer.

AN IMPENDING DESTRUCTION OF PERSON

Suffering is ultimately a personal matter. Patients sometimes report suffering when one does not expect it, or do not report suffering when one does expect it. Furthermore, a person can suffer enormously at the distress of another, especially a loved one.

In some theologies, suffering has been seen as bringing one closer to God. This "function" of suffering is at once its glorification and its relief. If, through great pain or deprivation, someone is brought closer to a cherished goal, that person may have no sense of having suffered but may instead feel enormous triumph. To an observer, however, only the deprivation may be apparent. This cautionary note is important because people are often said to have suffered greatly, in a religious context, when they are known only to have been injured, tortured, or in pain, not to have suffered.

Although pain and suffering are closely identified in the medical literature, they are phenomenologically distinct.[2] The difficulty of understanding pain and the problems of physicians in providing adequate relief of physical pain are well known.[3-5]

The greater the pain, the more it is believed to cause suffering. However, some pain, like that of childbirth, can be extremely severe and yet considered rewarding. The perceived meaning of pain influences the amount of medication that will be required to control it. For example, a patient reported that when she believed the pain in her leg was sciatica, she could control it with small doses of codeine, but when she discovered that it was due to the spread of malignant disease, much greater amounts of medication were required for relief. Patients can writhe in pain from kidney stones and by their own admission not be suffering, because they "know what it is"; they may also report considerable suffering from apparently minor discomfort when they do not know its source. Suffering in close relation to the intensity of pain is reported when the pain is virtually overwhelming, such as that associated with a dissecting aortic aneurysm. Suffering is also reported when the patient does not believe that the pain can be controlled. The suffering of patients with terminal cancer can often be relieved by demonstrating that their pain truly can be controlled; they will then often tolerate the same pain without any medication, preferring the pain to the side effects of their analgesics. Another type of pain that can be a source of suffering is pain that is not overwhelming but continues for a very long time.

In summary, people in pain frequently report suffering from the pain when they feel out of control, when the pain is overwhelming, when the source of the pain is unknown, when the meaning of the pain is dire, or when the pain is chronic.

In all these situations, persons perceive pain as a threat to their continued existence—not merely to their lives, but to their integrity as persons. That this is the relation of pain to suffering is strongly suggested by the fact that suffering can be relieved, in the presence of continued pain, by making the source of the pain known, changing its meaning, and demonstrating that it can be controlled and that an end is in sight.

It follows, then, that suffering has a temporal element. In order for a situation to be a source of suffering, it must influence the person's perception of future events. ("If the pain continues like this, I *will be* overwhelmed"; "If the pain comes from cancer, I *will* die"; "If the pain cannot be controlled, I *will not* be able to take it.") At the moment when the patient is saying, "If the pain continues like this, I will be overwhelmed," he or she is not overwhelmed. Fear itself always involves the future. In the case with which I opened this paper, the patient could not give up her fears of her sense of future, despite the agony they caused her. As suffering is discussed in the other dimensions of personhood, note how it would not exist if the future were not a major concern.

Two other aspects of the relation between pain and suffering should be mentioned. Suffering can occur when physicians do not validate the patient's pain. In the absence of disease, physicians may suggest that the pain is "psychological" (in the sense of not being real) or that the patient is "faking." Similarly, patients with chronic pain may believe after a time that they can no longer talk to others about their distress. In the former case the person is caused to distrust his or her perceptions of reality, and in both instances social isolation adds to the person's suffering.

Another aspect essential to an understanding of the suffering of sick persons is the relation of meaning to the way in which illness is experienced. The word "meaning" is used here in two senses. In the first, to mean is to signify, to imply. Pain in the chest may imply heart disease. We also say that we know what something means when we know how important it is. The importance of things is always personal and individual, even though meaning in this sense may be shared by others or by society as a whole. What something signifies and how important it is relative to the whole array of a person's concerns contributes to its personal meaning. "Belief" is another word for that aspect of meaning concerned with implications, and "value" concerns the degree of importance to a particular person.

The personal meaning of things does not consist exclusively of values and beliefs that are held intellectually; it includes other dimensions. For the same word, a person may simultaneously have a cognitive meaning, an affective or emotional meaning, a bodily meaning, and a transcendent or spiritual meaning. And there may be contradictions in the different levels of meaning. The nuances of personal meaning are complex, and when I speak of personal meanings I am implying this complexity in all its depth—known and unknown. Personal meaning is a fundamental dimension of personhood, and there can be no understanding of human illness or suffering without taking it into account.

A SIMPLIFIED DESCRIPTION OF THE PERSON

A simple topology of a person may be useful in understanding the relation between suffering and the goals of medicine. The features discussed below point the way to further study and to the possibility of specific action by individual physicians.

Persons have personality and character. Personality traits appear within the first few weeks of life and are remarkably durable over time. Some personalities handle some illnesses better than others. Individual persons vary in character as well. During the heyday of psychoanalysis in the 1950s, all behavior was attributed to unconscious determinants: No one was bad or good; they were merely sick or well. Fortunately, that simplistic view of human character is now out of favor. Some people do in fact have stronger characters and bear adversity better. Some are good and kind under the stress of terminal illness, whereas others become mean and offensive when even mildly ill.

A person has a past. The experiences gathered during one's life are a part of today as well as yesterday. Memory exists in the nostrils and the hands, not only in the mind. A fragrance drifts by, and a memory is evoked. My feet have not forgotten how to roller-skate, and my hands remember skills that I was hardly aware I had learned. When these past experiences involve sickness and medical care, they can influence present illness and medical care. They stimulate fear, confidence, physical symptoms, and anguish. It damages people to rob them of their past and deny their memories, or to mock their fears and worries. A person without a past is incomplete.

Life experiences—previous illness, experiences with doctors, hospitals, and medications, deformities and disabilities, pleasures and successes, miseries and failures—all form the nexus for illness. The personal meaning of the disease and its treatment arises from the past as well as the present. If cancer occurs in a patient with self-confidence from past achievements, it may give rise to optimism and a resurgence of strength. Even if it is fatal, the disease may not produce the destruction of the person but rather reaffirm his or her indomitability. The outcome would be different in a person for whom life had been a series of failures.

The intensity of ties to the family cannot be overemphasized; people frequently behave as though they were physical extensions of their parents. Events that might cause suffering in others may be borne without complaint by someone who believes that the disease is part of his or her family identity and hence inevitable. Even diseases for which no heritable basis is known may be borne easily by a person because others in the family have been similarly afflicted. Just as the person's past experiences give meaning to present events, so do the past experiences of his or her family. Those meanings are part of the person.

A person has a cultural background. Just as a person is part of a culture and a society, these elements are part of the person. Culture defines what is meant by masculinity or femininity, what attire is acceptable, attitudes toward the dying and sick, mating behavior, the height of chairs and steps, degrees of tolerance for odors and excreta, and how the aged and the disabled are treated. Cultural definitions have an enormous impact on the sick and can be a source of untold suffering. They influence the behavior of others toward the sick person and that of the sick toward themselves. Cultural norms and social rules regulate whether someone can be among others or will be isolated, whether the sick will be considered foul or acceptable, and whether they are to be pitied or censured.

Returning to the sculptor described earlier, we know why that young woman suffered. She was housebound and bedbound, her face was changed by steroids, she was masculinized by her treatment, one breast was scarred, and she had almost no hair. The degree of importance attached to these losses—that aspect of their personal meaning—is determined to a great degree by cultural priorities.

With this in mind, we can also realize how much someone devoid of physical pain, even devoid of "symptoms," may suffer. People suffer from what they have lost of themselves in relation to the world of objects, events, and relationships. We realize, too, that although medical care can reduce the impact of sickness, inattentive care can increase the disruption caused by illness.

A person has roles. I am a husband, a father, a physician, a teacher, a brother, an orphaned son, and an uncle. People are their roles, and each role has rules. Together, the rules that guide the performance of roles make up a complex set of entitlements and limitations of responsibility and privilege. By middle age, the roles may be so firmly set that disease can lead to the virtual destruction of a person by making the performance of his or her roles impossible. Whether the patient is a doctor who cannot doctor or a mother who cannot mother, he or she is diminished by the loss of function.

No person exists without others; there is no consciousness without a consciousness of others, no speaker without a hearer, and no act, object, or thought that does not somehow encompass others.[6] All behavior is or will be involved with others, even if only in memory or reverie. Take away others, remove sight or hearing, and the person is diminished. Everyone dreads becoming blind or deaf, but these are only the most obvious injuries to human interaction. There are many ways in which human beings can be cut off from others and then suffer the loss.

It is in relationships with others that the full range of human emotions finds expression. It is this dimension of the person that may be injured when illness disrupts the ability to express emotion. Furthermore, the extent and nature of a sick person's relationships influence the degree of suffering from a disease. There is a vast difference between going home to an empty apartment and going home to a network of friends and family after hospitalization. Illness may occur in one partner of a long and strongly bound marriage or in a union that is falling apart. Suffering from the loss of sexual function associated with some diseases will depend not only on the importance of sexual performance itself but also on its importance in the sick person's relationships.

A person is a political being. A person is in this sense equal to other persons, with rights and obligations and the ability to redress injury by others and the state. Sickness can interfere, producing the feeling of political powerlessness and lack of representation. Persons who are permanently handicapped may suffer from a feeling of exclusion from participation in the political realm.

Persons do things. They act, create, make, take apart, put together, wind, unwind, cause to be, and cause to vanish. They know themselves, and are known, by these acts. When illness restricts the range of activity of persons, they are not themselves.

Persons are often unaware of much that happens within them and why. Thus, there are things in the mind that cannot be brought to awareness by ordinary reflection. The structure of the unconscious is pictured quite differently by different scholars, but most students of human behavior accept the assertion that such an interior world exists. People can behave in ways that seem inexplicable and strange even to themselves, and the sense of powerlessness that the person may feel in the presence of such behavior can be a source of great distress.

Persons have regular behaviors. In health, we take for granted the details of our day-to-day behavior. Persons know themselves to be well as much by whether they behave as usual as by any other set of facts. Patients decide that they are ill because they cannot perform as usual, and they may suffer the loss of their routine. If they cannot do the things that they identify with the fact of their being, they are not whole.

Every person has a body. The relation with one's body may vary from identification with it to admiration, loathing, or constant fear. The body may even be perceived as a representation of a parent, so that when something happens to the person's body it is as though a parent were injured. Disease can so alter the relation that the body is no longer seen as a friend but, rather, as an untrustworthy enemy. This is intensified if the illness comes on without warning, and as illness persists, the person may feel increasingly vulnerable. Just as many people have an expanded sense of self as a result of changes in their bodies from exercise, the potential exists for a contraction of this sense through injury to the body.

Everyone has a secret life. Sometimes it takes the form of fantasies and dreams of glory; sometimes it has a real existence known to only a few. Within the secret life are fears, desires, love affairs of the past and present, hopes, and fantasies. Disease may destroy not only the public or the private person but the secret person as well. A secret beloved friend may be lost to a sick person because he or she has no legitimate place by the sickbed. When that happens, the patient may have lost the part of life that made tolerable an otherwise embittered existence. Or the loss may be only of a dream, but one that might have come true. Such loss can be a source of great distress and intensely private pain.

Everyone has a perceived future. Events that one expects to come to pass vary from expectations for one's children to a belief in one's creative ability. Intense unhappiness results from a loss of the future—the future of the individual person, of children, and of other loved ones. Hope dwells in this dimension of existence, and great suffering attends the loss of hope.

Everyone has a transcendent dimension, a life of the spirit. This is most directly expressed in religion and the mystic traditions, but the frequency with which people have intense feelings of bonding with groups, ideals, or anything larger and more enduring than the person is evidence of the universality of the transcendent dimension. The quality of being greater and more lasting than an individual life gives this aspect of the person its timeless dimension. The profession of medicine appears to ignore the human spirit. When I see patients in nursing homes who have become only bodies, I wonder whether it is not their transcendent dimension that they have lost.

THE NATURE OF SUFFERING

For purposes of explanation, I have outlined various parts that make up a person. However, persons cannot be reduced to their parts in order to be better understood. Reductionist scientific methods, so successful in human biology, do not help us to comprehend whole persons. My intent was rather to suggest the complexity of the person and the potential for injury and suffering that exists in everyone. With this in mind, any suggestion of mechanical simplicity should disappear from my definition of suffering. All the aspects of personhood—the lived past, the family's lived past, culture and society, roles, the instrumental dimension, associations and relationships, the body, the unconscious mind, the political being, the secret life, the perceived future, and the transcendent dimension—are susceptible to damage and loss.

Injuries to the integrity of the person may be expressed by sadness, anger, loneliness, depression, grief, unhappiness, melancholy, rage, withdrawal, or yearning. We acknowledge the person's right to have and express such feelings. But we often forget that the affect is merely the outward expression of the injury, not the injury itself. We know little about the nature of the injuries themselves, and what we know has been learned largely from literature, not medicine.

If the injury is sufficient, the person suffers. The only way to learn what damage is sufficient to cause suffering, or whether suffering is present, is to ask the sufferer. We all recognize certain injuries that almost invariably cause suffering: the death or distress of loved ones, powerlessness, helplessness, hopelessness, torture, the loss of a life's work, betrayal, physical agony, isolation, homelessness, memory failure, and fear. Each is both universal and individual. Each touches features common to all of us, yet each contains features that must be defined in terms of a specific person at a specific time. With the relief of suffering in mind, however, we should reflect on how remarkably little is known of these injuries.

THE AMELIORATION OF SUFFERING

One might inquire why everyone is not suffering all the time. In a busy life, almost no day passes in which one's intactness goes unchallenged. Obviously, not every challenge is a threat. Yet I suspect that there is more suffering than is known. Just as people with chronic pain learn to keep it to themselves because others lose interest, so may those with chronic suffering.

There is another reason why every injury may not cause suffering. Persons are able to enlarge themselves in response to damage, so that instead of being reduced, they may indeed grow. This response to suffering has encouraged the belief that suffering is good for people. To some degree, and in some persons, this may be so. If a leg is injured so that an athlete cannot run again, the athlete may compensate for the loss by learning another sport or mode of expression. So it is with the loss of relationships, loves, roles, physical strength, dreams, and power. The human body may lack the capacity to gain a new part when one is lost, but the person has it.

The ability to recover from loss without succumbing to suffering is sometimes called resilience, as though nothing but elastic rebound were involved, but it is more as though an inner force were withdrawn from one manifestation of a person and redirected to another. If a child dies and the parent makes a successful recovery, the person is said to have "rebuilt" his or her life. The term suggests that the parts of the person are structured in a new manner, allowing expression in different dimensions. If a previously active person is confined to a wheelchair, intellectual pursuits may occupy more time.

Recovery from suffering often involves help, as though people who have lost parts of themselves can be sustained by the personhood of others until their own recovers. This is one of the latent functions of physicians: to lend strength. A group, too, may lend strength: Consider the success of groups of the similarly afflicted in easing the burden of illness (for example, women with mastectomies, people with ostomies, and even the parents or family members of the diseased).

Meaning and transcendence offer two additional ways by which the suffering associated with destruction of a part of personhood is ameliorated. Assigning a meaning to the injurious condition often reduces or even resolves the suffering associated with it. Most often, a cause for the condition is sought within past behaviors or beliefs. Thus, the pain or threat that causes suffering is seen as not destroying a part of the person, because it is part of the person by virtue of its origin within the self. In our culture, taking the blame for harm that comes to oneself because of the unconscious mind serves the same purpose as the concept of karma in Eastern theologies; suffering is reduced when it can be located within a coherent set of meanings. Physicians are familiar with the question from the sick, "Did I do something that made this happen?"

It is more tolerable for a terrible thing to happen because of something that one has done than it is to be at the mercy of chance.

Transcendence is probably the most powerful way in which one is restored to wholeness after an injury to personhood. When experienced, transcendence locates the person in a far larger landscape. The sufferer is not isolated by pain but is brought closer to a transpersonal source of meaning and to the human community that shares those meanings. Such an experience need not involve religion in any formal sense; however, in its transpersonal dimension, it is deeply spiritual. For example, patriotism can be a secular expression of transcendence.

WHEN SUFFERING CONTINUES

But what happens when suffering is not relieved? If suffering occurs when there is a threat to one's integrity or a loss of a part of a person, then suffering will continue if the person cannot be made whole again. Little is known about this aspect of suffering. Is much of what we call depression merely unrelieved suffering? Considering that depression commonly follows the loss of loved ones, business reversals, prolonged illness, profound injuries to self-esteem, and other damages to personhood, the possibility is real. In many chronic or serious diseases, persons who "recover" or who seem to be successfully treated do not return to normal function. They may never again be employed, recover sexual function, pursue career goals, reestablish family relationships, or reenter the social world, despite a physical cure. Such patients may not have recovered from the nonphysical changes occurring with serious illness. Consider the dimensions of personhood described above, and note that each is threatened or damaged in profound illness. It should come as no surprise, then, that chronic suffering frequently follows in the wake of disease.

The paradox with which this paper began—that suffering is often caused by the treatment of the sick—no longer seems so puzzling. How could it be otherwise, when medicine has concerned itself so little with the nature and causes of suffering? This lack is not a failure of good intentions. None are more concerned about pain or loss of function than physicians. Instead, it is a failure of knowledge and understanding. We lack knowledge, because in working from a dichotomy contrived within a historical context far from our own, we have artificially circumscribed our task in caring for the sick.

Attempts to understand all the known dimensions of personhood and their relations to illness and suffering present problems of staggering complexity. The problems are no greater, however, than those initially posed by the question of how the body works—a question that we have managed to answer in extraordinary detail. If the ends of medicine are to be directed toward the relief of human suffering, the need is clear.

REFERENCES

1. Cassell E. Being and becoming dead. *Soc Res.* 1972; 39:528–42.

2. Bakan D. *Disease, pain and sacrifice: toward a psychology of suffering.* Chicago: Beacon Press, 1971.

3. Marks RM, Sachar EJ. Undertreatment of medical inpatients with narcotic analgesics. *Ann Intern Med.* 1973; 78:173–81.

4. Kanner RM, Foley KM. Patterns of narcotic drug use in a cancer pain clinic. *Ann NY Acad Sci.* 1981; 362:161–72.

5. Goodwin JS, Goodwin JM, Vogel AV. Knowledge and use of placebos by house officers and nurses. *Ann Intern Med.* 1979; 91:106–10.

6. Zaner R. *The context of self: a phenomenological inquiry using medicine as a clue.* Athens, Ohio: Ohio University Press, 1981.

AUTHOR'S ACKNOWLEDGMENTS

I am indebted to Rabbi Jack Bemporad; to Drs. Joan Cassell, Peter Dineen, Nancy McKenzie, and Richard Zaner; to Ms. Dawn McGuire; to the members of the Research Group on Death, Suffering, and Well-Being of the Hastings Center for their advice and assistance; and to the Arthur Vining Davis Foundation for support of the research group.

THE NATURE OF SUFFERING AND THE GOALS OF NURSING

**BETTY R. FERRELL, R.N., PH.D., F.A.A.N.
AND NESSA COYLE, N.P., PH.D., F.A.A.N.**

The article originally appeared as Ferrell BR, Coyle N. The nature of suffering and the goals of nursing. *Oncol Nurs Forum.* 2008;35:241–247. Copyright © 2008 Oncology Nursing Society. All rights reserved. Reprinted with permission.

EDITORS' INTRODUCTION

Betty R. Ferrell and Nessa Coyle are among the nation's leading researchers and educators on nursing and palliative care. In this article they identify unique characteristics of the nursing profession critical to the dignity and personhood of the seriously ill, including provision of intimate personal care of the body, listening, and presence at the bedside.

■ ■ ■

In a medical-surgical unit in a small hospital in the midwestern region of the United States, a patient's suffering is reduced by the night shift nurse. The older female patient has lung cancer. She was admitted two days prior with a bowel obstruction, likely the cumulative result of immobility, inadequate food and fluid intake, medication side effects, and progressive disease. Her uncontrollable nausea, vomiting, and pain over the past few days at home now are relieved by a nasogastric (NG) tube, IV fluids, and careful titration of analgesics. Having finally slept a few hours, the woman awakens in the middle of the night. Given the myriad tubes and wires attached to her body, she remains motionless, afraid to move. Still, her wakefulness stirs her exhausted daughter, who is wedged into a cold, hard reclining chair at her bedside.

Mother and daughter exchange mutual queries: "Are you okay?" "Why don't you go home?" the mother suggests. "This chair is fine," the daughter lies. The patient's husband went home after a few hours at the hospital. After fifty-five years of marriage, the angst of seeing his wife so miserably ill and the strangeness of the hospital world were enough to propel him home, despite the terrifying and total silence of an empty house. Mother and daughter reaffirm to each other that he is home asleep, but both know he is probably wide awake, sitting in his easy chair in the living room, sipping stale coffee, reading his Bible, and counting on God to come through. After all, God has come through many times before. He has faith. God will come through again.

The night nurse enters the room, careful not to turn on the bright lights even though she sees that both mother and daughter are awake. She performs the routine checks—NG tube functioning, IV dripping, urinary catheter draining. The same nurse was on duty when the woman was admitted the night before. Comparing her patient's distress then and her current relatively peaceful state, and given the goals of care, she decides to skip the routine vital signs. Instead, she asks the woman how she is doing. The woman politely answers, "Fine." She adds that she did not really know how poorly she had felt until she started to feel better. The nurse resists the urge to hurry out the door to the next patient and to continue her long list of tasks. It is hard to stand still. She sees the woman's cachectic body, she hears the flow of oxygen and the pulsing suction of the NG tube, and she feels the clammy coolness of the woman's arm as she gently touches it. The nurse knows well the signs of approaching death—too well. Death is a frequent visitor in the hospital.

Assured of her patient's comfort, the nurse speaks to the daughter: "You must be relieved your mother is not in pain now." The nurse says how wonderful the daughter's presence has been and acknowledges the daughter's exhaustion. As the daughter's eyes fill with tears, she finds herself grateful that the room is dark. In just two days, she will need to leave to pack her own daughter for college. On the airplane, she will reverse roles, become the mother, and somehow navigate that other—and almost as difficult—rite of passage. After the move to college is completed, her husband will drop her off at the closest airport so she can return to her mother. She has been praying a lot. She asks God whose idea this is—that she may lose her mother and daughter in the same week. Her faith usually is strong, but not this week. She has found her limit.

The nurse senses the quiet tears of the daughter, hidden from her mother's eyes as she lies next to her, staring at the dark ceiling. She asks the daughter if she would like some coffee. It is the mother who answers: "We are tea sippers." She describes how the two of them had "tea parties" all their lives. From the time the daughter was a little girl with a floral porcelain tea set to heartier mugs shared over monumental life decisions, the two have sipped tea. The pale and weak patient perks up and proclaims, "You know, we could have a tea party now!"

The nurse hesitates. The woman cannot have oral fluids because of the bowel obstruction. But given that the primary goal for her patient is comfort, and given the enormous pleasure the ritual would give them, the nurse decides to let her have a few sips of tea. The NG suction will keep the sips from becoming instant, violent nausea. In silence, all three women realize with profound grief that this tea party may well be the last. The nurse excuses herself and goes to her locker to get a "special stash" tea bag. No industrial hospital tea bag will do, not for this occasion.

She returns in a moment with a full cup for the daughter, another smaller cup and a straw for the patient. After a deliberate pause and then an intimate connection as the nurse's hand touches the daughter's hand and lingers, she offers the tea. She leaves only when she is certain that her patient is comfortable, careful to leave the lights off and to close the door quietly. The mother and daughter sip tea. In the stillness of the room, with only the intermittent sound of the suction machine, they are recipients of the sacred care of a nurse.

The case illustrates the nature of suffering and the goals of nursing. The story is, on one level, a very simple narrative of a common situation. On another level, it is a rich and deep portrayal of the work of nursing delivered at one of the most poignant moments in the lives of a mother and her daughter. The deep and profound experience of suffering is the focus of this paper.

CASSELL'S FOUNDATIONAL WORK ON THE NATURE OF SUFFERING

In 1982, Eric Cassell, M.D., published a seminal paper on suffering. The publication in the *New England Journal of Medicine* opened the door to what has become an ongoing professional conversation about suffering in health care settings. Cassell's original article later was expanded to a book, and his initial article has been cited internationally by professionals from many disciplines, challenging systems to respond not only to physical injury and disease but also to human suffering (Cassell, 1991).

The essence of Cassell's description is that suffering is "experienced by persons, not merely by bodies, and has its source in challenges that threaten the intactness of the person as a complex social and psychologic entity" (Cassell, 1982, p. 639). Cassell also asserted that suffering may include pain but is not limited to it and that the relief of suffering is an obligation of medicine. His comparisons of pain versus suffering and his exploration of the concept of meaning echo the historic themes of medicine and nursing. Although both disciplines have a historic mandate to relieve suffering, the current health care system often fails to uphold this basic duty. Nursing and medicine have become highly technical and often quite depersonalized.

Cassell's analysis of the meaning of illness is particularly relevant to nursing. He described personal meaning as a fundamental dimension of personhood and explained that the act of recognizing personal meaning is critical to understanding human illness and suffering. He also rebuked modern medicine for ignoring the transcendent dimension—the spirit of human life.

THE NEED FOR A UNIQUE ANALYSIS OF NURSING AND SUFFERING

Oncology nurses are the professionals most often available to patients and families as they experience cancer across all settings of care. From the acute onset of illness or the moment of diagnosis of cancer, individuals look to nurses for reassurance and understanding, as a human connection in the overwhelming reality of health care. Nurses who bear witness to suffering are a valuable voice to articulate lived experiences of people in their most vulnerable and broken states. The title of "nurse" is a broad category, including a spectrum of human beings as diverse as the patients they serve.

A night shift nurse caring for a seriously ill, complex patient with cancer may be a twenty-two-year-old new graduate with limited nursing or life experience. Yet she is the professional on the front line addressing the needs of a suffering patient. The day nurse who relieves the new graduate may be a fifty-five-year-old man with thirty years of cumulative professional and personal experiences of triumph, loss, relieving pain, and witnessing suffering. He also may bring to the bedside his own intense personal experience of the recent deaths of his parents.

Nursing as a profession often is recognized for addressing whole-person care (Beckstrand and Kirchhoff, 2005). Nurses often are similar to physicians, guilty of using a "fix it" approach to care (Jackson, 2003). They want to heal the wound, eliminate the pain, relieve the nausea, and increase function. Many oncology nurses, the authors included, were taught that a "good nurse" was one whose patients ate well and consumed sufficient fluids, had functioning bowels and bladders, breathed deeply, and ambulated independently—preferably by the end of the nurse's shift! Each of those aspects of physical care is important yet incomplete without attention to psychosocial and spiritual concerns. Sister Rosemary Donley (1991), a senior nursing scholar, wrote, "Spiritual dimensions of health care: Nursing's mission." Donley wrote, "Nursing response to suffering persons runs parallel to the religious tradition: accompaniment, meaning giving, and action" (p. 179). Yet she articulated concern that the art and mystery of healing have been lost as nurses have become part of a moneymaking, technologic system, not a sacred system. She described the crisis in health care as a crisis of meaning and values. Donley concluded that "concern with spiritual elements of care brings greater meaning to the work of nursing and a sense of participation in the realm of mystery and grace. When nurses, acting compassionately to alleviate suffering, also search with their patients for a spiritual meaning for the experience, there will be a rebuilding of trust in professional relationships. This restoration will have a positive effect on patients, nurses, and on the healthcare system itself" (p. 183).

Several studies in recent years have documented the lack of palliative care content in nursing curricula and nursing textbooks, and extensive reports from practicing nurses have highlighted the need for attention to end-of-life care (Ferrell, Virani, et al., 2005; Malloy et al., 2006; Paice et al., 2006). For some, nursing education (and thus the journey to "becoming" nurses) has been guided by a nursing process and a nursing care plan that often resembled a checklist of actions to restore the sick to health and the dependent to independence. For some, educational preparation has been void of philosophy, role modeling, or reward for behaviors such as compassion and presence. The focus on communication in nursing practice is sometimes reduced to "patient teaching," in which an informed nurse directs an uninformed patient regarding cancer treatment.

Yet communication is more than information and includes the art of listening and witnessing suffering. Somewhere on the journey to learning the art of "healing," many nurses have had the profound gift of witnessing true nursing by a seasoned and compassionate colleague. Watching a nurse who is fully present, who listens carefully and says little but provides the sufferer the opportunity of "voice" as described by Reich

(1989), is a true education. Reich described the skilled professional as helping the suffering person who may "scream in pain and suffer in silence" and said that, through listening and patiently waiting, nurses "give voice" to suffering. Such mentors teach that silencing or stifling the voice of suffering serves only to intensify it.

Researchers from Canada (Daneault et al., 2004) explored the nature of suffering and its relief through a qualitative study of twenty-six terminally ill patients with cancer. Their findings revealed that patients experienced suffering in the dimensions of physical, psychological, and social well-being. The content analysis of the interviews recognized three irreducible, core dimensions of suffering: (1) being subjected to violence, (2) being deprived and overwhelmed, and (3) living in apprehension.

In a similar study, nurse researchers from Finland explored suffering in patients with advanced cancer (Kuuppelomaki and Lauri, 1998). Their research found suffering to exist in the same three dimensions. Physical suffering included fatigue, pain, and side effects of chemotherapy. Psychological suffering, most commonly expressed as depression, was related to the physical changes resulting from the disease and overall debilitation as death became imminent. The physical and psychological effects of worsened disease caused withdrawal and isolation, hence the third dimension of social suffering. The study reinforced the inter-relatedness of the dimensions of suffering and the whole-person phenomenon.

The findings of the Canadian and Finnish researchers were very similar to a study by a nurse researcher in the United States who studied suffering in patients with lung cancer (Benedict, 1982). The similarities in the studies are interesting, as are the common descriptions of distress from patients across diverse countries and cultures. Such studies help nurses to understand patient experiences of suffering and to uncover sources of suffering.

METHODS USED FOR THIS WORK

Three sources of data have informed this descriptive paper on the nature of suffering and the goals of nursing. The first was descriptions of suffering as derived from the literature. The literature reviewed was selected based on searches of medical, nursing, ethics and theology, and other literature, guided primarily by course work and directed readings of the authors. The two authors are doctorally prepared nurses who each, several years postdoctorate, returned to formal study. The first author was completing a master's degree in theology, ethics, and culture, the second author a nondegree program in medical humanities.

The second source of data that informed this work was narrative data derived from interviews or written comments from patients, family caregivers, and nurses. The data were abstracted from several studies the authors had conducted and analyzed previously. The data were reevaluated from the perspective of suffering. Narrative data also were collected from nurses attending End-of-Life Nursing Education Consortium courses (www.aacn.nche.edu/ELNEC). The narrative data were interpreted with content analysis methods. The narratives of nurses, patients, and family members were analyzed to identify common themes and concepts related to suffering. This paper, intended for oncology clinicians, includes several case studies as a preferred method of conveying the analysis of suffering.

The third source of information for this work was the personal and professional experiences of the authors. Beverly Harrison (1985) and Carol Gilligan (1982), as well as many other feminist scholars, have acknowledged that personal reflection and experience are valued sources of scholarship. To embrace the depths of suffering requires scholarly inquiry, synthesis of the literature, and reflection on clinical experiences and the lived observations of those who suffer.

THE UNIQUE RELATIONSHIP OF THE PATIENT AND NURSE

Many health care professionals are involved with patients' suffering from illness, but this analysis addressed only the unique relationship of the patient and nurse. The features of the relationship are illustrated in the following case.

The case of Mrs. K. and the night-time encounter with a nurse illustrates the unique relationship of nurse and patient in a complex healthcare system. Mrs. K. was surrounded by many caregivers yet expressed her suffering only in an intimate, personal encounter with a nurse. In the darkness of her room, the patient shared her greatest fears, explained her life losses, requested help, and exposed her vulnerability as her physical body forced her to become a patient, thus betraying her role as caregiver for her spouse. The nurse became her confidante, the vessel for her anxiety, and the counselor for her spiritual distress.

Mrs. K. is a seventy-eight-year-old Polish woman currently hospitalized after a seizure and diagnosis of a brain tumor. She responded well to the acute care she received in the emergency department and intensive care unit and is now on the neuro-oncology floor of an academic medical center. She is being seen by four medical specialties as well as speech therapy, physical therapy, and occupational therapy. Now that her condition is stable, she is undergoing further diagnostic work to evaluate her cardiovascular status and to determine her overall health status for treatment planning. She has short-term memory loss, unsteady gait, elevated blood pressure, and some left-sided weakness as well as some difficulty with speech.

During the night shift, after a day that included encounters with no fewer than twenty different health care professionals, attendants, transporters, and visitors, Mrs. K. is found sobbing quietly by the night nurse. She denies pain but admits that the reality of the brain tumor "just hit me." She tearfully speaks for a few moments with the nurse, who softly strokes her hand and offers a tissue. As their eyes connect, Mrs. K.'s quiet sobs become intense. She clutches the nurse's hand, repeating intensely, "I have to get well . . . I have to get well."

After finally calming her, the nurse asks her to try to explain her fears and to specifically express what is of greatest concern. Mrs. K. says that she must return home this week

Continued

Continued

because she is the only caregiver for her husband, who has advanced prostate cancer. She shares that their son has come from another state but can stay only a few days and that he and his father do not get along; thus she is worried about what may be happening at home. She tells the nurse that she has promised her husband to be there for him as he has always been there for her, including a few years ago, when she was treated for breast cancer. She also shares that her fifty-year-old daughter died of breast cancer last year.

Mrs. K. asks the nurse to please try to convince the doctors to let her go home. She also asks the nurse whether a priest is ever in the hospital at night; she would like to see him. She explains that she cannot ask for a priest during the daytime when her husband might be visiting because he "no longer believes there can be a God."

Witnessing suffering is the everyday work of nurses. In every setting, across diseases, and in people of all ages, suffering is part of being human, often intensified when being human also involves being ill. This paper is intended to be a step toward supporting nurses who care constantly for those who suffer. Nursing scholars Kahn and Steeves (1994) captured the need for attention to suffering by writing, "One characteristic of nursing's development over the past decade is the discovery of its voice—the ability and willingness to express what nurses collectively know and understand about the nature of nursing practice. To continue the development of nursing's voice, it is crucial that we talk freely about what we know, including what we know about suffering" (p. 260).

THE CONTEXT OF CANCER

Analogous to the association of pain with suffering is the association of cancer with death. Despite advances in earlier detection, treatment, and survivorship, the words "you have cancer" are almost always viewed as a death sentence. The prevalence and visibility of cancer are two social factors in the fear of cancer diagnosis. Virtually everyone knows someone with cancer and has witnessed the sometimes devastating effects of the disease. Most people also know of someone who has died from cancer. Unfortunately, society often collectively remembers people who died in pain (Chochinov, 2006; Lin and Bauer-Wu, 2003).

Another major factor in the association of cancer with suffering is the recognition of the caustic effects of cancer treatments. Even with the best prognosis, the effects of surgery, chemotherapy, and radiation therapy are distressing and can be devastating. A legacy exists in which many people diagnosed with cancer are reminded of the public images of those who have died from the disease or of personal experiences of having witnessed cancer's effects and the effects of treatment on loved ones. In the authors' research related to women with ovarian cancer, an unfortunately large number of women shared stories of having witnessed their own mothers or grandmothers die from ovarian cancer and in agonizing pain (Ferrell, Cullinane, et al., 2005). Health care professionals must reverse this legacy so that future patients will have legacies of compassionate care and comfort.

SUFFERING IN CANCER SURVIVORSHIP

All phases of the cancer trajectory—diagnosis, treatment, remission, and recurrence—are associated with suffering. A common perception is that suffering is limited to advanced cancer or to the final months of life as the physical body declines and a living person becomes a dying person. The Institute of Medicine (2005) report From Cancer Patient to Cancer Survivor: Lost in Transition recognizes that more than ten million cancer survivors reside in the United States. The suffering of those individuals

Alan is a thirty-year-old Jewish man. He had a slight head injury during a tennis game and is seen in the emergency room. An X-ray reveals a mass in his brain that is believed to be a brain tumor. Alan says that although he has been raised in a very devout Jewish family grounded in multiple generations of religious life, his own faith diminished in early adulthood and his only affiliations at the temple are social in nature, void of any deep meaning. Having had what he described as a "dress rehearsal" for death, Alan becomes deeply involved in his faith and an active leader in the temple. As he returns to an active spiritual life, he encounters many others in his religious community who share a recent life-altering experience that led to their return to formal involvement in their faith. Participating in Rosh Hashanah for the first time after his illness touches him more profoundly than he ever would have imagined.

Alan says that a nursing assistant in the hospital radiology department was his "rabbi." The nursing assistant, Ben, also is Jewish and met Alan on his initial emergency visit when his mass was discovered. The men share humorous stories of growing up Jewish that Alan finds to be of great benefit as a distraction amidst the terrifying tests. In the weeks that follow, as Alan returns for more diagnostic tests, their conversations become more serious. Alan confides his growing remorse about having abandoned his family heritage. Ben becomes his "rabbi" as Alan practices on Ben what he plans to say to the temple rabbi about his return to the faith community. Ben mostly listens as Alan talks but also offers to pray for Alan.

After three additional weeks, which he describes as "torturous," Alan is told that the mass is benign and that he will require no further treatment. When Alan receives the biopsy report confirming the unexpected good news, he makes a trip back to the hospital just to thank Ben for his support. Still overwhelmed by the news, Alan says he needs another week to absorb it all, to get his emotions in check before going to his temple. He gives Ben a donation to his temple and asks Ben to pass it on as an offering of thanks.

across the trajectory from initial diagnosis, treatment, remission, and even long-term survival is enormous. Cancer caught at even the earliest stage, with the best treatment, leading to the best response, and with the most optimistic prognosis is . . . cancer (Charmaz, 1983). Health care providers often believe that if their care is good, then suffering can be avoided. Although suffering can be heard, validated, and diminished, it remains a common response to serious illness and death. The effects on family members of patients with cancer are equally distressing (Lewis and Deal, 1995; Morse and Fife, 1998; Northouse et al., 2002).

Awareness is growing that cancer survivorship may be a time of deep spiritual meaning (McClain-Jacobson et al., 2004). Surviving cancer may result in becoming closer to God or faith to "get through" treatment. Faith can offer protection against the enduring threat that cancer will return. A case illustration follows.

This case illustrates one of the many opportunities for health care professionals to be present to people during life crises as they face their own mortality and revisit their faith traditions. In this case, Ben's genuine compassion and sharing of mutual faith experiences were vital forces in Alan's weeks of suffering and now in his reevaluation of life priorities.

SUFFERING IN ADVANCED CANCER

Advanced cancer has served as a model for studying the concept of suffering. With more than 559,650 cancer deaths each year in the United States (American Cancer Society 2007), suffering in advanced cancer is all too common. Advances in the provision of cancer care, which offer excellent physical care and symptom management combined with psychological, social, and spiritual care, have allowed for the ability to minimize suffering to the extent possible.

Remarkable consistency exists in studies describing the experience of suffering in advanced cancer (Cherny, Coyle, and Foley, 1994; Chochinov et al., 2002). Researchers in diverse settings consistently have concluded that suffering exists across dimensions of physical, psychological and emotional, social and interpersonal, and spiritual and existential well-being (Battenfield, 1984; Benedict, 1982; Kuuppelomaki and Lauri, 1998; O'Connor, Wicker, and Germino, 1990). Coyle (2006) published an article titled "The Hard Work of Living in the Face of Death." The phenomenologic study captured the essence of simultaneously living with advanced cancer and facing the immediacy of death. The author described the hard work of tasks such as maintaining control, creating a system of support and safety, finding meaning, and creating a legacy.

Nurses play an essential role throughout the disease trajectory in reducing the suffering of cancer. Recognizing losses and speaking of them ranges from circumstances such as a patient's loss of hair after initial chemotherapy to the loss of a role when a patient becomes too weak to hold a grandchild. Suffering is acknowledged and sometimes reduced by the act of comforting as nurses give voice and a listening presence to the individual's suffering.

Nurses tend to the physical bodies of patients rendered weak by treatments and advancing disease and, in doing so, help restore a sense of dignity to people with ravaged bodies. Nurses also demonstrate caring to family members who will assume responsibility for the twenty-four-hour-a-day physical care of patients. Family members often observe nurses in their intimate care of patients and model that care. Observing nurses gently turning, massaging, or positioning patients can provide family caregivers with the confidence that they too can touch and care for their fragile loved ones. A participant in the study by Coyle (2006) described the care his family was able to provide after observing the nurse's care: "They clean my bottom for me and they do it with such grace and beauty, they don't make me feel like some sort of unhuman person. I am paralyzed, I need their strength, they don't turn away from me" (p. 270).

THE NATURE OF SUFFERING AND THE GOALS OF NURSING

Works by Cassell and others in the field of medicine inform the perspectives on suffering but are not sufficient to describe the goals of nursing. In reviewing lay and professional literature, the authors are struck by how often the relief of suffering is attributed to the medical profession alone. This likely represents a broader paradigm in which the relief of suffering is meant to equal the cure of disease—a biomedical perspective that implies that the only true relief of suffering comes from fixing, curing, eliminating, and making a person free from illness.

Nurses play a fundamental role in caring for those who suffer. The relief of suffering is at the core of nurses' work as a profession committed to the human response to illness or injury. Nurses also are dedicated to serving the most poor and vulnerable (Hughes, 2006). The care required may vary considerably, even among individuals with a similar diagnosis. For example, the suffering of a person with AIDS may be dramatically different from one case to another. A middle-class African American man with a dedicated partner and who lives in a comfortable environment with good access to health care is likely to experience a much different trajectory than a Caucasian, homeless drug addict whose physiologic experience of AIDS may be similar but whose life experience is not (Williams, 2004).

Nurses are intimately involved in whole-person care and are, apart from families, the witnesses most often present as people struggle with fundamental ethical concerns and spirituality in illness. Emerging fields of thought, such as feminist ethics and medical humanities, offer a broader paradigm beyond a single focus on cure.

Feminist ethics provides a perspective of women's experiences and women's ways of knowing, being, and doing. Feminine refers to women's unique voice and advocacy of an ethic of care, including concepts such as nurturance, compassion, and communication. Feminist refers to advancing beyond traditional patriarchal domination and examining the moral experiences and intuition of women. Feminist ethics address patterns of dominance and oppression and power structures that are a part of the tradition of health care and many other aspects of society (Welch, 2000). Medical humanities is an interdisciplinary field including humanities (for example, literature, ethics, history), social sciences (for example, anthropology, sociology), and arts (for example, film, visual arts) to bring a focus on human values and personalized care to medicine (Charon et al., 1995). The perspectives open the possibility that suffering often is not relieved, removed, or resolved but rather is witnessed, supported, accompanied, and borne with companionship and compassion (Potter, 2006).

Suffering often is viewed as an inherent part of illness, especially in serious or life-threatening disease. Illness that cannot be cured is a threat to human integrity because it reminds people that they have no ultimate control—that illness and death will persist. Yet in enduring illness, suffering can be transformative and provide meaning and ways of coping with chronic disease (Morse and Carter, 1996).

Many narratives about nurses are powerful depictions of unique circumstances, but most are profound in their simplicity. Nurses' work actually resembles rather ordinary people enduring very stressful circumstances. Nurses relate to suffering patients with an authentic and gentle approach. Caring nurses offer calm to terrified parents in intensive care units, assurance to families awaiting the outcomes of surgery, hope to patients receiving a first dose of chemotherapy, and consistent presence to patients in long-term care.

What is the nature of suffering by patients and families living through illness? What are the goals of nursing in responding to those needs? Although the questions are not answered easily, an attempt has been made to provide an initial schema of tenets that respond to the questions. The authors offer these tenets for future clinical inquiry and theoretical evaluation.

- Suffering is a loss of control that creates insecurity. Suffering people often feel helpless and trapped, unable to escape their circumstances.

- In most instances, suffering is associated with loss. The loss may be of a relationship, of some aspect of the self, or of some aspect of the physical body. The loss may be evident only in the mind of the sufferer, but it nonetheless leaves a person diminished and with a sense of brokenness.

- Suffering is an intensely personal experience.

- Suffering is accompanied by a range of intense emotions, including sadness, anguish, fear, abandonment, despair, and myriad other emotions.

- Suffering can be linked deeply to recognition of one's own mortality. When threatened by serious illness, people may fear the end of life. Conversely, for others, living with serious illness may result in a yearning for death.

- Suffering often involves asking the question "why?" Illness or loss may be seen as untimely and undeserved. Suffering people frequently seek to find meaning and answers for that which is unknowable.

- Suffering often is associated with separation from the world. Individuals may express intense loneliness and yearn for connection with others while also feeling intense distress about dependency on others.

- Suffering often is accompanied by spiritual distress. Regardless of religious affiliation, individuals experiencing illness may feel a sense of hopelessness. When life is threatened, people may conduct self-evaluation of what has been lived and what remains undone. Becoming weak and vulnerable and facing mortality may cause a person to reevaluate his or her relationship with a higher being.

- Suffering is not synonymous with pain but is closely associated with it. Physical pain is closely related to psychological, social, and spiritual distress. Pain that persists without meaning becomes suffering.

- Suffering occurs when an individual feels voiceless. This may occur when a person is unable to give words to his or her experience or when the person's "screams" are unheard.

Nurses are the confidants for patients who experience the personal threat of injury or serious illness. Nurses provide competent care for pain and other symptoms; in relieving physical problems, they also reduce psychological, social, and spiritual distress. The intimate care of the physical body offers nurses a special opportunity for healing "brokenness" and helping to restore a sense of integrity.

Nurses recognize that witnessing suffering is a part of their daily work, yet they seek to understand each person who is suffering as a unique individual. Nurses respond to suffering primarily through identifying its sources and offering presence. As witnesses to suffering, they serve as compassionate voices and recognize the human response to illness in the confusing and frequently depersonalized health care environment.

Nurses listen to patients, helping them to move beyond silent suffering to express their emotional distress. Their distress often includes expressions of sadness, loneliness, fear, helplessness, hopelessness, and a sense of brokenness. Nurses help to relieve distress and restore wholeness through human connection. Nurses respond to the spiritual distress of suffering, regardless of the suffering person's religious affiliation. Through the intimacy of caring, nurses also experience suffering and sometimes respond by seeking a balance of life and work and through deep spiritual reflection.

Nurses help patients to regain control in the face of illness and to cope with vulnerability and the uncertainty of life. As witnesses, nurses support patients in seeking meaning in distressing circumstances. Nurses accompany patients on their journeys; through such ongoing and intimate encounters, they support patients in confronting the weariness of living and dying.

REFERENCES

American Cancer Society. (2007). *Cancer facts and figures*. Atlanta, GA: Author.

Battenfield, B. L. (1984). Suffering: A conceptual description and content analysis of an operational schema. *Image— The Journal of Nursing Scholarship*, 16(2), 36–41.

Beckstrand, R. L., and Kirchhoff, K. T. (2005). Providing end-of-life care to patients: Critical care nurses' perceived obstacles and supportive behaviors. *American Journal of Critical Care*, 14(5), 395–403.

Benedict, S. (1989). The suffering associated with lung cancer. *Cancer Nursing*, 12(1), 34–40.

Cassell, E. J. (1982). The nature of suffering and the goals of medicine. *New England Journal of Medicine*, 306(11), 639–645.

Cassell, E. J. (1991). *The nature of suffering and the goals of medicine*. Oxford, United Kingdom: Oxford University Press.

Charmaz, K. (1983). Loss of self: A fundamental form of suffering in the chronically ill. *Sociology of Health and Illness*, 5(2), 168–195.

Charon, R., Banks, J. T., Connelly, J. E., Hawkins, A. H., Hunter, K. M., Jones, A. H., et al. (1995). Literature and medicine: Contributions to clinical practice. *Annals of Internal Medicine*, 122(8), 599–606.

Cherny, N. I., Coyle, N., and Foley, K. M. (1994). Suffering in the advanced cancer patient: A definition and taxonomy. *Journal of Palliative Care*, 10(2), 57–70.

Chochinov, H. M. (2006). Dying, dignity, and new horizons in palliative end-of-life care. *CA: A Cancer Journal for Clinicians*, 56(2), 84–103.

Chochinov, H. M., Hack, T., Hassard, T., Kristjanson, L. J., McClement, S., and Harlos, M. (2002). Dignity in the terminally ill: A cross-sectional, cohort study. *Lancet*, 360(9350), 2026–2030.

Coyle, N. (2006). The hard work of living in the face of death. *Journal of Pain and Symptom Management*, 32(3), 266–274.

Daneault, S., Lussier, V., Mongeau, S., Paille, P., Hudon, E., Dion, D., et al. (2004). The nature of suffering and its relief in the terminally ill: A qualitative study. *Journal of Palliative Care*, 20(1), 7–11.

Donley, R. (1991). Spiritual dimensions of health care: Nursing's mission. *Nursing and Health Care*, 12(4), 178–183.

Ferrell, B., and Coyle, N. (2008). *The nature of suffering and the goals of nursing*. New York: Oxford University Press.

Ferrell, B. R., Cullinane, C. A., Ervin, K., Melancon, C., Uman, G. C., and Juarez, G. (2005). Perspectives on the impact of ovarian cancer: Women's views of quality of life. *Oncology Nursing Forum*, 32(6), 1143–1149.

Ferrell, B. R., Virani, R., Grant, M., Rhome, A., Malloy, P., Bednash, G., et al. (2005). Evaluation of the End-of-Life Nursing Education Consortium undergraduate faculty training program. *Journal of Palliative Medicine*, 8(1), 107–114.

Gilligan, C. (1982). *In a different voice: Psychological theory and women's development*. Cambridge, MA: Harvard University Press.

Harrison, B. W. (1985). *Making the connections: Essays in feminist social ethics*. Boston: Beacon Press.

Hughes, A. (2006). Poor, homeless, and underserved populations. In B. R. Ferrell and N. Coyle (Eds.), *Textbook of palliative nursing* (pp. 661–670). New York: Oxford University Press.

Institute of Medicine. (2005). *From cancer patient to cancer survivor: Lost in transition*. Washington, DC: National Academies Press.

Jackson, C. (2003). *The gift to listen, the courage to hear*. Minneapolis, MN: Augsburg Fortress.

Kahn, D. L., and Steeves, R. H. (1994). Witnesses to suffering: Nursing knowledge, voice, and vision. *Nursing Outlook*, 42(6), 260–264.

Kuuppelomaki, M., and Lauri, S. (1998). Cancer patients' reported experiences of suffering. *Cancer Nursing*, 21(5), 364–369.

Lewis, F. M., and Deal, L. W. (1995). Balancing our lives: A study of the married couple's experience with breast cancer recurrence. *Oncology Nursing Forum*, 22(6), 943–953.

Lin, H. R., and Bauer-Wu, S. M. (2003). Psycho-spiritual well-being in patients with advanced cancer: An integrative review of the literature. *Journal of Advanced Nursing*, 44(1), 69–80.

Malloy, P., Ferrell, B. R., Virani, R., Uman, G., Rhome, A. M., Whitlatch, B., et al. (2006). Evaluation of end-of-life nursing education for continuing education and clinical staff development educators. *Journal for Nurses in Staff Development*, 22(1), 31–36.

McClain-Jacobson, C., Rosenfeld, B., Kosinski, A., Pessin, H., Cimino, J. E., and Breitbart, W. (2004). Belief in an afterlife, spiritual well-being and end-of-life despair in patients with advanced cancer. *General Hospital Psychiatry*, 26(6), 484–486.

Morse, J. M., and Carter, B. (1996). The essence of enduring and expressions of suffering: The reformulation of self. *Scholarly Inquiry for Nursing Practice*, 10(1), 43–60.

Morse, S. R., and Fife, B. (1998). Coping with a partner's cancer: Adjustment at four stages of the illness trajectory. *Oncology Nursing Forum*, 25(4), 751–760.

Northouse, L .L., Mood, D., Kershaw, T., Schafenacker, A., Mellon, S., Walker, J., et al. (2002). Quality of life of women with recurrent breast cancer and their family members. *Journal of Clinical Oncology*, 20(19), 4050–4064.

O'Connor, A. P., Wicker, C. A., and Germino, B. B. (1990). Understanding the cancer patient's search for meaning. *Cancer Nursing*, 13(3), 167–175.

Paice, J. A., Ferrell, B. R., Virani, R., Grant, M., Malloy, P., and Rhome, A. (2006). Graduate nursing education regarding end-of-life care. *Nursing Outlook*, 54(1), 46–52.

Potter, M. (2006). Loss, suffering, bereavement, and grief. In M. L. Matzo and D. W. Sherman (Eds.), *Palliative care nursing: Quality care to the end of life* (2nd ed., pp. 273–315). New York: Springer Publishing.

Reich, W. T. (1989). Speaking of suffering: A moral account of compassion. *Soundings*, 72(1), 83–108.

Welch, S. D. (2000). *A feminist ethic of risk* (revision). Minneapolis, MN: Fortress Press.

Williams, B. R. (2004). Dying young, dying poor: A sociological examination of existential suffering among low-socioeconomic-status patients. *Journal of Palliative Medicine*, 7(1), 27–37.

6

DEATH: "THE DISTINGUISHED THING"

DANIEL CALLAHAN

This article originally appeared as Callahan D. Death: "The Distinguished Thing." *Improving End of Life Care: Why Has It Been So Difficult?* Hastings Center Special Report, vol. 35, no. 6., 2005. All rights reserved. Reprinted with permission.

EDITOR'S INTRODUCTION

Daniel Callahan was a prescient voice of reason decades in advance of our growing recognition of the profligate waste and harm caused by the routine application of technology to forestall death at any cost. In this essay, Callahan discusses the implicit belief driving modern medicine that, with enough research, death itself could (and should) be defeated. His challenge to this uniquely American technology and research imperative must be tackled if we are—get the health care system reform we need.

■ ■ ■

Faced with his imminent death, Henry James is reported to have said, "So it has come at last, the distinguished thing." Distinguished? That seems an odd term to use, but James was a master at choosing the right word, and he may have seen better than most of us what death is all about. My dictionary defines "distinguished" as "having an air of distinction, dignity, or eminence." Yet there is dissent from that judgment. The late theologian Paul Ramsey contended that there could be no death with dignity. Death is too profound a blow to our selfhood, to everything good about our existence. James or Ramsey?

For at least forty years now—Ramsey notwithstanding—a massive effort has been under way to bring about death with dignity. The leading techniques have been the use of advance directives, hospice and palliative care, and improved end-of-life education for physicians, nurses, and other health care workers. As the *Hastings Center Report* 1995 special supplement on the SUPPORT study indicated, that effort achieved only a mixed success; a decade later, this report describes progress since then but points to the long road for creating real and lasting improvement.

There has always been some ambiguity in that effort. James and Ramsey, for instance, seem to be talking about the meaning and place of death in human life, not about what kind of care is desirable at the end of life. Ramsey was no opponent of those efforts to improve end-of-life care. He objected to the sentimentalizing of death: even the best end-of-life care could not sugarcoat death's fundamental offense. Was he right? Unless it is possible to work out some reasonably satisfactory answer to that question, my guess is that the care of the dying will remain seriously hamstrung. I sometimes get the impression that recent efforts to improve that care are managing, perhaps inadvertently, to evade dealing with death itself, focusing instead on palliative techniques and strategies.

I want to get at the core question here—that of the appropriate relationship between the care of the dying and our stance toward death itself—by proposing some historical ways these two issues have either been blended or separated.

My point of departure is the premodern era, most plausibly described in the French historian Philippe Ariès's fine 1977 book *The Hour of Our Death*. He detailed "the persistence of an attitude toward death that remained unchanged for thousands of years, an attitude that expressed a naïve acceptance of destiny and nature." He called that "the tame death" and showed how it was accompanied by practices at the end of life that stressed death's public impact—the loss to the community of an individual's life, underscored by rituals of mourning that made the same point. How people died and the meaning of death were inextricably blended.

Though Ariès specified no particular time at which that long era ended, I believe it wound down in the 1950s and 1960s. By then postwar medical progress, rapidly enriched with lifesaving drugs and technologies, was in full flower and eagerly embraced. Medicine could finally do something about death, and doctors were quick to take up the new arms in a new cause, that of aggressively fighting to save lives, now a plausible effort.

No quarter was to be given. I recall in the 1960s arguing with physicians, educated in the postwar years, who told me that they had a moral duty to save life at all costs. The quality of life, the actual prognosis, or the pain induced by zealous treatment were all but irrelevant. The technological imperative to use every possible means to save life was combined with the sanctity-of-life principle in what seemed the perfect marriage of medicine and morality.

Then came the backlash, beginning in the late 1960s. Often bitter complaints about useless but painful treatments, about abandonment at the end of life, and about death in a cocoon of tubes and monitors began to turn the tide.

These complaints led to reform efforts that focused on means to improve end-of-life care. What was left out of these efforts was a coming to grips with the meaning and place of death. What Ariès had called a "naïve acceptance of destiny and nature" was put to one side—but nothing, seemingly, was put in its place.

That gap was soon filled. President Nixon in 1970 declared war on cancer, and the National Institutes of Health was soon on a roll. Gradually, almost imperceptibly, there emerged what I think of as the great schism in medicine. On one side was palliative care, seeking to bring back into clinical practice the relief of pain and suffering as one of the highest goals of medicine. That kind of care, as initially understood, required that both doctor and patient accept death as an unavoidable part of life. On the other side was an ever-expansive medical research drive, the sworn and well-financed enemy of death and illness of every stripe. That research drive is the implacable foe of an old-fashioned, anachronistic fatalism which held, as fixed human wisdom, that many bodily miseries, but especially death, just have to be endured. Death is now not to be accepted but eliminated.

There is no easy way to reconcile these two faces of medicine. The research push treats death as a contingent, accidental event that can be done away with, one disease at a time. Research advocates can hardly contain their enthusiasm for the great possibilities that lie ahead. Think only of the campaign for stem cell research, with its promissory note of cures for heart disease, Alzheimer's, Parkinson's, diabetes—just about everything except athlete's foot.

That kind of zeal spills over into clinical practice. Force-fed by research turned into technology and undergirded by medical education and clinical acculturation, good medicine saves lives. It does not give up. It refuses to negotiate with death. Why should anyone accept, at least in principle, a death that researchers believe will someday be cured—any more than AIDS should be tolerated when, someday, a vaccine will work? In the meantime, innovative technologies can provide a few more days, weeks, maybe months of life, than were possible even a few years ago. Every physician has his miracle story. Go for it!

I once asked a visibly dying friend, someone who had taught medical ethics for thirty years, why he had agreed to one more round of chemotherapy for his recurrent pancreatic cancer, leaving his mouth so full of sores he could speak only with great pain. "They talked me into it," he said. His oncologist probably talked himself into it as well. Death came quickly after that, the treatment useless. But how else to proceed, the true believer might ask, to gain the progress that is possible? If that chemotherapy trial failed, the next one may succeed; or at least the one after that one.

But is there an inconsistency in helping someone die well when death is on its way while simultaneously seeking a cure that will benefit future patients dying from the same disease? There is no logical inconsistency, narrowly understood, but there is a powerful psychological clash. It pits the value of accepting death when a particular death is unavoidable against rejecting death as a matter of principle for a research-ambitious medicine.

———

It may well be that still another stage is beginning to appear. If the "naïve acceptance of destiny and nature" has been put to one side—for a time, with no other clear view of death to put in its place—such a view may now be coming into focus. It might be called the Denial of Death II, to invoke Ernest Becker's 1973 book *The Denial of Death*. By that phrase I mean not a refusal to look death in the face, to hide it away, which was Becker's point, but to incrementally whittle away at its supposed inevitability, and to return to the treatment aggressiveness of the 1950s and 1960s.

Part of this new stage is motivated by the research imperative, which is steadily gaining ground, and part by a combination of other influences, each of them more incremental than decisive in nature but, taken together, strong in their aggregate force. Let me give some examples of those influences, each of which drives a wedge between the care of the dying and the place of death in life. My evidence is, on the whole, anecdotal, and the items I note may not be all that telling; but this is what I see and hear.

The advanced edges of the palliative care movement, I have been told, have quietly been dropping the notion that its patients must have accepted death if it is to succeed in caring for them; it seems to be embracing a cautious neutrality on that point. At the same time, a new compromise with death has been proposed in some territory between acceptance and rejection: the teaming up, for instance, of an oncologist and a palliative care specialist to treat a terminally ill patient who teeters on the borderline between hope for life and acceptance of death.

Those (like myself) who are ready to accept death as biologically inevitable are being labeled either "mortalists" or "apologists." Some of us have sunk pretty low, I suppose. In this climate, abetted by industry marketing and media hype of one breakthrough after another, should we be surprised that physicians complain about inflated patient expectations, or that many patients or their families want aggressive treatment without limits when faced with death? Should we be surprised that some consider the death of Terri Schiavo, defined as simply disabled and thus not beyond the reach of medical care, as nothing less than murder? Religious conservatives and disability advocates often now team up to call into question the motives of those seeking an acquiescence in death, attributing it to moral insensitivity, to a denigration of those with diminished capacities, or to a crude desire to cut costs by eliminating the expensively burdensome. They are adding a new instability to an already complicated situation.

I do not mean to suggest that end-of-life care is burdened simply by medicine's profound ambivalence about death, intensified by a public that shares some of that ambivalence. No doubt advance directives have never had the impact hoped for because most people resist facing up to their eventual death (even the preparation of ordinary wills is widely neglected). Education and publicity can make a dent in the otherwise poor figures (less than 25 percent have advance directives by most accounts), but the fact that most deaths are not seen up close and occur for the most part in old age does not push the reality of death in one's face the way it once did. If you don't want to think about it, there are lots of ways to look in other directions.

No less important, it seems, is what I call the multiple-variable problem. Just as health care reform in the United States is stymied by a large number of competing interests and a plethora of subversive variables, end-of-life care has its own excess of variables. Even with the best will in the world and advance directives (or surrogates) in place, much can go wrong: disagreements between doctor and patient, doctor and doctor, family and patient, family and doctor, hospital and medical cultures (some favorable and some cool to advance directives), and so on.

The Schiavo case illustrates the point. Had she or had she not clearly stated her desires? Who had her best interests at heart, her husband or her parents? Even if recovery was unlikely, was it at least possible, and might some further treatments have made a difference? We all have our answers to those questions, but the point is that it was not hard to pick a fight. There are many cases that do not rise to the sad and unseemly level of the Schiavo fight. Many people will conclude that it is vitally important to have clear advance directives or a dependable surrogate, while others, unwisely and unhappily, seem to have concluded that there is some kind of plot afoot to do in patients in a persistent vegetative state or with other disabilities. There is no such plot (though surely some insensitivity here and there), but advance directives do not guarantee you will get what you want, only that they may increase the likelihood you will.

———

The question left hanging is: How should medicine and its practitioners think about death and locate it in the human life cycle? There is no doubt that the nature of dying has changed, and no less doubt that medicine has been encouraged to grab death by the throat and not to let go—even as our biology one way or another continues to conspire to bring us down. I believe Paul Ramsey was profoundly wrong in holding that there can be no death with dignity. The weakest sense of dignity in the context of dying focuses on the loss of control, that of life's trajectory leading irreversibly downhill, the body falling apart, marked by incontinence, pain, humiliation, dependence upon others for our very existence. One ceases to be the person one once was and wanted to be, with a new physical (if not necessarily psychological) identity taking its place, not one to be admired or to be proud of.

I call that "dignity" in the weak sense, not because physical identity is unimportant but because, as many survivors of genocide, starvation, death camps, and severe disability have shown, there is more to a human life than the state of the body. The serious sense of a loss of dignity I understand to be the supposed ultimate insult that death brings to life, which was what Ramsey had in mind: I live, therefore I am.

I have never understood why someone should feel that way. Surely from the viewpoint of species welfare, death is no evil. It is a condition of constant species renewal (though I grant that species vitality does not do much for me as an individual). But death does not seem to me to be an evil if it comes at the end of a long life, one marked by a completion, or near it, of those aims that mark a full life. It is no accident that weeping is ordinarily absent at the funeral of an elderly person. Almost all of us know old people who, while still enjoying life, profess themselves ready to die and seem to mean it. It is hard to see indignity in a death marked by that acceptance. Of course there are many others, not yet old, not yet with a full life behind them, who will be ambivalent, and some will not want to give up, at least not at once. Advance directives can have an important place for them; and when they are ready to go, palliative care will usually be needed. One can only hope they will die in the hands of physicians and nurses who will understand their plight and their needs.

Considerable progress has been made during the past three decades in improving the care of the dying. But there remain some old obstacles, familiar from the start, and some that are not many years old. Physicians unwilling to give up and indifferent to patient desires are still with us, just as soon-to-be patients resistant to advance directives are still with us. There is unfinished work here to be done. Forces on the scientific side that treat death as the great enemy, not to be tolerated, and on the ideological side, seeing snares and delusions in end-of-life care, create the new obstacles.

How our society responds to those two forces will make a great deal of difference; if we are not careful, we could reverse the progress made to improve end-of-life care thus far. In the end, we die, and it is not an evil that our biology has made it so. We can and will argue about the timing and the details, about acceptable and unacceptable deaths. That is right and proper. Difficult decisions will never run out. But if we hedge our bets about the inevitability of death, waffling and dreaming—a fresh science-driven embrace of the denial of death—then we are likely to face worse lives and, when it comes, worse deaths.

7

ACCESS TO HOSPICE CARE: EXPANDING BOUNDARIES, OVERCOMING BARRIERS

A summary of the report prepared by the Hastings Center and the National Hospice Work Group, March–April 2003

BRUCE JENNINGS, TRUE RYNDES, CAROL D'ONOFRIO, AND MARY ANN BAILY

This summary originally appeared as a special supplement to the *Hastings Center Report* as Jennings B, Ryndes T, D'Onofrio C, Baily MA. *Access to hospice care: expanding boundaries, overcoming barriers.* The Hastings Center, 2003, March–April, Suppl:S3–7, S9–13, S15–21. Copyright © 2003, The Hastings Center. All rights reserved. Reprinted with permission.

EDITORS' INTRODUCTION

This influential report assesses the barriers to good palliative care from the perspective of social justice, access, and fairness in public policy. It calls for expansion in access to hospice and palliative care based on patients' and families' need, not prognosis. Its thinking underlies the momentum of the recent growth in the palliative care continuum beyond the six-month prognosis constraints of the Medicare hospice benefit.

■ ■ ■

In recent years, widely publicized research studies have documented a litany of seemingly intractable problems with the quality of care given to Americans at the end of their lives—inadequate pain control, inadequate counseling and family support, inadequate compassion or human presence. A comprehensive new report issued by the Hastings Center, a leading bioethics research center in Garrison, N.Y., confirms those previous findings while identifying new opportunities for overcoming high levels of preventable suffering at the end of life. A major thrust of its recommended solutions lies in a surprising but familiar direction: making greater use of America's 3,400 existing providers of hospice care.

Access to Hospice Care: Expanding Boundaries, Overcoming Barriers, a report drawn from a three-year study of hospice access and values issues conducted by the Hastings Center and the National Hospice Work Group, a voluntary association of progressive hospices, was published as a special supplement accompanying the March/April 2003 issue of the bioethics journal *The Hastings Center Report.*

The purpose of the study was to contribute to the broad goal of improving end-of-life care by addressing specific problems in access to and delivery of hospice care. Its distinctive contribution is to pay explicit attention to the human values involved in hospice care policy and practice. The report examines the problem of hospice access from the perspective of social justice, equity or fairness and makes an ethical case for equitable access on the basis of the vulnerability of the population served, the moral importance of meeting their needs and the values upon which comprehensive, high-quality hospice care is constructed (see pages S13–S17 of the full report).

The report also offers a new vision of hospice, one that holds firm to many of the traditions and values of the past but finds new and more flexible ways to deliver care. The model of traditional hospice care as an independent and specialized service will gradually be transformed into a more comprehensive model in which hospice becomes the coordinating center for a range of services and types of expertise that can be accessed by patients. In the authors' new vision, America's hospices will play an expanded role in addressing more of the supportive and symptom-relief needs of patients confronting life-limiting illnesses and their families for longer periods and in a wider variety of settings and contexts.

To achieve this ambitious goal, policies must change, and powerful cultural taboos surrounding death and dying must be overcome. What's needed are a national program of professional education about hospice and palliative care and a massive social marketing campaign regarding hospice programs' abilities to address and resolve many of the most widely held fears about the end of life.

CHALLENGES OF END-OF-LIFE SUFFERING

Death is an inevitable aspect of the human condition. Dying badly is not. But the problems of dying badly are often social in nature, reflecting the way America's health care system is organized and financed. While the acceptance and utilization of hospice care has grown in recent years, more than a million Americans die each year of chronic, life-limiting illnesses without receiving hospice services.

Some of the "barriers" to hospice actually result from misunderstandings and misinformation, while others have sources that are structural, financial, regulatory, cultural and even "self-imposed" (by hospices themselves). The cultural issues—taboos, denial of death, avoidance of painful subjects—are major contributors to the problem, but so, too, are unfairly restrictive government policies. (See pages S27–S38 of the full report.)

Specifically, the hospice access problem takes four forms:

1. Some dying patients never get referred to hospice;

2. Other patients are referred to hospice only in the final days of their lives (nationally, more than a third of patients spend less than seven days enrolled in hospice);

3. Some aspects of hospice's care management are needed much earlier than the last six months of life, and

4. Cultural differences and barriers contribute to an inequitable distribution of hospice services while hospices' efforts to overcome these barriers have not been entirely successful (see pages S39–S43 of the full report).

CHARACTERISTICS OF HOSPICE VALUED BY CONSUMERS

The success of the hospice movement is attributed to its demonstrations of trustworthiness to patients and families. Its nonprofit origins and early reliance on volunteers secured the support of community members, and its special value to those made vulnerable by profound illness was reinforced by the following characteristics of care:

1. Responses to the human consequences of profound illness (palliative care management). (See pages S44–S48 of the full report.) Hospice staff responds to the need for comfort, safety, choice and support experienced by dying patients and their families as their conditions change and they move from one care setting to another.

2. Continuity of caregiving. (See page S49 of the full report.) Hospice staff maintains a coherent vision of what is preferred by and effective for patients and their families as care shifts to new settings and providers.

3. Response to evolving community needs. (See pages S48–S49 of the full report.) Hospice leaders have expanded a philosophy of care originally based on the needs of white, middle-class adults with cancer. Hospices now serve people with many other diseases, as well as children, persons living in difficult service areas such as prisons and the rural "outback," and the community's bereaved.

The report recommends freeing America's hospice providers from existing regulatory, financial and cultural constraints so that their expertise can be applied more broadly in new settings and contexts. The authors also note that new palliative care providers and innovative palliative demonstration projects have much to offer to the evolving landscape of end-of-life care in America, particularly in collaboration with hospices.

The existing organizational infrastructure of hospice programs is a national resource of continuing value and viability for patients and families as they move from one setting to the next. But hospice must develop new organizational forms if it is to continue providing the essential components of trustworthiness: palliative care management, continuity of caregiving and responsiveness to the changing needs of its patients, families and community. The challenge is to find new practical approaches to hospice care, correcting policies and practices that have become unduly restrictive.

Dying persons, their families and loved ones, and society as a whole are diminished by the current failure to respect the autonomy and dignity of the person with a life-threatening illness, to respond to that person's suffering, or to offer care, compassion and vigilance at the end of life. When so many die without the support of good hospice or palliative care, America has not met its obligation to the most vulnerable in society and has not kept faith with its highest moral ideals.

A just increase in access to hospice care should take place principally in three ways:

1. By making it easier for more chronically ill people to be eligible for hospice admission;

2. By lengthening the average time patients spend in hospice care, primarily through expanded services and earlier referral; and

3. By maintaining both high-quality palliative care and good stewardship of scarce resources through a rigorous care management system that follows patients at home and in institutions.

APPROACHING JUST ACCESS: RECOMMENDATIONS

The recommendations contained in *Access to Hospice Care* (see pages S53–S56 of the full report) identify a realistic but challenging course for the future of hospice in America. They require patience, political leadership, broad debate, willingness to compromise and openness to new ideas. They also require further research and increased understanding of why the health care system behaves as it does and how various new practices may affect the needs and well-being of dying patients and their families. The report recommends:

1. Health care leaders, policy makers and key stakeholder groups must come to consensus on the definition of palliative care and develop a framework for greater accountability in palliative care delivery in concert with financing mechanisms. As was done with hospices in the early 1980s, this consensus process would be achieved in part through a national field survey of services that call themselves "palliative care" to determine which elements the services have in common and how they qualitatively differ. A foundation for the process would come from the exhaustive NHPCO [National Hospice and Palliative Care Organization] Standards of Hospice Care/Robert Wood Johnson Foundation Precepts of Palliative Care. A national forum would also be convened, bringing together key constituencies to establish a definition for palliative care to provide the framework for delivery, standards of care and reimbursement and to draft a position paper articulating the conclusions.

2. Public policy should expand the scope of hospice services. Congress should approve a series of demonstration projects to advance hospice access for patients who do not yet qualify for traditional hospice care and to foster and promote access to hospice's palliative care management through innovative community relationships.

3. Policymakers should act immediately to bring about policy reform of the absolute application of an individual's prognosis as a primary criterion for reimbursement of services. The federal Center for Medicare and Medicaid Services (CMS) and its contract fiscal intermediaries should take steps to protect hospices, referring physicians, and patients from regulatory misinterpretations by establishing a statistically accurate definition of terminal prognosis. Such a definition would recognize the relevance of prognosis as a population measure, not an individual one, consistent with the wide literature addressing the fallibility of medical prognostication on individual patients.

4. Expand access and delivery of hospice to dying persons residing in long-term care facilities. Modifying Medicare's Part A and RUG reimbursement systems could help support hospice care for residents of long-term care facilities without causing financial penalty to the nursing home or the resident/family unit. CMS and state departments of health should also adopt a common survey process for hospice patients in nursing homes so that patients' wishes for end-of-life care are not subordinated to clinically and personally harmful regulatory requirements, such as the enforcement of feedings among dying patients.

5. Leaders in the hospice community and in mainstream medicine must promote hospice-hospital partnerships in order to meet current and projected needs of the rapidly expanding volume of chronically and terminally ill patients. Leadership groups in hospice and palliative care should work with palliative care physicians and administrators of hospices and hospitals to construct a regulatory reform agenda that would enable improved outcomes for hospitalized patients in need of hospice and palliative care. Ongoing studies of maturing hospital/hospice models are also needed, while a surgeon general's report on the quality of dying in America could provide the proper venue for viewing care of the dying as a public health issue.

6.   Develop telemedicine to expand access to palliative care. The imminent collision between the burgeoning senior population and decreasing numbers of health care providers will dramatically alter how care is provided to the chronically and terminally ill. Therefore, CMS or some other appropriate government agency should move quickly to fund multisite telehospice demonstration projects in which centrally located palliative care specialists can interact at a moment's notice with rural hospice staff, family caregivers in varied geographical settings, and staff in nonhospice inpatient settings.

7.   Engage the business community. Good care of dying Americans is clearly a workforce issue because it relates to productivity of employees as patients and as caregivers. Therefore, the major national hospice foundations, in concert with community hospices, should assist the business community in understanding the economic value associated with support to employees who are caregivers as well as the benefits associated with proactive responses to employees who become chronically ill or bereaved.

8.   Develop educational programs to "reintroduce" hospice and palliative care to the public in light of their new capabilities, flexibility and accessibility. Population-wide educational and outreach programs could emphasize that hospice is no longer just about death and dying, with more positive messages about the benefits of hospice programs: comfort, safety, choice and support in responding to the life consequences associated with illness and disability.

SOCIAL, LEGAL, AND ETHICAL ISSUES

George J. Annas, "The Health Care Proxy and the Living Will"
Timothy E. Quill, "Terri Schiavo: A Tragedy Compounded"

THE HEALTH CARE PROXY
AND THE LIVING WILL

GEORGE J. ANNAS, J.D., M.P.H.

This article originally appeared as Annas GJ. Sounding board: the health care proxy and the living will. *N Engl J Med.* 1991:324;1210–1213. Copyright © Massachusetts Medical Society. All rights reserved. Reprinted with permission.

EDITORS' INTRODUCTION

This article heralded the December 1991 advent of mandatory provision of information on advance care planning to all patients admitted to U.S. hospitals, nursing homes, hospices, and HMOs serving Medicare or Medicaid beneficiaries. George J. Annas describes the hopes tied to this new law and anticipates many of the limitations that later were demonstrated on the failure of this mechanism to influence decisions at the bedside.

■ ■ ■

American medicine is awash in forms: insurance forms, disability forms, informed-consent forms, and forms for various examinations, to name just a few. Forms can help make the practice of medicine more efficient, but they can also make it more routinized, impersonal, and bureaucratic. Congress and the President have decreed that beginning December 1, 1991, all hospitals, nursing facilities, hospice programs, and health maintenance organizations that serve Medicare or Medicaid patients must provide all their new adult patients with written information describing the patient's rights under state law to make decisions about medical care, including their right to execute a living will or durable power of attorney.[1] New forms will be routinely added to the practice of medicine. Their purpose is to help implement a right that has been universally recognized: the right to refuse any and all medical interventions, even life-sustaining interventions. The challenge is to use these forms to foster communication between doctor and patient, as well as respect for the patient's autonomy.

HISTORICAL CONTEXT

The term "living will" was coined by Luis Kutner in 1969 to describe a document in which a competent adult sets forth directions regarding medical treatment in the event of his or her future incapacitation.[2] The document is a will in the sense that it spells out the person's directions. It is "living" because it takes effect before death. Public interest in this document has always been high, and a national organization, Concern for Dying, has devoted most of its resources for the past twenty years to educating the public and professionals about the living will. A sister organization, Society for the Right to Die (which is in the process of merging with Concern for Dying to form the National Council for Death and Dying), simultaneously devoted its primary efforts to encouraging states to pass legislation giving formal legal recognition to the living will.

In 1976 the country's attention focused on the case of Karen Ann Quinlan, a young woman in a persistent vegetative state, and her parents' attempts to have her ventilator removed so she could die a natural death.[3] The New Jersey Supreme Court granted the parents' petition and held that an "ethics committee" could grant all parties concerned legal immunity for their actions.[3] The court did this because it believed that it was the fear of legal liability that prevented Quinlan's physicians from honoring her parents' request. Her story prompted the enactment of the nation's first living-will statute, California's Natural Death Act, in 1976. The California statute is very narrow. A legally enforceable declaration can be executed only fourteen days or more after a person is diagnosed as having a terminal illness, defined as one that will cause the patient's death "imminently," whether or not life-sustaining procedures are continued. Thus, even though this statute was inspired by her story, it would not have helped Quinlan, because she was not terminally ill.

By 1991, more than forty states had enacted living-will statutes. All these laws provide immunity to physicians and other health care professionals who follow the patient's wishes as expressed in a living will. Virtually all of them also suffer from four major shortcomings, however: they are applicable only to those who are "terminally ill"; they limit the types of treatment that can be refused, usually to "artificial" or "extraordinary" therapies; they make no provision for the person to designate another person to make decisions on his or her behalf or set forth the criteria for such decisions; and there is no penalty if health care providers do not honor these documents.[4,5]

ADDRESSING THE LIMITATIONS OF THE LIVING WILL

These problems led to calls for second-generation legislation on the living will.[4] Other shortcomings were also noted. Living wills require a person to predict accurately his or her final illness or injury and what medical interventions might be available to postpone death, and living wills require physicians to make decisions on the basis of their interpretation of a document, rather than a discussion of the treatment options with a person acting on behalf of the patient. The proposed solution to these problems was not to modify the living will but to replace it with another form, one assigning a durable power of attorney to a designated person (known, in this context, as appointing a health care proxy).[6,7] The person named in the document (also called the health care proxy) is variously known as the attorney, the agent, the surrogate, or the proxy—four terms that are synonyms in this context.

Every state has a durable-power-of-attorney law that permits persons to designate someone to make decisions for them if they become incapacitated.[8] Although these statutes were enacted primarily to permit the agent to make financial decisions, no court has ever invalidated a durable power of attorney specifically designed to enable the designated person to make health care decisions. In the recent *Cruzan* case—in which Nancy Cruzan's parents, basing their attempt on their daughter's previous statements, sought to have her tube feeding discontinued after she had been left in a persistent vegetative state by an automobile accident—Justice Sandra Day O'Connor advised citizens to employ this device. In her concurring opinion, O'Connor observed that the decision in *Cruzan* "does not preclude a future determination that the Constitution requires the States to implement the decisions of a duly appointed surrogate."[9,10] The *Cruzan* case itself, which involved facts essentially identical to those in *Quinlan,* gave impetus to the concept of a health care proxy, just as the *Quinlan* case had previously increased interest in the living will. Physicians are legally and ethically bound to respect the directions of a patient set forth in a living will, but living wills are limited because no one can accurately foretell the future, and interpretation may be difficult.[11] Attempts to make the living will less ambiguous by developing comprehensive checklists with alternative scenarios may be too confusing and abstract to be useful to either patients or health care providers, although opinions on this differ.[12, 13]

THE MOVE TO DESIGNATE HEALTH CARE PROXIES

Although new laws are not necessary in any state (because of existing laws regarding the assignment of a durable power of attorney), the current trend in the United States is for states to enact additional proxy laws that specifically deal with health care. Such laws generally specify the information that must be included in the proxy form and the standards on which treatment decisions must be based and grant good-faith immunity for all involved in carrying out the treatment decision. Two of the best-written proxy laws have recently become effective in New York (in January 1991) and Massachusetts (in December 1990).[14] The New York law is based on a recommendation of the New York State Task Force on Life and the Law, and that group's statement of its rationale is still the best introduction to the concept of the health care proxy.[15] The Massachusetts proxy law is largely modeled on the New York law.

The heart of both laws (and all proxy laws) is the same: to enable a competent adult (the "principal") to choose another person (the "proxy" or "agent") to make treatment decisions for him or her if he or she becomes incompetent to make them. The agent has the same authority to make decisions that the patient would have if he or she were still competent. Instead of having to decipher a document, the physician is able to discuss treatment options with a person who has the legal authority to grant or withhold consent on behalf of the patient. The manner in which the agent must exercise this authority is also crucial. The agent must make decisions that are consistent with the wishes of the patient, if these are known, and otherwise that are consistent with the patient's best interests.

Proxy laws also permit the principal to limit the authority of the agent in the document (for example, by not granting authority to refuse cardiopulmonary resuscitation or tube feeding), but the more limitations the principal puts on the agent, the more the document appointing a health care proxy resembles a living will. In addition, because every limitation is subject to interpretation, the likelihood that a dispute will arise about the meaning of the document is increased. One compromise is to give the agent blanket authority to make decisions and to detail one's values and wishes with as much precision as possible in a private letter to the agent. The agent could use this letter when it was relevant to the actual decision and keep it private when it was not relevant.[16]

IMPLEMENTING LAWS REGARDING HEALTH CARE PROXIES

The goal of appointing a proxy is to simplify the process of making decisions and to make it more likely that the patient's wishes will be followed—not to complicate existing problems. If hospitals and hospital lawyers cooperate, this goal will be attained, because the vast majority of physicians will welcome the ability to discuss treatment options with a person chosen by the patient who has the legal authority to give or withhold consent.[7] Hospitals can help their patients by making a simple proxy form available, by educating their medical, nursing, and social service staffs about the laws governing health care proxies, and by supporting decisions made by the agents. Hospitals can impede the process of making good decisions, however, if they concentrate on the paperwork rather than on the way in which decisions are made. Some Massachusetts attorneys, for example, have already drafted a thirteen-page, single-spaced proxy form that is all but unintelligible to nonlawyers. Others have begun to explore and to catalogue all the reasons why physicians and hospitals might want to seek judicial review before honoring the decision of a health care agent. Neither of these strategies is constructive. The use of complex forms and obstructive strategies makes it likely that treatment decisions will actually be made by the hospital's lawyers and the agent's lawyers, not by the agent and the physician. If this happens, the trend to designating a health care agent will be frustratingly counterproductive, since, instead of encouraging a focus on the patient and the patient's wishes, where it belongs, the new proxy forms will add another layer of bureaucracy and another outsider to the decision process.

The most useful form for both patients and providers is a simple one-page document that sets forth all necessary information in easily comprehensible language. The one-page form in the Appendix [at the end of this chapter], which is easily understood and meets all the requirements of the new Massachusetts proxy law (as well as those of the New York law), was developed by a broad-based task force made up of representatives of all the major health care organizations in the state, including the Massachusetts Medical Society, the Massachusetts Hospital Association, the Massachusetts Nurses Association, the Massachusetts Federation of Nursing Homes, and the Massachusetts Department of Public Health as well as the Massachusetts Executive Office of Elder Affairs and the Massachusetts Bar Association. The degree of cooperation in its development was virtually unprecedented and may provide a model for future efforts.

ADDING TO THE DOCUMENT DESIGNATING A PROXY

Perhaps out of concern for efficiency, some commentators have advocated combining an organ-donor form with the form designating a health care proxy.[10] This is a serious error for at least two reasons. First, much effort has been expended over the past twenty years to separate the issues of organ donation and treatment decisions in the public's mind, since the main reason people do not sign organ-donor cards is that they believe doctors might "do something to me before I'm really dead."[17] Tying organ donation to treatment refusals that might lead to death only heightens this concern and is likely to lead people to use neither form. Second, the proxy form takes effect when the patient becomes incompetent; in contrast, the organ-donor form takes effect only on the patient's death. The health care agent can have nothing to say about organ donation, because the agent can make only treatment decisions, an authority that dies with the patient. Organ donation is laudable, but it is not related to the designation of a health care agent, and the principal should authorize donation on a separate form designed for that purpose.

Organ-donor forms may teach another lesson as well. No physician in the United States will honor an organ-donor form over the objections of the patient's family. Similarly, physicians have difficulty honoring a patient's living will over the family's objections. Because it identifies a person with legal authority to talk with the physician, the health care proxy is likely to be a more effective mechanism to implement the patient's wishes.

It should be stressed that forms naming a health care proxy do not substantively change existing law; they merely make it procedurally easier for a person to designate an agent who is authorized to make whatever health care decisions the person could legally make if competent, and they give health care providers legal immunity for honoring such decisions. The patient can, for example, give the agent the authority to refuse any and all medical care, but the agent has no more legal authority than the principal to insist on assisted suicide or to demand a lethal injection. The naming of an agent also solves the problem of a dispute among family members concerning treatment, since the agent has the legal and ethical right and responsibility to make the decision. When a long-lost relative arrives and demands that "everything be done or I'll sue," the physician can refer that person to the agent rather than have to try to achieve a consensus.

LIMITS OF THE CONCEPT OF THE HEALTH CARE PROXY

Only competent adults who actually execute a document can name a health care agent. Since fewer than 10 percent of Americans have either living wills or organ-donor cards, few may use this mechanism. It has no application to children, the mentally retarded, or others unable to appreciate the nature and consequences of their decisions. Treatment decisions for these groups will continue to be governed by the vague "best interests" standard, which is the functional equivalent of "reasonable medical care," "appropriate medical care," or "indicated medical care." The document will also be of limited use in the emergency department, although in rare cases the health care agent may arrive with the principal and there may be time for consultation and informed consent before a specific intervention is tried. Nor will the document solve problems of futility. Physicians will retain the right not to offer treatment that is contraindicated, useless, or futile.

THE RESPONSIBILITY OF PHYSICIANS

I have encouraged members of both the Boston Bar Association and the Massachusetts Bar Association to make health care proxy forms available to the public and their clients free of charge as a public service. Many have agreed. It will also be useful to the public if physicians make such forms available to their patients and encourage them to fill them out. Physicians may also be more comfortable about relying on the decisions of the designated agent if patients are willing to discuss their choice of agent with the physician, although this is not a requirement. Any form that is used must be written in language that both patients and health care providers can easily understand; the form need not be written by a lawyer and should not require a lawyer to interpret.

Like soldiers in past wars, Americans serving in the Persian Gulf wrote their wills. This time, however, many also wrote living wills or executed durable powers of attorney. As one reporter observed, "In the process, the soldiers had to clarify ambiguous personal relationships, chart out their children's lives, and, in some cases, confront their own mortality for the first time."[18] Designating a health care agent gives us all the opportunity to confront our mortality and to determine who among our friends and relatives we want to make treatment decisions on our behalf when we are unable to make them ourselves. A clear focus on these substantive issues, rather than on forms or formalities, could help patients feel more secure that their wishes regarding medical treatment will be respected and could help health care professionals be more secure that the treatment decisions made for incompetent patients actually reflect the patients' wishes. These are certainly worthy goals.

APPENDIX: A MODEL HEALTH CARE PROXY FOR USE IN MASSACHUSETTS

I, _____ , residing at
         (principal—print your name)

_____ ,
   (street)   (city or town)   (state)

appoint as my Health Care Agent _____
            (name of person you choose as agent)

of _____ .
  (street)   (city or town)   (state)   (phone)

Optional: If my agent is unwilling or unable to serve, then I appoint as my alternate _____
          (name of person you choose as alternate)

of _____ .
  (street)   (city or town)   (state)   (phone)

My agent shall have the authority to make all health care decisions for me, subject to any limitations I state below, if I am unable to make decisions myself. My agent's authority becomes effective if my attending physician determines in writing that I lack the capacity to make or to communicate health care decisions. My agent is then to have the same authority to make health care decisions as I would if I had the capacity to make them, *except* (here list the limitations, *if any*, you wish to place on your agent's authority):

I direct my agent to make decisions on the basis of my agent's assessment of my personal wishes. If my personal wishes are unknown, my agent is to make decisions on the basis of my agent's assessment of my best interests. Photocopies of this Health Care Proxy shall have the same force and effect as the original.

Signed _____

Complete only if principal is physically unable to sign: I have signed the principal's name above at his or her direction in the presence of the principal and two witnesses.

_____
               (name)

_____
              (street)

_____
    (city or town)   (state)

Witness Statement

We, the undersigned, each witnessed the signing of this Health Care Proxy by the principal or at the direction of the principal and state that the principal appears to be at least 18 years of age, of sound mind, and under no constraint or undue influence. Neither of us is named as the health care agent or alternate in this document.

In our presence this _____ day of _____ , 199 _____ .

Witness 1 _____   Witness 2 _____
        (signature)   (signature)

Name (print) _____   Name (print) _____

Address _____   Address _____

_____   _____

REFERENCES

1. 42 U.S.C. 1395 cc (a) (1) et. seq. (as amended Nov. 1990).

2. Kutner L. Due process of euthanasia: the living will a proposal. *Indiana Law J* 1969; 44:539.

3. In re Quinlan, 70 N.J. 10, 355 A.2d 647 (1976).

4. Legal Advisors Committee, Concern for Dying. The right to refuse treatment: a model act. *Am J Public Health* 1983; 73:918–21.

5. Annas GJ. *The rights of patients: the basic ACLU guide to patient rights*. 2nd ed. Carbondale, Ill.: Southern Illinois University Press, 1989:196–255.

6. Veatch RM. *Death, dying, and the biological revolution: our last quest for responsibility*. New Haven, Conn.: Yale University Press, 1976:184–6.

7. Relman AS. Michigan's sensible "living will." *N Engl J Med* 1979; 300:1270–2.

8. Sabatino CP. *Health care powers of attorney*. Chicago: American Bar Association, 1990.

9. *Cruzan* v. *Director, Missouri Dept. of Health*, 110 S. Ct. 2841 (1990).

10. Annas GJ. Nancy Cruzan and the right to die. *N Engl J Med* 1990; 323:670–3.

11. Danis M, Southerland LI, Garrett JM, et al. A prospective study of advance directives for life-sustaining care. *N Engl J Med* 1991; 324:882–8.

12. Emanuel LL, Emanuel EJ. The medical directive: a new comprehensive advance care document. *JAMA* 1989; 261:3288–93.

13. Emanuel LL, Barry MJ, Stoeckle JD, Ettelson LM, Emanuel EJ. Advance directives for medical care—a case for greater use. *N Engl J Med* 1991; 324:889–95.

14. Mass. G.L. c. 201D.

15. *Life-sustaining treatment: making decisions and appointing a health care agent*. New York: New York State Task Force on Life and the Law, 1987.

16. Rosenthal E. Filling the gap where a living will won't do. *New York Times*. January 17, 1991:B9.

17. *Organ transplantation: issues and recommendations: report of the Task Force on Organ Transplantation*. Washington, D.C.: Department of Health and Human Services, 1986:38.

18. Margolick, D. Connecticut army reservists learn to write a will. *New York Times*. February 4, 1991:B1.

9

TERRI SCHIAVO

A Tragedy Compounded

TIMOTHY E. QUILL, M.D.

This article first appeared as Quill T. Terri Schiavo—a tragedy compounded. *New Engl J Med.* 2005:352; 16:1630–1633.

EDITORS' INTRODUCTION

Timothy E. Quill has been writing about the hardest questions in medicine for over twenty years, including assisted dying, the ethical obligations of physicians to patients, and overcoming barriers to quality care for the dying. The media and political circus surrounding the debate and the legal proceedings in the case of Terri Schiavo, a young women in a vegetative state for fifteen years, exemplifies the deeply felt and persistent American conflict between the right to withdraw life-sustaining therapy based on a surrogate's knowledge of the patient's wishes and an assessment of his or her best interests versus the view that every effort should be made to sustain life, no matter what the circumstances.

■ ■ ■

The story of Terri Schiavo should be disturbing to all of us. How can it be that medicine, ethics, law, and family could work so poorly together in meeting the needs of this woman who was left in a persistent vegetative state after having a cardiac arrest? Ms. Schiavo had been sustained by artificial hydration and nutrition through a feeding tube for fifteen years, and her husband, Michael Schiavo, was locked in a very public legal struggle with her parents and siblings about whether such treatment should be continued or stopped. Distortion by interest groups, media hyperbole, and manipulative use of videotape characterized this case and demonstrate what can happen when a patient becomes more a precedent-setting symbol than a unique human being.

Let us begin with some medical facts. On February 25, 1990, Terri Schiavo had a cardiac arrest, triggered by extreme hypokalemia brought on by an eating disorder. As a result, severe hypoxic-ischemic encephalopathy developed, and during the subsequent months she exhibited no evidence of higher cortical function. Computed tomographic scans of her brain eventually showed severe atrophy of her cerebral hemispheres, and her electroencephalograms were flat, indicating no functional activity of the cerebral cortex. Her neurologic examinations were indicative of a persistent vegetative state, which includes periods of wakefulness alternating with sleep, some reflexive responses to light and noise, and some basic gag and swallowing responses, but no signs of emotion, willful activity, or cognition.[1] There is no evidence that Ms. Schiavo was suffering, since the usual definition of this term requires conscious awareness that is impossible in the absence of cortical activity. There have been only a few reported cases in which minimal cognitive and motor functions were restored three months or more after the diagnosis of a persistent vegetative state due to hypoxic-ischemic encephalopathy; in none of these cases was there the sort of objective evidence of severe cortical damage that was present in this case, nor was the period of disability so long.[2]

Having viewed some of the highly edited videotaped material of Terri Schiavo and having seen other patients in a persistent vegetative state, I am not surprised that family members and others unfamiliar with this condition would interpret some of her apparent alertness and movement as meaningful. In 2002, the Florida trial court judge conducted six days of evidentiary hearings on Ms. Schiavo's condition, including evaluations by four neurologists, one radiologist, and her attending physician. The two neurologists selected by Michael Schiavo, a court-appointed "neutral" neurologist, and Ms. Schiavo's attending physician all agreed that her condition met the criteria for a persistent vegetative state. The neurologist and the radiologist chosen by the patient's parents and siblings, the Schindler family, disagreed and suggested that Ms. Schiavo's condition might improve with unproven therapies such as hyperbaric oxygen or vasodilators—but had no objective data to support their assertions. The trial court judge ruled that the diagnosis of a persistent vegetative state met the legal standard of "clear and convincing" evidence, and this decision was reviewed and upheld by the Florida Second District Court of Appeal. Subsequent appeals to the Florida Supreme Court and the U.S. Supreme Court were denied a hearing.

So what was known about Terri Schiavo's wishes and values? Since she unfortunately left no written advance directive, the next step would be to meet with her closest family members and try to understand what she would have wanted under these medical circumstances if she could have spoken for herself, drawing on the principle of "substituted judgment." Some families unite around this question, especially when there is a shared vision of the patient's views and values. Other families unravel, their crisis aggravated by genuine differences of opinion about the proper course of action or preexisting fault lines arising from long-standing family dynamics.

Here Ms. Schiavo's story gets more complex. Michael Schiavo was made her legal guardian under Florida law, which designates the spouse as the decision maker above other family members if a patient becomes irreversibly incapacitated and has not designated a health care proxy. After three years of trying traditional and experimental therapies, Mr. Schiavo accepted the neurologists' diagnosis of an irreversible persistent vegetative state. He believed that his wife would not want to be kept alive indefinitely in her condition, recalling prior statements that she had made, such as "I don't want to be kept alive on a machine." The Schindler family, however, did not accept the diagnosis of a persistent vegetative state, believing instead that Ms. Schiavo's condition could improve with additional rehabilitative treatment.

The relationship between Mr. Schiavo and the Schindler family began breaking down in 1993, around the time that a malpractice lawsuit revolving around the events that led to Ms. Schiavo's cardiac arrest was settled. In 1994, Mr. Schiavo attempted to refuse treatment for an infection his wife had, and her parents took legal action to require treatment. Thus began wide-ranging, acrimonious legal and public-opinion battles that eventually involved multiple special-interest groups who saw this case as a cause célèbre for their particular issue. Michael Schiavo was criticized for being motivated by financial greed, and his loyalty to his wife was questioned because he now lives with another woman, with whom he has two children. The Schindlers were criticized for not accepting the painful reality of their daughter's condition and for expressing their own wishes and values rather than hers.

The right of competent patients to refuse unwanted medical treatment, including artificial hydration and nutrition, is a settled ethical and legal issue in this country—based on the right to bodily integrity. In the Nancy Cruzan case, the Supreme Court affirmed that surrogate decision makers have this right when a patient is incapacitated, but it said that states could set their own standards of evidence about patients' own wishes.[3] Although both the Schiavo and Cruzan cases involved the potential withdrawal of a feeding tube from a patient in a persistent vegetative state, the family was united in believing that Nancy Cruzan would not want to be kept alive in such a state indefinitely. Their challenge, under Missouri law, was to prove to the court in a clear and convincing manner that this would have been Nancy Cruzan's own wish. The Schiavo case raises much more challenging questions about how to define family and how to proceed if members of the immediate family are not in agreement.

The relevant Florida statute requires "clear and convincing evidence that the decision would have been the one the patient would have chosen had the patient been competent or, if there is no indication of what the patient would have chosen, that the decision is in the patient's best interest." Since there is no societal consensus about whether a feeding tube is in the "best interest" of a patient in a persistent vegetative state, the main legal question to be addressed was that of Terri Schiavo's wishes. In 2001, the trial court judge ruled that clear and convincing evidence showed that Ms. Schiavo would have chosen not to receive life-prolonging treatment under the circumstances that then applied. This ruling was also affirmed by the Florida appeals court and denied a hearing by the Florida Supreme Court. When Terri Schiavo's feeding tube was removed for the second time, in 2003, the Florida legislature created Terri's Law to override the court decision, and the tube was again reinserted. This law was subsequently ruled an unconstitutional violation of the separation of powers.

On March 18, 2005, Ms. Schiavo's feeding tube was removed for a third time. The U.S. Congress then passed an "emergency measure" that was signed by the President in an effort both to force federal courts to review Ms. Schiavo's case and to create a legal mandate to have her feeding tube reinserted yet again. The U.S. District Court in Florida denied the emergency request to reinsert the feeding tube, and this decision was upheld on appeal. Multiple subsequent legal appeals were denied, and Ms. Schiavo died on March 31, 2005, thirteen days after the feeding tube was removed.

This sad saga reinforces my personal belief that the courts—though their involvement is sometimes necessary—are the last place one wants to be when working through these complex dilemmas. Although I did not examine her, from the data I reviewed I have no doubt that Terri Schiavo was in a persistent vegetative state and that her cognitive and neurologic functions were unfortunately not going to improve. Her life could have been further prolonged with artificial hydration and nutrition, and there is some solace in knowing that she was not consciously suffering. I also believe that both her husband and her family, while seeing the situation in radically different ways, were trying to do what was right for her. Her family and the public should be reassured and educated that dying in this way can be a natural, humane process (humans died in this way for thousands of years before the advent of feeding tubes).[4]

In considering such profound decisions, the central issue is not what family members would want for themselves or what they want for their incapacitated loved one, but rather what the patient would want for himself or herself. The New Jersey Supreme Court that decided the case of Karen Ann Quinlan got the question of substituted judgment right: If the patient could wake up for fifteen minutes and understand his or her condition fully, and then had to return to it, what would he or she tell you to do? If the data about the patient's wishes are not clear, then in the absence of public policy or family consensus, we should err on the side of continued treatment even in cases of a persistent vegetative state in which there is no hope of recovery. But if the evidence is clear, as the courts found in the case of Terri Schiavo, then enforcing life-prolonging treatment against what is agreed to be the patient's will is both unethical and illegal.

Let us hope that future courts and legislative bodies put aside all the special interests and distractions and listen carefully to the patient's voice as expressed through family members and close friends. This voice is what counts the most, and in the Terri Schiavo case, it was largely drowned out by a very loud, self-interested public debate.

REFERENCES

1. Jennett B. *The vegetative state: medical facts, ethical and legal dilemmas*. New York: Cambridge University Press, 2002.

2. The Multi-Society Task Force on PVS. Medical aspects of the persistent vegetative state. *N Engl J Med* 1994; 330:1499–508, 1572–9. [Erratum, *N Engl J Med* 1995; 333:130.]

3. Gostin LO. Life and death choices after Cruzan. *Law Med Health Care* 1991; 19:9–12.

4. Ganzini L, Goy ER, Miller LL, Harvath TA, Jackson A, Delorit MA. Nurses' experiences with hospice patients who refuse food and fluids to hasten death. *N Engl J Med* 2003; 349:359–65.

RESEARCH INTO END-OF-LIFE CARE

SUPPORT Principal Investigators, "A Controlled Trial to Improve Care for Seriously Ill Hospitalized Patients: The Study to Understand Prognoses and Preferences for Outcomes and Risks of Treatments (SUPPORT)"

Karen E. Steinhauser, Nicholas A. Christakis, Elizabeth C. Clipp, Maya McNeilly, Lauren McIntyre, and James A Tulsky, "Factors Considered Important at the End of Life by Patients, Family, Physicians, and Other Care Providers"

John E. Wennberg, Elliott S. Fisher, Thérèse A. Stukel, Jonathan S. Skinner, Sandra M. Sharp, and Kristen K. Bronner, "Use of Hospitals, Physician Visits, and Hospice Care During Last Six Months of Life Among Cohorts Loyal to Highly Respected Hospitals in the United States"

Joan M. Teno, Brian R. Clarridge, Virginia Casey, Lisa C. Welch, Terrie Wetle, Renee Shield, and Vincent Mor, "Family Perspectives on End-of-Life Care at the Last Place of Care"

10

A CONTROLLED TRIAL TO IMPROVE CARE FOR SERIOUSLY ILL HOSPITALIZED PATIENTS

The Study to Understand Prognoses and Preferences for Outcomes and Risks of Treatments (SUPPORT)

THE SUPPORT PRINCIPAL INVESTIGATORS

This article originally appeared as Study to Understand Prognoses and Preferences for Outcomes and Risks of Treatments (SUPPORT) Principal Investigators. A controlled trial to improve care for seriously ill hospitalized patients: the study to understand prognoses and preferences for outcomes and risks of treatments (SUPPORT). *JAMA.* 1995;274(20);1591–1598. Copyright © 1995, American Medical Association. All rights reserved. Reprinted with permission.

EDITORS' INTRODUCTION

This seminal and large randomized trial proved that the provision of information on prognosis and patient preferences has no impact on care received by patients with advanced chronic illness in American teaching hospitals. Hospitalized patients experienced protracted pain and other symptoms that were largely untreated. Families faced bankruptcy and other major stressors. Communication about what was happening and realistic options for care did not occur. The multiple publications resulting from this study provided the evidence demonstrating the urgent need for reliable access to quality palliative care.

■ ■ ■

Public health and clinical medicine during this century have given Americans the opportunity to live longer and more productive lives, despite progressive illness. For some patients, however, this progress has resulted in prolonged dying, accompanied by substantial emotional and financial expense.[1] Many Americans today fear they will lose control over their lives if they become critically ill, and their dying will be prolonged and impersonal.[2] This has led to an increasingly visible right-to-die movement. Two years after voters in California and Washington State narrowly defeated referenda on physician-assisted euthanasia, Oregon voters approved physician prescription of lethal medications for persons with a terminal disease.[3,4] Physicians and ethicists have debated when to use cardiac resuscitation and other aggressive treatments for patients with advanced illnesses.[5,6] Many worry about the economic and human cost of providing life-sustaining treatment near the end of life.[7-9]

In response, professional organizations, the judiciary, consumer organizations, and a president's commission have all advocated more emphasis on realistically forecasting outcomes of life-sustaining treatment and on improved communication between physician and patient.[2,10-16] Statutes requiring informed consent and communication, like the Patient Self-Determination Act,[17] have been passed. Advance care planning and effective ongoing communication among clinicians, patients, and families are essential to achieve these goals. Previous studies indicate, however, that communication is often absent or occurs only during a crisis.[18-20] Physicians today often perceive death as failure,[1] they tend to be too pessimistic regarding prognoses,[21] and they provide more extensive treatment to seriously ill patients than they would choose for themselves.[22]

Phase I of the Study to Understand Prognoses and Preferences for Outcomes and Risks of Treatments (SUPPORT) confirmed barriers to optimal management and shortfalls in patient-physician communication.[23,24] The phase II intervention sought to address these deficiencies by providing physicians with accurate predictive information on future functional ability,[25] survival probability for each day up to six months,[26] and patient preferences for end-of-life care; a skilled nurse augmented the care team to elicit patient preferences, provide prognoses, enhance understanding, enable palliative care, and facilitate advance planning. We hypothesized that increased communication and understanding of prognoses and preferences would result in earlier treatment decisions, reductions in time spent in undesirable states before death, and reduced resource use. This article describes the effect of the SUPPORT intervention on five specific outcomes: physician understanding of patient preferences; incidence and time of documentation of do-not-resuscitate (DNR) orders; pain; time spent in an intensive care unit (ICU), comatose, or receiving mechanical ventilation before death; and hospital resource use (Figure 10.1).

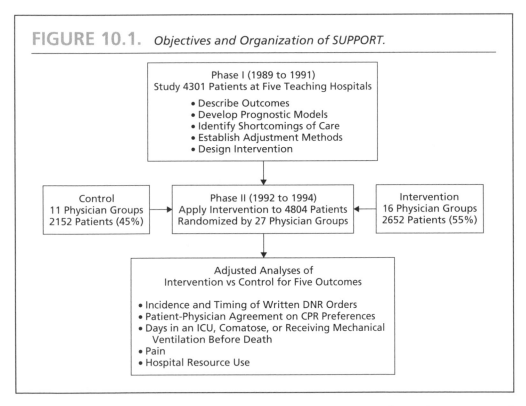

FIGURE 10.1. *Objectives and Organization of SUPPORT.*

Overall schematic presentation of phases I and II of the Study to Understand Prognoses and Preferences for Outcomes and Risks of Treatment (SUPPORT) project, 1989 to 1994. DNR indicates do not resuscitate; CPR, cardiopulmonary resuscitation; and ICU, intensive care unit.

METHODS

Phase I was a prospective observational study that described the process of decision making and patient outcomes. Phase II was a cluster randomized controlled clinical trial to test the effect of the intervention. Enrollment, data collection, and interviewing were virtually identical during the two phases.[21,23–28]

Enrollment

Qualified patients were in the advanced stages of one or more of nine illnesses: acute respiratory failure, multiple organ system failure with sepsis, multiple organ system failure with malignancy, coma, chronic obstructive lung disease, congestive heart failure, cirrhosis, metastatic colon cancer, and non–small cell lung cancer. Patients were excluded if they were younger than eighteen years, were discharged or died within forty-eight hours of qualifying for the study, were admitted with a scheduled discharge within seventy-two hours, did not speak English, were admitted to the psychiatric ward, had acquired immunodeficiency syndrome, or were pregnant or sustained an acute burn, head, or other trauma (unless they later developed acute respiratory failure or multiple organ system failure).[26,28] Nurses trained in the SUPPORT eligibility criteria reviewed hospital admissions and ICU patients daily to identify newly qualified patients.

Phase I enrolled patients from June 1989 to June 1991, and phase II enrolled patients from January 1992 through January 1994. Patients were recruited from five medical centers: Beth Israel Hospital, Boston, Mass; MetroHealth Medical Center, Cleveland, Ohio; Duke University Medical Center, Durham, NC; Marshfield Clinic/St Joseph's Hospital, Marshfield, Wis; and the University of California at Los Angeles Medical Center. An independent committee monitored potential adverse events, including six-month mortality for intervention patients and changes in patient satisfaction with medical care. Mortality follow-up to six months was complete for all phase I patients. In phase II, 22 patients (0.5 percent) were unavailable for follow-up at a median of eighty days.

Data Collection Methods

Data collection was based on both concurrent and retrospective medical record reviews and on interviews with patients, patient surrogates (defined as the person who would make decisions if the patient was unable to do so), and patients' physicians.

Medical Record–Based Data We collected physiological indicators of disease severity,[29,30] length of stay, a modified version of the Therapeutic Intervention Scoring System,[31] and comorbidities from the medical records on days 1, 3, 7, 14, and 25. The permanent medical record was retrospectively reviewed for discussions or decisions concerning eighteen important issues, such as the use of dialysis, withdrawal from a ventilator, and DNR orders. Reliability testing on 10 percent of the medical records showed at least 90 percent agreement on abstracted data.

Interview Data Patients and their designated surrogates were interviewed in the hospital between days 2 and 7 (median, day 4) and again between days 6 and 15 (median, day 12) after study enrollment, whether or not the patient remained hospitalized. The surrogate was interviewed four to ten weeks after the patient's death. Among the 45 percent of patients who were able to communicate, the response rate for the first interview was 85 percent. The surrogate response rate for the first interview was 87 percent. For the second-week interviews, the patient response rate was 71 percent and the surrogate response rate was 78 percent. The interviews collected information on patient demographics, functional status, self-assessed quality of life, communication with physicians, frequency and severity of pain, satisfaction with medical care,[32] and the patient's preferences for cardiopulmonary resuscitation (CPR). When a patient interview was not possible, the surrogate's responses were substituted, a strategy that mirrors clinical practice. Important elements of the patient/surrogate questionnaires were retested for reliability. Initial and repeat responses had greater than 80 percent agreement.

The most senior available physician acknowledging responsibility for the patient's medical decisions was interviewed in the first and second weeks after patient enrollment (median, days 3 and 11, respectively). In both interviews, we asked the physician's understanding of the patient's preferences for CPR. In the second interview, physicians assigned to the intervention were queried about its influence on the patient's care. Physician response rates were 86 percent for the first interview and 82 percent for the second interview.

Phase II Intervention

Presented with early findings from phase I documenting substantial shortcomings in communication, decision making, and outcomes,[23,24] physicians at the participating institutions voiced interest in attempting change. Physician leaders and study investigators at the sites met to discuss how decision making could be improved to more closely reflect both probable outcomes and patient preferences and ways to improve patient, family, and physician communication. Physicians suggested that communication could improve if there were more reliable and prompt information generated by the study and if study personnel would make it more efficient to have conversations. In response to these suggestions, the phase II intervention aimed to improve communication and decision making by providing timely and reliable prognostic information, by eliciting and documenting patient and family preferences and understanding of disease prognosis and treatment, and by providing a skilled nurse to help carry out the needed discussions, convene the meetings, and bring to bear the relevant information. The elements of the intervention and their timing are presented in Table 10.1.

In each case, the nurse was free to shape her role so as to achieve the best possible care and outcome. For example, she sometimes engaged in extensive emotional support. Other times, she mainly provided information and ensured that all parties heard one another effectively. All of the nurses' involvement required approval of the attending physicians. In virtually all cases, the physician approval came with no limits. Physicians were free, however, to limit the intervention in any way that they felt was best for the patient, and there was no requirement for them to share or discuss the information with the patient or family or to allow the nurse's involvement to continue. The nurse was identified on her badge and in the consent process as part of a research effort, but she had the role and appearance of a typical clinical specialist.

TABLE 10.1. Content, Recipient, and Timing of Phase II SUPPORT Intervention[a]

	Content	Provided to	Timing
FEEDBACK of PHASE I RESULTS			
	Benchmarking information describing phase I incidence of patient-physician communication, pain, and timing of DNR order	All intervention physicians	Early phase II
Prognostic Information			
	Survival time estimates for up to 6 mos[26]	Intervention physicians and medical records	Study days 2, 4, 8, 15, and 26
	Prognosis for outcome for CPR if needed[26]	Intervention physicians and medical records	Study day 2
	Survival estimates, enhanced by physician[26]	Intervention physicians and medical records	Study day 4
	Prognosis, probability of severe disability, at 2 months[25]	Intervention physicians and medical records	Study day 8
Interview Information			
	Patient and surrogate report of prognosis, preferences about CPR, advance directives, quality of life, information desires, and pain	Intervention physicians and medical records	First and second study weeks
	Interview on knowledge of preferences[b]	Intervention physicians	Study day 10
Nurse Involvement			
	Explaining prognostic estimates and interview reports	Patient, family, staff, intervention physicians, and medical records	Study day 3 and continuously until death or 6 months

Content	Provided to	Timing
Enhancing understanding of likely outcomes/preferences	Patient, family, staff, intervention physicians, and medical records	Study day 3 and continuously until death or 6 months
Eliciting and documenting preferences/advance directives	Patient, family, staff, intervention physicians, and medical records	Study day 3 and continuously until death or 6 months
Assessing pain and enabling treatment	Patient, family, staff, intervention physicians, and medical records	Study day 3 and continuously until death or 6 months
Voicing patient/family preferences and values	Patient, family, staff, intervention physicians, and medical records	Study day 3 and continuously until death or 6 months
Convening meetings, negotiating agreements	Patient, family, staff, intervention physicians, and medical records	Study day 3 and continuously until death or 6 months
Encouraging planning for future decisions	Patient, family, staff, intervention physicians, and medical records	Study day 3 and continuously until death or 6 months

[a]SUPPORT indicates Study to Understand Prognoses and Preferences for Outcomes and Risks of Treatment; DNR, do not resuscitate; CPR, cardiopulmonary resuscitation; and ICU, intensive care unit.
[b]Physician interview on day 10 was for evaluation, not part of the intervention.

Randomization To limit contamination, patients were assigned to intervention or control (usual care) status based on the specialty of their attending physician. Physician specialties were divided into five groups: internal medicine, pulmonology/medical ICU, oncology, surgery, and cardiology. We used a cluster randomization scheme to assign the intervention randomly to twenty-seven physician group-site combinations, restricted by the conditions that 50 percent to 60 percent of patients would be assigned intervention status, and that at least one intervention and one control physician specialty group be at each of the five study institutions. This resulted in eleven physician specialty groups assigned to control and sixteen assigned to the intervention (see Figure 10.1). Analyses were based on allocation to intervention (that is, intention to treat), irrespective of whether a given patient received the intervention. Investigators were blinded to the phase II results during data collection.

Analytic Methods Five measures were chosen to evaluate the intervention: (1) The timing of written DNR orders was analyzed with a log-normal regression model to prepare Kaplan-Meier predicted median time until the first DNR order was written. If a DNR order was not written, DNR order timing was censored at the day of death or hospital discharge. (2) Patient and physician agreement on preferences to withhold resuscitation was based on the first interview of the patient (or surrogate if the patient was unable to be interviewed) and the responsible physician. Agreement was defined as a response to forgo resuscitation from both patient and physician, analyzed with binary logistic regression, and applied to all interviewed patients or surrogates who had matching physician interviews. (3) Days spent in an ICU, receiving mechanical ventilation, or comatose before death were analyzed using ordinary least-squares regression (after taking the log of 0.5 plus the number of days) and only included phase II patients who died during the index hospitalization. (4) Frequency and severity of pain analyses were based on all patients or surrogates interviewed in the second week with a combined measure (moderate or severe pain all, most, or half the time) and analyzed using a single, ordinal logistic regression model. (5) Hospital resource use was defined as the log of the product of the average Therapeutic Intervention Scoring System rating and length of hospital stay after the second day of the study. In regression analyses on phase I data, this measure closely estimated hospital bills across the five study institutions (Pearson $R^2 = 0.93$ on log product). We used ordinary least-squares regression to model the log of resource use, which was then converted to 1993 dollars. This method allows comparisons of groups and institutions across time without having to adjust for varying hospital billing practices.

Power and Safety Calculations

Power calculations based on phase I data indicated greater than 90 percent power ($\alpha = .05$) to detect a one-day decrease in days until a DNR order was written, a 5 percent increase in the proportion of physicians and patients agreeing on a DNR order, a 20 percent decrease in undesirable days, a 10 percent decrease in reported pain, and a 5 percent decrease in resource use. Effects of the intervention on mortality rates were quantified by the estimated intervention, control hazard ratio from adjusted Cox models.[33]

Adjustment Methods for Phase II Results

Because patients were assigned to intervention or control status based on a limited number of specialty groups, the resulting cohorts might be unbalanced in patient baseline risk factors. Furthermore, practice patterns among the physician specialty groups in phase I differed substantially. We controlled for these expected preintervention differences using baseline multivariable risk scores that were derived by generating models to predict phase I outcomes, each of which incorporated interactions between physician specialty and hospitals. Observed imbalances in phase II baseline patient characteristics were also adjusted using a propensity score that corrected for selection bias associated with being assigned to intervention status.[34] Further details on the construction of both of these risk scores are available on request. Imputation methods for missing data have been published.[25] Finally, we simulated the phase II randomization scheme on the phase I data to evaluate secular trends. To adjust for multiple outcomes, our methods prespecified adjusting confidence intervals (CIs) using the method of Hochberg and Benjamini[35] if more than one *P* value was less than .05. All statistical analyses were done with UNIX S-Plus, version 3.2 software[36] and the Design library.[37]

RESULTS

Phase I Observations

Phase I enrolled 4,301 patients (Figure 10.1) with a median age of sixty-five years and other characteristics summarized in Table 10.2. The mean predicted six-month survival probability was 52 percent with an actual six-month survival probability of 48 percent (Table 10.2). Thirty-one percent of phase I patients with interviews preferred that CPR be withheld, but only 47 percent of their physicians accurately reported this preference during the first interview. Nearly half (49 percent) of the 960 phase I patients who indicated a desire for CPR to be withheld did not have a DNR order written during that hospitalization. Nearly one-third of these patients (278 [29 percent]) died before discharge.

Among all phase I patients who died during the index hospitalization (n = 1,150), 79 percent died with a DNR order, but 46 percent of these orders were written within two days of death. Among all phase I deaths, the median number of days spent in an ICU, comatose, or receiving mechanical ventilation was eight, more than one-third (38 percent) spent at least ten days in an ICU, and 46 percent received mechanical ventilation within three days of death. In the second week, 22 percent of patients reported being in moderate to severe pain at least half the time. In interviews conducted after a patient died, surrogates indicated that 50 percent of all conscious phase I patients who died in the hospital experienced moderate or severe pain at least half the time during their last three days of life.

We found substantial variation in the five outcomes among physician specialty groups and across the five institutions. Across institutions, the median number of days spent in an ICU before death varied from five to nine. The proportion of patients reporting moderate to severe pain at least half the time varied by a factor of 2.7, from 12 percent to 32 percent across study institutions. The predicted median number of days until a DNR order was written for a standard patient varied by a factor of 3.5, from seventy-three days for patients on a surgical service to twenty-two for oncology. One study institution had a predicted median time until DNR was written for a standard patient of twenty-eight days, and another institution had a predicted median time of forty-nine days. Agreement on DNR varied from 8 percent for cardiology patients to 24 percent for oncology patients and from a low of 8 percent at one study institution to a high of 27 percent at another. The median number of days spent in an ICU before death ranged from fourteen in the surgical specialties to five for patients in pulmonary/ICU and oncology services.

TABLE 10.2. Characteristics of 9,105 SUPPORT Patients, 1989 to 1994[a]

	Total Phase I (n = 4,301)	Phase II (n = 4,804)	Control Group (n = 2,152)	Intervention Group (n = 2652)
Median Age, y	65	65	64	66
Sex, % female	43.0	44.3	43.0	45.4
Race, %				
White	79.5	79.0	82.1	77
Black	15.3	15.4	11.5	19
Other	5.3	5.6	6.4	5.0
Annual income, <$11,000, %	59.1	53.1	48.9	57
Education, high school or more, %	53.4	59.0	63.2	56
Primary insurance, %				
Private	29.2	29.6	32.7	27.1
Medicare	53.8	56.0	53.5	57.9
Medicaid	11.8	10.8	11.2	10.6
None	5.3	3.6	2.6	4.4
Disease class, %				
Acute organ system failure[b]	42.9	49.6	52.8	47
Chronic disease[c]	34.4	28.8	25.0	31.8
Nontraumatic coma	5.7	7.3	5.9	8.4
Cancer[d]	16.9	14.4	16.3	12.9
Mean ADL Scale Score[e,f]	1.6	1.5	1.5	1.5
Median APS of APACHE III[e,g]	33	32	32	32
Support 6-month mean survival estimate[e]	0.52	0.52	0.51	0.52
Hospital mortality, %	26.7	25.2	24.6	25.6
6-month mortality, %	48.0	45.6	43.8	47.1
Median hospital charges, in thousands of dollars	21	29	33	27

[a]SUPPORT indicates Study to Understand Prognoses and Preferences for Outcomes and Risks of Treatment.
[b]Includes acute respiratory failure and multiple organ system failure with or without sepsis.
[c]Includes end-stage cirrhosis and acute exacerbations of severe congestive heart failure or severe chronic obstructive pulmonary disease.
[d]Includes colon cancer with liver metastases and stage III or stage IV non–small cell lung cancer.
[e]Measured on the third study day.
[f]ADL indicates activities of daily living score from 0 to 7, with each point representing an impairment in basic function, reflecting patient status two weeks before admission.
[g]APS indicates acute physiology score; and APACHE III, Acute Physiology, Age, Chronic Health Evaluation III.[29] The APS varies from 0 to 252, with a higher score indicating greater physiological instability and risk of death.

Phase II Demographics

Phase II enrolled 4,804 patients, 2,152 assigned to usual medical care and 2,652 assigned to intervention status (Figure 10.1). Their characteristics were generally similar to those of phase I patients (Table 10.2).

Delivery of the Intervention Ninety-five percent of intervention patients received one or more patient-specific components of the intervention. The SUPPORT nurse was involved in the care of all but 133 patients, and 75 of these were patients who died or were discharged on the day of enrollment. The SUPPORT nurse communicated with the physician in virtually all cases. She talked directly with the patient or family in most cases (for example, with 84 percent concerning prognosis, 77 percent about pain, 63 percent about likely outcomes or resuscitation, and 73 percent concerning written advance directives). For patients in the hospital for seven or more days after qualifying for the study, the median number of SUPPORT nurse contacts with the patient, family, or physician was four and the mean was six. Documentation in the progress notes of discussions about patients' preferences with regard to resuscitation was increased from 38.5 percent in phase I to 50.3 percent among phase II intervention patients.

The patient's physician received at least one prognostic report for 94 percent of patients, and the report was put in the medical record of 80 percent. The patient's physician received at least one printed report of patient or surrogate understanding and preferences in 78 percent of cases.

No physician refused to receive the printed reports or to have them shared with other professional staff. The physicians for 43 patients refused to allow the SUPPORT nurse to have contact with the patient and family, and seven patients or surrogates refused to speak with the SUPPORT nurse.

Effect of Intervention on Outcomes The prevalence or timing of documentation of DNR orders for the 2,534 intervention patients was the same as for the 2,208 control patients (adjusted ratio of median time, 1.02; 95 percent CI, 0.90 to 1.15) (Table 10.3).

TABLE 10.3. **Effect of the SUPPORT Phase II Intervention on Five Outcomes: Intervention Group Versus Control Group, 1992 to 1994**

	Adjusted Ratio (95% CI)
Median time until DNR order was written, d	1.02 (0.90-1.15)
DNR agreement, %	1.22 (0.99-1.49)
Undesirable states, median d	0.97 (0.87-1.07)
Pain, %	1.15 (1.00-1.33)
Resource use, median 1993 dollars	1.05 (0.99-1.12)

[a]SUPPORT indicates Study to Understand Prognoses and Preferences for Outcomes and Risks of Treatment; DNR, do not resuscitate; and CI, confidence interval.

There was a small association of the intervention with improved patient-physician DNR agreement for the 1,480 intervention patients who had patient or surrogate and matching physician interviews, compared with 1,159 control patients (adjusted ratio, 1.22; 95 percent CI, 0.99 to 1.49). The number of days spent in an ICU, comatose, or receiving mechanical ventilation before death for the 680 intervention patients who died in the hospital was the same as for the 530 control patients (adjusted ratio of median days, 0.97; 95 percent CI, 0.87 to 1.07). Reported pain increased for the 1,677 intervention patients and surrogates interviewed in the second week, compared with the control group (adjusted ratio, 1.15; 95 percent CI, 1.00 to 1.33) (Table 10.3). There was no change in hospital resources used for 2,593 intervention patients not dead or discharged before the third study day compared with 2,129 control patients (adjusted ratio of average resource use, 1.05; 95 percent CI, 0.99 to 1.12).

The unadjusted differences between intervention and control patients for median days until the first DNR order was written were large, especially for patients with colon cancer and non–small cell lung cancer for whom the median number of days until a written DNR order was 80 percent lower in intervention patients. Adjustment for baseline imbalances reduced much of the difference in each category (Table 10.4). The differences that persist in the cancer category are of uncertain importance, being one among multiple comparisons and being based on a small number of patients (Table 10.4).

Figure 10.2 illustrates the secular trends of each outcome in the phase II intervention and control groups, as well as in phase I, using simulations of the physician specialty groupings used in phase II. None of the five outcomes changed significantly during the five years of the study. The differences between those who would have been assigned to intervention and control in phase I persisted throughout the SUPPORT study, unaffected by time or by the intervention.

Communication and Preferences

The intervention did not change the unadjusted proportion of patients or surrogates reporting a discussion about CPR; 37 percent of control patients and 40 percent of intervention patients reported discussing their preference. Of patients who did not have such a discussion, 41 percent of each group said they would like to discuss CPR. Seventeen percent of control patients and 20 percent of intervention patients changed their resuscitation preferences to forgo CPR by the second week after enrollment, and 39 percent of control patients and 41 percent of intervention patients reported having a discussion about their prognosis with a physician. Of those who did not discuss their prognosis, 44 percent of control patients and 42 percent of intervention patients reported that they would like to have such a discussion.

Physician's Perspective on Intervention

In the second physician interview, 59 percent acknowledged receiving the prognostic reports and 34 percent acknowledged receiving the preference reports. Fifteen percent reported discussing this specific information with patients or families. Nearly a quarter of respondents (22 percent) said they thought the SUPPORT nurses' involvement improved patient care.

TABLE 10.4. Effect of the SUPPORT Intervention on Five Outcomes Within the Major Disease Categories[a]

	Unadjusted Outcomes				Adjusted Outcomes			
	Acute Respiratory or Multiple System Failure	Acute Exacerbation of Cirrhosis, COPD, or CHF	Coma	Advanced Lung or Colon Cancer	Acute Respiratory or Multiple System Failure	Acute Exacerbation of Cirrhosis, COPD, or CHF	Coma	Advance Lung or Colon Cancer
Median time until DNR order was written, d								
Control	46	40	10	58	38	41	8	40
Intervention	34	45	10	14	41	50	10	21
DNR agreement, %								
Control	11	13	33	17	8	8	25	18
Intervention	13	14	21	32	9	10	18	26
Undesirable states, median d								
Control	10	9.5	6	1	11	7	6.5	1
Intervention	9	4	6	0	10	4	7	1
Pain, %								
Control	17	16	5	21	17	16	9	20
Intervention	17	18	9	23	18	16	12	26
Resource use, median 1993 dollars								
Control	36,800	9,000	26,900	5,700	32,700	9,100	20,900	5,100
Intervention	36,300	8,100	19,500	5,600	33,400	8,900	22,000	6,100

[a]SUPPORT indicates Study to Understand Prognoses and Preferences for Outcomes and Risks of Treatments; COPD, chronic obstructive pulmonary disease; CHF, congestive heart failure; and DNR, do not resuscitate.

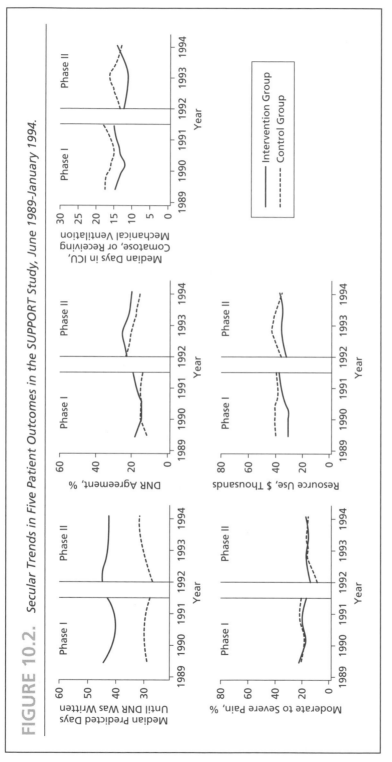

FIGURE 10.2. *Secular Trends in Five Patient Outcomes in the SUPPORT Study, June 1989–January 1994.*

The horizontal axes represent the years of SUPPORT. The time between phase I and phase II is represented by a space. The intervention and control group lines have been smoothed nonparametrically. The phase II results represent the actual impact of the trial, and the phase I results are the baseline or historical differences. There were no significant differences in intervention patients between phases I and II, and after adjustment, no significant differences were noted between phase II control and intervention patients for the five main outcomes. DNR indicates do not resuscitate; CPR, cardiopulmonary resuscitation; and ICU, intensive care unit.

Safety Monitoring

After adjusting for baseline differences, the six-month mortality for phase II control patients was the same as for intervention patients (adjusted relative hazard, 0.95; 95 percent CI, 0.87 to 1.04). Both control (68 percent) and intervention (69 percent) patients or surrogates rated their care as excellent or very good.

COMMENT

Findings from phase I of SUPPORT documented many shortcomings of care. The SUPPORT patients were all seriously ill, and their dying proved to be predictable, yet discussions and decisions substantially in advance of death were uncommon. Nearly half of all DNR orders were written in the last two days of life. The final hospitalization for half of patients included more than eight days in generally undesirable states: in an ICU, receiving mechanical ventilation, or comatose. Families reported that half of the patients who were able to communicate in their last few days spent most of the time in moderate or severe pain. Based on a study in a defined population at our Wisconsin site, we estimate that patients meeting SUPPORT criteria account for approximately 400,000 admissions per year in the United States and that another 925,000 people are similarly ill but would not meet SUPPORT entry requirements of being hospitalized or in intensive care.[38] Patients with SUPPORT illnesses and severity account for about 40 percent of persons dying in the defined population.

Building on the findings in phase I, observations of others,[1–16,23,24,39–45] the opinions of physicians at the five sites, and the marked variation in their baseline practices, the phase II intervention aimed to make it easier to achieve better decision making for these seriously ill patients. The intervention gave physicians reliable prognostic information and timely reports of patient and surrogate perceptions, the two most important factors cited recently by physicians when considering life-support decisions for critically ill patients.[44] The intervention nurse also undertook time-consuming discussions, arranged meetings, provided information, supplied forms, and did anything else to encourage the patient and family to engage in an informed and collaborative decision-making process with a well-informed physician (Table 10.1).

The intervention was limited by its application to a diverse group of physicians and patients, all of whom had to comply voluntarily. The intervention had to be perceived as helpful, polite, and appropriate. As an initial attempt to change outcomes for seriously ill patients, we did not seek authority to be coercive or more than minimally disruptive. As designed, however, the intervention was vigorously applied. The SUPPORT nurses were committed, energetic, and highly trained. They engaged in the care of virtually all our patients, and nearly everyone had printed reports delivered promptly.

Because we thought that changes in the decision-making processes that were not reflected in improved patient outcomes would not be worth much expense, we specified five outcomes, each indicating an important improvement in patient experience, as the main targets of the intervention.

The intervention had no impact on any of these designated targets (Tables 10.3 and 10.4). Furthermore, even though the targeted outcomes are objectives of much ethical and legal writing and of some explicit social policy (such as informed consent statutes, the Patient Self-Determination Act, and guidelines on pain),[10-17] there were no secular trends toward improvement for intervention or control patients during the five years of SUPPORT data collection (Figure 10.2).

These results raise fundamental questions about the intent and design of this trial. Do patients and physicians see the documented shortcomings as troubling? Can enhanced decision making improve the experience of seriously ill and dying patients? Were the inevitable limitations of this project too great to draw strong conclusions?

Because there was no movement toward what would seem to be better practices, one could conclude that physicians, patients, and families are fairly comfortable with the current situation. Certainly, most patients and families indicated they were satisfied, no matter what happened to them. Physicians have their established patterns of care, and while they were willing to have the SUPPORT nurse present and carrying on conversations, physician behavior appeared unchanged. Perhaps physicians and patients in this study acknowledged problems with the care of seriously ill patients as a group. However, when involved with their own situation or engaged in the care of their individual patients, they felt they were doing the best they could, were satisfied they were doing well, and did not wish to directly confront problems or face choices.[46,47]

The study certainly casts a pall over any claim that, if the health care system is given additional resources for collaborative decision making in the form of skilled professional time, improvements will occur. In phase II of SUPPORT, improved information, enhanced conversation, and an explicit effort to encourage use of outcome data and preferences in decision making were completely ineffectual, despite the fact that the study had enough power to detect small effects.

It is possible that the intervention would have been more effective if implemented in different settings, earlier in the course of illness, or with physician leaders rather than nurses as implementers. Perhaps it would have been effective if continued for more time or tested at later end points.[48] However, the overall results of this study are not encouraging. No pattern emerged that implied that the intervention was successful for some set of patients or physicians or that its impact increased over time. The five hospitals had been chosen for their diversity and their willingness to undertake a substantial and controversial challenge. Yet none showed a tendency toward improvement in these outcomes.

SUPPORT did demonstrate, however, that issues this complex can be studied with sufficient scientific rigor to be confident of the findings. We achieved good interview response rates among seriously ill patients, their families, and physicians, widespread acceptance of the intervention in diverse hospitals, and high-quality data. Consent and confidentiality issues were complex but amenable to solution. The analytic issues required application of relatively novel approaches, but they proved effective. The study also demonstrated the need for such methods when performing evaluations of complex interventions in seriously ill patients. We would have concluded that the intervention positively influenced all outcomes had we not had phase I results for baseline adjustment and phase II control patients to evaluate secular trends (Table 10.4 and Figure 10.2).

In conclusion, we are left with a troubling situation. The picture we describe of the care of seriously ill or dying persons is not attractive. One would certainly prefer to envision that, when confronted with life-threatening illness, the patient and family would be included in discussions, realistic estimates of outcome would be valued, pain would be treated, and dying would not be prolonged. That is still a worthy vision.[2,49] However, it is not likely to be achieved through an intervention such as that implemented by SUPPORT. Success will require reexamination of our individual and collective commitment to these goals, more creative efforts at shaping the treatment process, and, perhaps, more proactive and forceful attempts at change.

REFERENCES

1. Callahan D. *The Troubled Dream of Life: Living With Mortality*. New York, NY: Simon & Schuster; 1993.

2. McCue JD. The naturalness of dying. *JAMA*. 1995; 273:1039–1043.

3. Annas GJ. Death by prescription: the Oregon initiative. *N Engl J Med*. 1994; 301:1240–1243.

4. Brown D. Medical community still divided on Oregon's assisted suicide law. *Washington Post*. November 13, 1994: A20.

5. Tomlinson T, Brody H. Futility and the ethics of resuscitation. *JAMA*. 1990; 264:1276–1280.

6. Blackhall LJ. Must we always use CPR? *N Engl J Med*. 1987; 317:1281–1285.

7. Wanzer SH, Federman, DD, Adelstein SJ, et al. The physician's responsibility toward hopelessly ill patients. *N Engl J Med*. 1989; 320:884–849.

8. Ginzberg E. The high cost of dying. *Inquiry*. 1980; 17:293–295.

9. Hill TP, Shirley D. *A Good Death*. Reading, Mass: Addison-Wesley; 1992.

10. President's Commission for the Study of Ethical Problems in Medicine and Biomedical and Behavioral Research. *Deciding to Forego Life-Sustaining Treatment*. Washington, DC: US Government Printing Office; 1983.

11. Hastings Center. *Guidelines on the Termination of Life-Sustaining Treatment and the Care of the Dying*. New York, NY: Hastings Center; 1987.

12. Coordinating Council on Life-Sustaining Medical Treatment Decisions by the Court. *Guidelines for State Court Decision Making in Authorizing or Withholding Life-Sustaining Medical Treatment*. Williamsburg, Va: West Publishing Company; 1991.

13. *Cruzan v. Director, Missouri Dept of Health*. 110 SCt 284, 1990:2855–2856.

14. Council on Ethical and Judicial Affairs. Guidelines for the appropriate use of do-not-resuscitate orders. *JAMA*. 1991; 265:1868–1871.

15. American Thoracic Society Bioethics Task Force. Withholding and withdrawing life-sustaining therapy. *Ann Intern Med*. 1991; 115:478–485.

16. Cancer Pain Relief and Palliative Care. *Report of a WHO Expert Committee, Technical Report 804*. Geneva, Switzerland: World Health Organization; 1990.

17. Omnibus Budget Reconciliation Act of 1990 (OBRA-90), Pub L 101– 508, §§4206 and 4751 (Medicare and Medicaid, respectively), 42 USC §§ 1395cc(a)(I)(Q), 1395mm(c)(8), 1395cc(f), 1396a(a)(57), 1396a(a)(58), and 1396a(w) (supp 1991).

18. Bedell SE, Delbanco TL. Choices about cardiopulmonary resuscitation in the hospital. *N Engl J Med*. 1984; 310:1089–1093.

19. Katz J. *The Silent World of Doctor & Patient*. New York, NY: Free Press; 1986.

20. Blackhall LJ, Cobb J, Moskowitz MA. Discussions regarding aggressive care with critically ill patients. *J Gen Intern Med*. 1989; 4:399–402.

21. Arkes HR, Dawson NV, Speroff T, et al. The covariance decomposition of the probability score and its use in evaluating prognostic estimates. *Med Decis Making*. 1995; 15:120–131.

22. Molloy DW, Guyatt G, Alemayehu E, McIloy W. Treatment preferences, attitudes toward advance directives, and concerns about health care. *Humane Med.* 1991; 7:285–290.

23. Teno JM, Lynn J, Phillips RS, et al. Do formal advance directives affect resuscitation decisions and the use of resources for seriously ill patients? *J Clin Ethics.* 1994; 5:23–30.

24. Teno JM, Hakim RB, Knaus WA, et al. Preferences for CPR: physician-patient agreement and hospital resource use. *J Gen Intern Med.* 1995; 10:179–186.

25. Wu AW, Damiano AM, Lynn J, et al. Predicting future functional status for seriously ill hospitalized adults. *Ann Intern Med.* 1995; 122:342–350.

26. Knaus WA, Harrell FE, Lynn J, et al. The SUPPORT prognostic model: objective estimates of survival for seriously ill hospitalized adults. *Ann Intern Med.* 1995; 122:191–203.

27. Lynn J, Knaus WA. Background for SUPPORT. *J Clin Epidemiol.* 1990; 43(suppl): 1S–4S.

28. Murphy DJ, Knaus WA, Lynn J. Study population in SUPPORT. *J Clin Epidemiol.* 1990; 43(suppl): 11S–28S.

29. Knaus WA, Wagner DP, Draper EA, et al. The APACHE III prognostic system. *Chest.* 1991; 100:1619–1636.

30. Knaus WA, Draper EA, Wagner DP, Zimmerman JE. APACHE II: a severity of disease classification system. *Crit Care Med.* 1985; 13:818–829.

31. Cullen DJ, Civetta JM, Briggs BA, Ferrara LC. Therapeutic Intervention Scoring System. *Crit Care Med.* 1974; 2:57–60.

32. Ware JE Jr, Synder MK, Wright WR, Davies AR. Defining and measuring patient satisfaction with medical care. *Eval Program Plann.* 1983; 6:247–263.

33. Cox DR. Regression models and life tables. *J Royal Stat Society B.* 1972; 34:187–220.

34. Cook EF, Goldman L. Performance of tests of significance based on stratification by a multivariate confounder score or by a propensity score. *J Clin Epidemiol.* 1989; 42:317–324.

35. Hochberg Y, Benjamini Y. More powerful procedures for multiple significance testing. *Stat Med.* 1990: 811–818.

36. Statistical Sciences. *S-Plus Users Manual, Version 3.2.* Seattle, Wash: StatSci, MathSoft Inc; 1993.

37. Harrell FE. *Design: S-Plus functions for biostatistical/epidemiologic modeling, testing, estimation, validation, graphics, prediction, and typesetting.* 1994. Available on the Internet at lib.stat.cmu.edu.

38. Layde PM, Broste SK, Desbiens N, et al. Generalizability of clinical studies conducted at tertiary care medical centers. *J Clin Epidemiol.* In press.

39. Covinsky KE, Goldman L, Cook EF, et al. The impact of serious illness on patients' families. *JAMA.* 1994; 272:1839–1844.

40. Wachter RM, Luce JM, Hearst N, Lo B. Decisions about resuscitation: inequities among patients with different but similar prognosis. *Ann Intern Med.* 1989; 111:525–532.

41. Davidson KW, Hackler C, Caradine DR, McCord RS. Physicians' attitudes on advance directives. *JAMA.* 1989; 262:2415–2419.

42. Brody DS, Miller SM, Lerman CE, et al. Patient perception of involvement in medical care. *J Gen Intern Med.* 1989; 4:506–511.

43. Uhlmann RF, Pearlman RA, Cain KC. Physicians' and spouses' predictions of elderly patients' resuscitation preferences. *J Gerontol.* 1988; 43: M115–M121.

44. Cook DJ, Guyatt GH, Jaeschke R, et al. Determinants in Canadian health care workers of the decision to withdraw life support from the critically ill. *JAMA.* 1995; 273:703–708.

45. Danis M, Patrick DL, Southerland LI, et al. Patients' and families' preferences for medical intensive care. *JAMA.* 1988; 260:797–802.

46. Tversky A, Shafir E. Choice under conflict: the dynamics of deferred decision. *Psychol Sci.* 1992; 3:358–361.

47. Redelmeir DA, Shafir E. Medical decision making in situations that offer multiple alternatives. *JAMA*. 1995; 273:302–305.

48. Greco PJ, Eisenberg JM. Changing physician's practices. *N Engl J Med*. 1993; 329:1271–1274.

49. Nuland, S. *How We Die: Reflections on Life's Final Chapter*. New York, NY: Alfred A Knopf Inc; 1994.

ACKNOWLEDGMENTS

The SUPPORT Principal Investigators. Alfred F. Connors Jr., M.D., and Neal V. Dawson, M.D., Metro-Health Medical Center, Cleveland, Ohio; Norman A. Desbiens, M.D., Marshfield (Wis) Medical Research Foundation; William J. Fulkerson Jr., M.D., Duke University Medical Center, Durham, NC; Lee Goldman, M.D., M.P.H., Beth Israel Hospital, Boston, Mass; William A. Knaus, M.D., George Washington University Medical Center, Washington, DC; Joanne Lynn, M.D., Dartmouth Medical School, Hanover, NH; and Robert K. Oye, M.D., University of California at Los Angeles Medical Center.

National Coordinating Center. William A. Knaus, M.D., George Washington University Medical Center, Washington, DC, and Joanne Lynn, M.D., Dartmouth Medical School, Hanover, NH (co-principal investigators); Marilyn Bergner, Ph.D. (deceased), and Anne Damiano, Sc.D., Johns Hopkins University, Baltimore, M.D.; Rosemarie Hakim, Ph.D., George Washington University Medical Center; Donald J. Murphy, M.D., Presbyterian–St. Luke's Medical Center, Denver, Colo; Joan Teno, M.D., and Beth Virnig, Ph.D., Dartmouth Medical School; Douglas P. Wagner, Ph.D., George Washington University Medical Center; and Albert W. Wu, M.D., M.P.H., and Yutaka Yasui, Ph.D., Johns Hopkins University (co-investigators); Detra K. Robinson, M.A., George Washington University Medical Center (chart abstraction supervisor); Barbara Kreling, B.A., George Washington University Medical Center (survey coordinator); Jennie Dulac, B.S.N., R.N., Dartmouth Medical School (intervention implementation coordinator); Rose Baker, M.S.Hyg., George Washington University Medical Center (database manager); and Sam Holayel, B.S., Thomas Meeks, B.A., Mazen Mustafa, M.S., and Juan Vegarra, B.S. (programmers).

National Statistical Center, Duke University Medical Center, Durham, NC. Carlos Alzola, M.S., and Frank E. Harrell Jr., Ph.D.

Beth Israel Hospital, Boston, Mass. Lee Goldman, M.D., M.P.H. (principal investigator); E. Francis Cook, Sc.D., Mary Beth Hamel, M.D., Lynn Peterson, M.D., Russell S. Phillips, M.D., Joel Tsevat, M.D., Lachlan Forrow, M.D., Linda Lesky, M.D., and Roger Davis, Sc.D. (co-investigators); Nancy Kressin, M.S., and Jean-marie Solzan, B.A. (interview supervisors); Ann Louise Puopolo, B.S.N., R.N. (chart abstractor supervisor); Laura Quimby Barrett, B.S.N., R.N., Nora Bucko, B.S.N., R.N., Deborah Brown, M.S.N., R.N., Maureen Burns, B.S.N., R.N., Cathy Foskett, B.S.N., R.N., Army Hozid, B.S.N., R.N., Carol Keohane, B.S.N., R.N., Colleen Martinez, B.S.N., R.N., Dorcie McWeeney, B.S.N., R.N., Debra Melia, B.S.N., R.N., Shelley Otto, M.S.N., R.N., Kathy Sheehan, B.S.N., R.N., Alice Smith, B.S.N., R.N., and Lauren Tofias, M.S., R.N. (chart abstractors); Bernice Arthur, B.A., Carol Collins, B.A., Mary Cunnion, B.A., Deborah Dyer, B.A., Corinne Kulak, B.S., Mary Michaels, B.A., Maureen O'Keefe, B.A., Marian Parker, A.B., M.B.A., Lauren Tuchin, B.A., Dolly Wax, B.A., and Diana Weld, B.A. (interviewers); Liz Hiltunen, M.S., R.N., C.S., Georgie Marks, M.S., M.Ed., R.N., Nancy Mazzapica, M.S.N, R.N., and Cindy Medich, M.S., R.N. (SUPPORT nurse clinicians); and Jane Soukup, M.S. (analyst/data manager).

Duke University Medical Center, Durham, NC. William J. Fulkerson Jr., M.D. (principal investigator); Robert M. Califf, M.D., Anthony N. Galanos, M.D., Peter Kussin, M.D., and Lawrence H. Muhlbaier, Ph.D. (co-investigators); Maria Winchell, M.S. (project director); Lee Mallatratt, R.N. (chart abstractor supervisor); Ella Akin, B.A. (interviewer supervisor); Lynne Belcher, R.N., Elizabeth Buller, B.S.N., R.N., Eileen Clair, R.N., Laura Drew, B.S.N., R.N., Libby Fogelman, B.S.N., R.N., Dianna Frye, B.S.N., R.N., Beth Fraulo, B.S.N., R.N., Debbie Gessner, B.S.N., R.N., Jill Hamilton, B.S.N., R.N., Kendra Kruse, B.S.N., R.N., Dawn Landis, B.S.N., R.N., Louise Nobles, B.S.N., R.N., Rene Oliverio, B.S.N., R.N., and Carroll Wheeler, B.S.N., R.N. (chart abstractors); Nancy Banks, M.A., Steven Berry, B.A., Monie Clayton, Patricia Hartwell, M.A.T., Nan Hubbard, Isabel Kussin, B.A., Barbara Norman, B.A., Jackie Noveau, B.S.N.,

Heather Read, B.A., and Barbara Warren, M.S.W (interviewers); Jane Castle, M.S.N., R.N., Beth Fraulo, B.S.N., R.N., Rene Oliverio, B.S.N., R.N., and Kathy Turner, M.S.N., R.N. (SUPPORT nurse clinicians); and Rosalie Perdue (data manager).

MetroHealth Medical Center, Cleveland, Ohio. Alfred F. Connors Jr., M.D., and Neal V. Dawson, M.D. (co-principal investigators); Claudia Coulton, Ph.D., C. Seth Landefeld, M.D., Theodore Speroff, Ph.D., and Stuart Youngner M.D. (co-investigators); Mary J. Kennard, M.S.N., and Mary Naccaratto, M.S.N. (chart abstractor supervisors); Mary Jo Roach, Ph.D. (interviewer supervisor); Maria Blinkhorn, R.N., Cathy Corrigan, R.N.C., Elsie Geric, R.N., Laura Haas, R.N., Jennifer Harn, R.N., Julie Jerdonek, R.N., Marilyn Landy, R.N., Elaine Marino, R.N., Patti Olesen, R.N., Sherry Patzke, R.N., Linda Repas, R.N., Kathy Schneeberger, R.N., Carolyn Smith, R.N., Colleen Tyler, R.N., and Mary Zenczak, R.N. (chart abstractors); Helen Anderson, B.A., Pat Carolin, Cindy Johnson, B.A., Pat Leonard, B.A., Judy Leuenberger, Linda Palotta, B.A., and Millie Warren (interviewers); Jane Finley, R.N., Toni Ross, R.N., Gillian Solem, M.S.N., and Sue Zronek, R.N. (SUPPORT nurse facilitators); and Sara Davis, B.S. (data manager).

Marshfield Medical Research Foundation/St Joseph's Hospital, Marshfield, Wis. Norman A. Desbiens, M.D. (principal investigator); Steven Broste, M.S., and Peter Layde, M.D., M.Sc. (co-principal investigators); Michael Kryda, M.D., Douglas J. Reding, M.D., and Humberto J. Vidaillet Jr., M.D. (co-investigators); Marilyn Follen, R.N., M.S.N. (project manager and chart abstractor supervisor); Patsy Mowery, B.B.A. (interviewer supervisor); Barbara E. Backus, Debra L. Kempf, B.S.N., Jill M. Kupfer, Karen E. Maassen, L.P.N., Jean M. Rohde, L.P.N., Nancy L. Wilke, and Sharon M. Wilke, L.P.N. (chart abstractors); Elizabeth A. Albee, B.A., Barbara Backus, Angela M. Franz, B.S., Diana L. Henseler, Juanita A. Herr, Irene Leick, Carol L. Lezotte, B.S., and Laura Meddaugh (interviewers); Linda Duffy, R.N., M.S.N., Debrah Johnson, R.N., B.S.N., Susan Kronenwetter, R.N., B.S.N., and Anne Merkel, R.N., B.S.N. (SUPPORT nurse facilitators).

University of California at Los Angeles Medical Center. Robert K. Oye, M.D. (principal investigator); Paul E. Bellamy, M.D. (co-principal investigator); Jonathan Hiatt, M.D., and Neil S. Wenger, M.D., M.P.H. (co-investigators); Margaret Leal-Sotelo, M.S.W. (project director and interviewer supervisor); Darice Moranville-Hawkins, R.N., M.N., Patricia Sheehan, R.N., Diane Watanabe, M.S., and Myrtle C. Yamamoto, R.N. (chart abstractor supervisors); Allison Adema, R.N., Ellen Adkins, R.N., Ann Marie Beckson, R.N., Mona Carter, R.N., Ellen Duerr, R.N., Ayam El-Hadad, R.N., M.N., Ann Farber, R.N., M.A., Ann Jackson, R.N., John Justice, R.N., and Agnes O'Meara, R.N. (chart abstractors); Lee Benson, Lynette Cheney, Carlo Medina, and Jane Moriarty (interviewers); Kay Baker, R.N., M.N., Cleine Marsden, R.N., M.N., and Kara Watne, R.N., M.P.H. (clinical nurse liaisons); and Diane Goya, M.A. (data manager).

Steering Committee. Alfred F. Connors Jr., M.D. (chair), Norman Desbiens, M.D., William J. Fulkerson Jr., M.D., Frank E. Harrell Jr., Ph.D., William A. Knaus, M.D., Joanne Lynn, M.D., Robert K. Oye, M.D., and Russell S. Phillips, M.D.

National Advisory Committee. Charles C. J. Carpenter, M.D. (chair), Brown University/The Miriam Hospital, Providence, RI; Ronald A. Carson, Ph.D., University of Texas, Galveston; Don E. Detmer, M.D., University of Virginia, Charlottesville; Donald E. Steinwachs, Ph.D., The Johns Hopkins University, Baltimore, Md; Vincent Mor, Ph.D., Brown University; Robert A. Harootyan, M.S., M.A., American Association of Retired Persons, Washington, DC; Alex Leaf, M.D., Massachusetts General Hospital, Boston; Rosalyn Watts, Ed.D., R.N., University of Pennsylvania, Philadelphia; Sankey Williams, M.D., Hospital of the University of Pennsylvania; and David Ransohoff, M.D., University of North Carolina at Chapel Hill.

The SUPPORT Project was sponsored by the Robert Wood Johnson Foundation.

We are grateful for the contribution of the SUPPORT nurse clinicians and chart and interview supervisors and staff whose dedicated efforts ensured the high quality of the data. We also are grateful for the contributions of the patients, surrogates, and physicians who participated in the interviews and intervention.

11

FACTORS CONSIDERED IMPORTANT AT THE END OF LIFE BY PATIENTS, FAMILY, PHYSICIANS, AND OTHER CARE PROVIDERS

KAREN E. STEINHAUSER, PH.D., NICHOLAS A. CHRISTAKIS, M.D., PH.D., M.P.H, ELIZABETH C. CLIPP, PH.D., M.S., R.N., MAYA MCNEILLY, PH.D., LAUREN MCINTYRE, PH.D., AND JAMES A. TULSKY, M.D.

Steinhauser KE, Christakis NA, Clipp EC, McNeilly M, McIntyre L, Tulsky, JA. Factors considered important at the end of life by patients, family, physicians, and other care providers. *JAMA*. 2000;284(19):2476–2482. Copyright © 2000, American Medical Association. All rights reserved. Reprinted with permission.

EDITORS' INTRODUCTION

These researchers attempt to answer the question "What do patients want?" Perhaps surprisingly, given the routine application of aggressive life-prolonging technologies, patients with terminal illness list relief of symptoms such as pain, preparation for death, achieving a sense of completion, and being treated as a "whole " person as among their highest priorities for care at this stage of life.

■ ■ ■

Dying patients confront complex and unique challenges that threaten their physical, emotional, and spiritual integrity. The Study to Understand Prognosis and Preferences for Outcomes and Risks of Treatments (SUPPORT) documented that many patients die prolonged and painful deaths, receiving unwanted, expensive, and invasive care.[1] Patients' emotional suffering at the end of life can be profound, yet physicians are too frequently ill equipped to address this suffering.[2,3] In response, medical societies, health care organizations, and the public have identified improved end-of-life care as a high national priority. The American Medical Association and the Institute of Medicine have outlined goals for improved care of the dying, and the Robert Wood Johnson Foundation has devoted millions of dollars to public education on this issue through the Last Acts initiative.[4-6]

These efforts depend, in part, on certain presumptions regarding how dying patients and their families define quality at the end of life. During the latter part of the twentieth century, advances in biomedical technology propelled us to see a "good" death as one involving the fight against disease. Partly in response to this view, the modern hospice movement emerged, redefining a good death as one that included acceptance and closure, most often at home. Unfortunately, empirical support for a notion of a good death that might best structure end-of-life care is lacking, as is a comprehensive understanding about how the definition of a good death might vary across relevant constituencies.

Empirical evidence defining a good death would assist efforts to improve end-of-life care by documenting the breadth of preferences of dying patients and their families. Such data would provide clinicians with information to help guide patients through this challenging and uncertain time. Therefore, we investigated what patients, family members, physicians, and others consider to be important attributes at the end of life.

METHODS

This study was a cross-sectional, stratified random national survey of seriously ill patients, recently bereaved family members, physicians, and other care providers (nurses, social workers, chaplains, and hospice volunteers).

Subjects

Patients were randomly selected from the national Veterans Affairs (VA) Patient Treatment File database using *International Classification of Diseases, Ninth Revision* diagnostic codes for a variety of advanced chronic illnesses (lung, colon, gastric, esophageal, pancreatic, head and neck, and lymphatic cancer; end-stage renal disease; advanced chronic obstructive pulmonary disease; and congestive heart failure). All patients had been hospitalized for these diagnoses within the prior year. Family members were randomly selected from national samples of relatives of VA patients who had died six months to one year earlier. We chose this period so that family members would be past the immediate stages of grief, yet the death would not be so distant that the risk of retrospective bias would be introduced.[7-10] Patient and family samples reflected the racial/ ethnic and socioeconomic composition of VA patients. However, we oversampled female patients (20 percent).

Individuals involved in end-of-life care were randomly selected from membership lists of national professional associations (American College of Physicians–American Society of Internal Medicine, American Nurses Association, National Association of Social Workers, Association of Professional Chaplains, and National Hospice Volunteers). The sample composition reflects the demographic profile of each association's membership.

We mailed surveys to 500 subjects from each of the four groups (total potential n = 2,000). Sample size was calculated to provide adequate power to detect differences among groups. We used several well-established techniques to maximize response rates and data quality.[11,12] Participants who did not respond to the initial survey within five weeks received a second survey that included return postage. In the first wave only, we provided a nominal financial incentive. Survey completion time was less than fifteen minutes. The institutional review boards of the Durham VA and Duke University Medical Centers, Durham, NC, approved the study.

Measurements

The survey asked respondents to rate the importance of forty-four attributes of experience at the end of life (survey available at http://hsrd.durham.med.va.gov /pmepc/ Program.html). Survey items were generated on the basis of twelve previously conducted focus groups and in-depth interviews with patients, family members, physicians, and other care providers in which participants were asked to define attributes of a good death.[13] Participants rated the importance of each item on a 5-point scale: strongly disagree, disagree, neither agree nor disagree, agree, and strongly agree. Respondents also were presented with the nine items most frequently identified in the focus groups and asked to rank-order them from 1 (most important) to 9 (least important). The rank sum for each respondent for the nine items was constrained to be 45; tied ranks were permitted.

Analysis

We examined the distribution of responses for all forty-four items, including frequency, mean, median, and range. For descriptive parsimony, we collapsed the five response categories into three: agree, disagree, and neither agree nor disagree. Based on natural breaks in the distribution of the data, items for which more than 70 percent of respondents in all four groups chose "agree" or "strongly agree" were identified as having substantial agreement. We used χ^2 and, when appropriate, Fisher exact tests of independence to compare responses among groups. We also assessed mean rank score for the nine ranked items and conducted Friedman tests to examine whether rankings within groups were different than would be expected by chance alone. Wilcoxon tests were used to examine the significance of specific response differences among groups.

To identify independent correlates of four selected attributes with the most varied ratings of importance, we conducted multivariate exploratory analyses of factors associated with item response. We used logistic regression to model the likelihood of responding "disagree" or "neither agree nor disagree" versus "agree" for a given item. We used a stepwise procedure to identify covariates strongly associated with response. Our final models also included variables in which we had a substantive interest, regardless of their precise significance level. Each question was initially evaluated in the pooled sample using the same set of covariates. We present odds ratios (ORs) and 95 percent confidence intervals (CIs) only for significant covariates. Because income and education were strongly associated with role, socioeconomic status effects on the full sample could not be evaluated; hence, the effects of income and education on patient and bereaved family member responses were tested in separate analyses. Exploratory analyses revealed no differences in patients' responses by diagnosis; therefore, it was excluded from the multivariate models. Because only female patients were oversampled, we present results of unweighted analyses. In analyses not shown, we also modeled items as a three-category response variable, using multinomial logistic regression. Because the results were nearly identical, we report the less cumbersome binary models. Statistical analyses were conducted using SAS Version 8.0 software (SAS Institute Inc, Cary, NC).

RESULTS

Of the 2,000 mailed surveys, 1,885 potential subjects could be reached (that is, had not moved or died). We received responses from 340 (77 percent) of 444 patients, 332 (71 percent) of 465 bereaved family members, 361 (74 percent) of 486 physicians, and 429 (88 percent) of 490 other care providers (120 chaplains [96 percent], 105 hospice volunteers [84 percent], 107 social workers [86 percent], and 97 nurses [78 percent]), for a total of 1462 participants. The average age of respondents was fifty-seven years; 51 percent were men and 82 percent were white (Table 11.1). Nonrespondents did not differ from respondents with regard to sex, race/ethnicity, diagnosis, or geographic location.

Ratings of Attribute Importance

Based on responses to the survey, we classified the forty-four attributes into three categories: (1) items with strong agreement regarding importance among the entire sample (>70 percent of every group agreed that the attribute is important); (2) items with strong agreement regarding importance (<70 percent among patients but less agreement among physicians); and (3) items with broad response variation among the entire sample (that is, large percentages of respondents agreeing, disagreeing, and neither agreeing nor disagreeing that the item is important).

Attributes Rated As Important Among All Participants   Twenty-six survey items displayed strong agreement in all four groups (Table 11.2). Of the twenty-six items, five were associated with symptoms or personal care: freedom from pain, freedom from anxiety, freedom from shortness of breath, being kept clean, and having physical touch. Four items related to preparation for the end of life: having financial affairs in order, feeling prepared to die, believing that one's family is prepared for one's death, and knowing what to expect about one's physical condition. Three items related to achieving a sense of completion about one's life: saying good-bye to important people, remembering personal accomplishments, and resolving unfinished business. Two items involved decisions about treatment preferences: having treatment preferences in writing and naming someone to make decisions in the event that one cannot. Seven items were associated with what focus group participants in a prior study[13] called "being treated as a whole person": maintaining one's dignity, maintaining a sense of humor, having a physician who knows one as a whole person, presence of close friends, not dying alone, and having someone who will listen. Finally, five items were linked to patients' relationships with health care professionals: receiving care from one's personal physician, trusting one's physician, having a nurse with whom one feels comfortable, knowing that one's physician is comfortable talking about death and dying, and having a physician with whom one can discuss personal fears.

Attributes Important Among Patients   The second category included items that were consistently rated as important among patients (>70 percent) but were significantly less important to physicians ($P < .001$) (Table 11.3). These included being mentally aware, having funeral arrangements planned, feeling that one's life was complete, not being a burden to family or society, being able to help others, coming to peace with God, and praying. These differences persisted after conducting multivariate analyses controlling for sex, race/ethnicity, socioeconomic status, household composition, religion, and religiosity (data available on request).

TABLE 11.1. Demographics of Survey Participants[a]

Characteristics	Patients (n = 340)	Bereaved Family Members (n = 332)	Physicians (n = 361)	Other Care Providers (n = 429)	Overall (n = 1,462)
Sex, male	78.2	21.3	81.7	27.3	51
Age, mean, y	68	62	52	51	57
Race/ethnicity					
African American	15.6	11.3	1.4	3.3	7.4
American					
Asian American	2.5	1.3	10.3	0.5	3.6
American					
White	69	77.8	80.4	94.8	81.6
Latino	2.8	2.8	2.8	0.7	2.2
Native American	8.6	6.3	0.3	0	3.4
American					
Other	1.5	0.6	4.7	0.7	1.9
Education					
Less than high school	30.4	22	NA	0	15.8
High school	44.2	48.3	NA	3.5	29.3
Associate of arts degree	10.1	9.6	NA	3.7	7.4
Bachelor's degree	5.8	9.9	NA	8.7	8.2
Graduate degree	9.5	10.2	100	84.1	39.3
Annual income, $					
0–9999	29.7	22.7	. . .	. . .	26.3
10,000–19,999	40.9	24.1	. . .	. . .	32.8
20,000–34,999	19.8	19.9	. . .	. . .	10.4
35,000–49,999	6.6	14.3	. . .	. . .	10.4
$\geq$50,000	3	18.9	. . .	. . .	10.7

Characteristics	Patients (n = 340)	Bereaved Family Members (n = 332)	Physicians (n = 361)	Other Care Providers (n = 429)	Overall (n = 1,462)
Religion					
Protestant	60.3	61.9	33.9	62.4	54.7
Roman Catholic	24.8	23.8	24.3	18.9	22.7
Jewish	1.5	0.6	18.1	5	6.5
Muslim	0	0	2.5	0	0.6
Other	3.6	5.1	9	3.5	5.3
No religion	9.7	8.6	12.1	10.2	10.2
Living arrangement					
With spouse	40.6	18.9	33.2	41.3	34
With parent	2.8	2.3	0.9	1.8	1.9
With child	20.8	35.4	55	43.1	36.7
Alone	35.8	43.4	10.9	30.6	24.5
Marital status					
Married	47.9	34.9	86.6	75.1	62.7
Widowed	17.6	50	2.8	3.3	17
Divorced/separated	27.9	11.1	3.1	10.8	12.9
Never married	6.7	4	7.5	10.8	7.5
Importance of faith					
Very important	61.3	72.3	47.5	81.1	66.2
Somewhat important	32	23.4	39.9	15.8	27.4
Not at all important	6.7	4.4	12.6	3.1	6.6
Attend religious service					
More than once a week	8.4	13.1	4	16.1	10.7
Every week	16.2	25.9	22.7	38.1	26.5
2–3 times a month	8.4	10.9	12.5	12.5	11.2
Once a month	15	9.3	18.1	7.1	12.2

(*continued overleaf*)

TABLE 11.1. **Demographics of Survey Participants**[a] *(Continued)*

Characteristics	Patients (n = 340)	Bereaved Family Members (n = 332)	Other Care Physicians (n = 361)	Providers (n = 429)	Overall (n = 1,462)
Once or twice a year	28.7	21.4	25.2	17.7	23
Never	23.4	19.2	17	8.5	16.4
General health					
Excellent	0.6	9.3	54.7	38.4	27.3
Very good	4.9	24.5	28.8	44.1	26.9
Good	20.7	37.9	14.5	14.4	21.2
Fair	41.7	23.6	1.4	2.8	16.1
Poor	32	4.7	0.6	0.2	8.6
Overall mood					
Not at all depressed	32.1	42.8	75.1	73	57.3
Slightly depressed	40.1	35.3	21.5	24.2	29.8
Moderately depressed	16.5	15	3.4	1.9	8.6
Quite depressed	8	5.3	0	0.5	3.2
Extremely depressed	3.4	1.6	0	0	1.1
Been with someone in their last hour of life	60.1	77.3	97.2	94.4	83.3

[a]All data except age are reported as percentages. NA indicates not applicable; ellipses, that physicians and other care providers were not asked to report their income.

Attributes With Broad Response Variation Among All Participants A final category comprised ten items with a broad distribution of responses among the four groups. These items included attributes relating to treatment preferences, preparation, and completion or spirituality (Table 11.4). For example, the groups showed wide response variation regarding the importance of knowing the timing of death. A slight majority of the sample agreed with the importance of meeting with a clergy member, having a chance to talk about the meaning of death, and discussing spiritual beliefs with one's physician. However, a sizable percentage of each group disagreed or neither agreed nor disagreed about the importance of these items (Table 11.4). Compared with patients, bereaved family members more frequently agreed with and physicians less frequently agreed with the importance of meeting with clergy.

TABLE 11.2. **Attributes Rated as Important by More Than 70 Percent of All Participants**

Participants Who Agreed That Attribute Is Very Important at End of Life, %

Attributes	Patients (n = 340)	Bereaved Family Members (n = 332)	Physicians (n = 361)	Other Care Providers (n = 429)
Be kept clean	99	99	99	99
Name a decision maker	98	98	98	99
Have a nurse with whom one feels comfortable	97	98	91	98
Know what to expect about one's physical condition	96	93	88	94
Have someone who will listen	95	98	99	99
Maintain one's dignity	95	98	99	99
Trust one's physician	94	97	99	97
Have financial affairs in order	94	94	91	90
Be free of pain	93	95	99	97
Maintain sense of humor	93	87	79	85
Say goodbye to important people	90	92	95	99
Be free of shortness of breath	90	87	93	87
Be free of anxiety	90	91	90	90
Have physician with whom one can discuss fears	90	91	94	93
Have physician who knows one as a whole person	88	92	92	95
Resolve unfinished business with family or friends	86	85	87	97
Have physical touch	86	94	90	97
Know that one's physician is comfortable talking about death and dying	86	85	93	97
Share time with close friends	85	91	91	96
Believe family is prepared for one's death	85	88	83	90

(continued overleaf)

TABLE 11.2. **Attributes Rated as Important by More Than 70 Percent of All Participants** (Continued)

Participants Who Agreed That Attribute Is Very Important at End of Life, %

Attributes	Patients (n = 340)	Bereaved Family Members (n = 332)	Physicians (n = 361)	Other Care Providers (n = 429)
Feel prepared to die	84	81	79	87
Presence of family	81	95	95	96
Treatment preferences in writing	81	85	73	90
Not die alone	75	93	84	88
Remember personal accomplishments	74	80	78	91
Receive care from personal physician	73	77	82	82

TABLE 11.3. **Attributes Rated as Important by More Than 70 Percent of Patients But Not Physiciansa**

Attributes	Participants Who Agreed That Attribute Is Very Important at End of Life, %	
	Patients	Physicians
Be mentally aware	92	65
Be at peace with God	89	65
Not be a burden to family	89	58
Be able to help others	88	44
Pray	85	55
Have funeral arrangements planned	82	58
Not be a burden to society	81	44
Feel one's life is complete	80	68

$P < .001$ for all comparisons.

TABLE 11.4. Attributes with Broad Variation among Participants Regarding Importance at End of Life

Attributes	Patients, %			Bereaved Family Members, %			Physicians, %			Other Care Providers, %		
	Agree	Disagree	Neither	Agree	Disagree	Neither	Agree	Disagree	Neither	Agree	Disagree	Neither
Use all available treatments no matter what the chance of recovery	48	31	22	38	44	18	7	81	12	5	83	12
Not be connected to machines	64	16	20	63	17	20	50	9	41	61	10	30
Know the timing of one's death	39	22	39	49	16	35	26	29	46	35	18	47
Control the time and place of one's death	40	24	35	38	22	40	36	25	39	44	25	30
Discuss personal fears	61	11	28	80	4	16	88	1	11	94	1	5
Die at home	35	12	53	30	16	54	44	5	51	46	2	52
Be with one's pets	37	18	45	47	10	44	42	8	50	73	2	24
Meet with a clergy member	69	7	24	83	1	17	60	4	36	70	1	30
Have a chance to talk about the meaning of death	58	9	33	72	3	26	66	5	29	86	1	12
Discuss spiritual beliefs with one's physician	50	13	37	54	7	39	49	10	41	51	7	42

Multivariate Analyses

Multivariate models were created controlling for role, sex, race/ethnicity, income, education, religion, religiosity, being present during the last hour of someone's life, household composition, self-reported health status, and, for patients, diagnosis. Only ORs that were significant are presented herein.

Use of All Available Treatments   Physicians (OR, 0.1; 95 percent CI, 0.1–0.2) and other care providers (OR, 0.08; 95 percent CI, 0.04–0.14) were significantly less likely than patients to agree with the importance of using all available treatments no matter what the chance of recovery, whereas bereaved family members were equally likely to agree (OR, 0.8; 95 percent CI, 0.6–3.3). African American (OR, 3.3; 95 percent CI, 2.0–4.0) and other nonwhite ethnic groups (OR, 2.5; 95 percent CI, 1.4–3.3) were significantly more likely than white participants to agree with the importance of using all available treatments. Persons who had not been present during the last hour of another person's life were also more likely to agree (OR, 1.7; 95 percent CI, 1.0–2.5). Sex, religion, and the other variables were not associated with the response to this question. Among patients and bereaved family members, respondents with more education (bachelor's degree, OR, 0.5; 95 percent CI, 0.30.8; graduate/professional degree, OR, 0.4; 95 percent CI, 0.2–0.9 versus no college) and higher annual income ($20,000–$40,000, OR, 1.0; 95 percent CI, 0.6–1.7; ≥ $50,000, OR, 0.3; 95 percent CI, 0.2–0.8 versus < $20,000) were significantly less likely to agree with the importance of use of all available treatments.

Controlling Time and Place of Death   Religiosity was the only covariate significantly associated with preference for controlling the time and place of death. Participants who considered faith or spirituality not at all important were significantly more likely (OR, 1.7; 95 percent CI, 1.1–2.0) than were those who considered it very important to agree with the importance of such control.

Dying at Home   Other care providers (OR, 1.7; 95 percent CI, 1.1–2.0) were significantly more likely to agree with the importance of dying at home, compared with patients. Physicians (OR, 1.4; 95 percent CI, 1.0–2.0) and bereaved family members (OR, 0.8; 95 percent CI, 0.6–1.3) were not significantly different from patients. Roman Catholic (OR, 1.4; 95 percent CI, 1.02.0) and "other" respondents were significantly less likely than Protestants (the reference point) or Jews (OR, 0.8; 95 percent CI, 0.5–1.3) to disagree. Separate logistic analyses showed no significant covariates among patients and families.

Talking About the Meaning of Death   Physicians (OR, 2.0; 95 percent CI, 1.3–2.5), other care providers (OR, 1.7; 95 percent CI, 1.1–2.0), and bereaved family members (OR, 1.7; 95 percent CI, 1.1–2.7) were significantly more likely than patients to agree that talking about the meaning of death is important. Those for whom faith or spirituality was not at all (OR, 0.3; 95 percent CI, 0.2–0.5) or somewhat (OR, 0.4; 95 percent CI,

0.3–0.6) important were significantly less likely than those for whom spirituality was very important to agree that this attribute was important. Among patients and family members, women were significantly more likely to agree with talking about the meaning of death (OR, 2.0; 95 percent CI, 1.3–2.5).

Ranking Attributes

We measured the mean rank scores for the nine preselected attributes, with 1 being most important and 9 being least important (Table 11.5). Friedman tests were significant ($P <$ .001), suggesting that the rankings by each group were different than would be expected by chance alone. Freedom from pain was ranked as most important (that is, received the lowest mean score) by patients (3.07), bereaved family members (2.99), physicians (2.36), and other care providers (2.83). Coming to peace with God and presence of family were ranked second or third in importance in all groups. For patients and families, the difference between the ranking of freedom from pain and being at peace with God was trivial (0.09 and 0.12 difference, respectively), suggesting that these items are nearly identical in importance for both groups. Physicians' mean score difference between the items was 2.46; other care providers had a difference of 0.88 in mean score ($P <$ .001). Of note, dying at home received the least important relative ranking by all groups except other care providers, who ranked it second to last.

TABLE 11.5. **Mean Rank Scores of 9 Preselected Attributes[a]**

Attributes	Patients	Bereaved Family Members	Physicians	Other Care Providers
Freedom from pain	3.07 (1)	2.99 (1)	2.36 (1)	2.83 (1)
At peace with God	3.16 (2)	3.11 (2)	4.82 (3)	3.71 (3)
Presence of family	3.93 (3)	3.30 (3)	3.06 (2)	2.90 (2)
Mentally aware	4.58 (4)	5.41 (5)	6.12 (7)	5.91 (7)
Treatment choices followed	5.51 (5)	5.27 (4)	5.15 (5)	5.14 (5)
Finances in order	5.60 (6)	6.12 (7)	6.35 (8)	7.41 (9)
Feel life was meaningful	5.88 (7)	5.63 (6)	5.02 (4)	4.58 (4)
Resolve conflicts	6.23 (8)	6.33 (8)	5.31 (6)	5.38 (6)
Die at home	7.03 (9)	6.89 (9)	6.78 (9)	7.14 (8)

[a]Attributes are listed in the mean rank order based on patient response. Numbers in parentheses are mean rank order, with lowest rank score (1) indicating most important attribute and highest rank score (9) indicating least important. Friedman tests were significant at $P <$ .001, suggesting that rankings by each group were different from what would be expected by chance alone.

COMMENT

Our results reveal areas of strong agreement and variation among end-of-life care participants' definitions of what constitutes a good death. More than half of the survey items
showed consensus among all four groups. For example, in concert with previous findings in the palliative care literature, survey participants overwhelmingly endorsed pain
and symptom management.[14-16] Regardless of role, respondents also converged on the
importance of preparation for the end of life. These findings echo the results of a recent
study that showed that many patients wish to plan ahead for their own deaths and support
the importance of prognostication in clinical practice.[17-20] Additionally, respondents
expressed a strong preference for having an opportunity to gain a sense of completion
in their lives. Life review, saying good-bye, and resolving unfinished business provide
both patients and their families with an opportunity for human development at the end
of life.[21] Finally, all groups advocated strong relationships between patients and health
care professionals that emphasized more than just the patient's disease.

Results of this study also highlight one of the challenges of comprehensive end-
of-life care: attending to aspects of care that are not intuitively important to clinicians
but are critical to patients and their families. For example, in contrast with physicians,
patients strongly endorsed the importance of being mentally aware. When forced to
choose between attributes (Table 11.5), patients ranked pain control higher than mental
awareness; however, the mean rank difference was only 1.51. In contrast, the average
difference between the same items among physicians was 3.76, suggesting physicians
may be more willing than patients to sacrifice lucidity for analgesia. Similarly, other care
providers generally emphasize what patients need to receive, but our results indicate that
being able to help others is central to patients' conceptions of quality at the end of life.[13]
Finally, patients highly valued attention to spirituality; in particular, the importance of
coming to peace with God and praying. Rank-ordered responses showed that coming
to peace with God and pain control were nearly identical in importance for patients and
bereaved family members.

Perhaps the most interesting findings of our study are items for which there was
broad response variation within and across all groups. They serve as a reminder that
there is no one definition of a good death; quality end-of-life care is a dynamic process
that is negotiated and renegotiated among patients, families, and health care professionals, a process moderated by individual values, knowledge, and preferences for
care. We choose to illustrate this point with discussion of four critical issues raised in
the survey.

Consistent with previous research,[22,23] African Americans had higher odds than
white participants of wanting all available treatments, which may reflect a preference
for life-sustaining treatment or distrust of the predominantly white medical culture.[22]
The disagreement by physicians and other care providers with use of all available
treatments may reflect greater familiarity with life-sustaining treatments. In one study,
patients were less likely to want cardiopulmonary resuscitation after receiving additional
information about the procedure.[24] In addition, despite many patients valuing use of
all treatments, most disagreed with the importance of being connected to machines. In
contrast, physicians equate these interventions and disagreed with both.

Respondents displayed broad variation in their desire to control time and place of death. Those with less religiosity were most likely to want control.

Given the strong public support for the hospice movement and its emphasis on home care, we expected to find overwhelming preference for dying at home.[25] However, fewer than half of all participants in our sample agreed that this was an important attribute in quality of dying. Moreover, dying at home was consistently ranked least in importance among nine selected attributes. Religion and role were associated with a preference for dying at home. Recently, Fried and colleagues demonstrated a similar preference among older adults.[26] The notion of dying at home may be romantic among health care professionals who want to provide a good death. However, as symptoms accelerate in the last twenty-four to forty-eight hours, some patients and families may feel overwhelmed by concerns about symptom control or a dead body in the home and therefore prefer a skilled care environment.[26] Therefore, although for many patients an appropriate goal is to allow them to die at home, this should not be assumed.

While we anticipated that religiosity and female sex would be associated with a desire to talk about the meaning of death, we did not expect that physicians, other care providers, and bereaved family members would be more likely to agree with its importance than were patients. Similarly, patients as a group were least likely to rate discussing personal fears as important. All groups lacked consensus in assigning importance to meeting with clergy and discussing spiritual beliefs with one's physician. Spirituality, however, was clearly important to patients, as illustrated by their strong consensus surrounding the need for coming to peace with God and praying. These findings suggest that for some patients, issues of faith that are resolved with oneself are more important than social or interpersonal expressions of spirituality.[27]

This study has several limitations. Patients and family members were recruited from VA medical centers; therefore, generalizations to other groups should be made cautiously. However, participants' preferences reflected death in a variety of settings, and patients and families participating in the study represented broad age, educational, and socioeconomic ranges. The individuals comprising other care providers are a diverse group and are not necessarily expected to form a cohesive whole. However, given their role in end-of-life care, it is important to determine their viewpoints, although future studies should evaluate differences within these groups.

CONCLUSIONS

The results of this survey suggest that for patients and families, physical care is expectedly crucial but is only one component of total care. Whereas physicians tend to focus on physical aspects, patients and families tend to view the end of life with broader psychosocial and spiritual meaning, shaped by a lifetime of experiences. While physicians' biomedical focus is a natural outgrowth of medical care that emphasizes the physical self, physicians should recognize patients' other needs and facilitate means for them to be addressed. Physicians also should recognize that there is no one definition of a good death. Quality care at the end of life is highly individual and should be achieved through a process of shared decision making and clear communication that acknowledges the values and preferences of patients and their families.

Patients, families, and care providers each play a critical role in shaping the experience at the end of life. As our cultural lexicon of death and dying expands, further research is needed to define both the common ground and areas for negotiation as participants gather to construct quality at the end of life. A challenge to medicine is to design flexible care systems that permit a variety of expressions of a good death.

REFERENCES

1. SUPPORT Principal Investigators. A controlled trial to improve care for seriously ill hospitalized patients. *JAMA.* 1995; 274:1591–1598.

2. Wanzer S, Federman D, Adelstein S, et al. The physician's responsibility toward hopelessly ill patients: a second look. *N Engl J Med.* 1989; 320:844–849.

3. Garvin J, Chapman C. Clinical management of dying patients. *West J Med.* 1995; 163:268–277.

4. Council on Scientific Affairs, American Medical Association. Good care of the dying patient. *JAMA.* 1996; 275:474–478.

5. Field M, Cassel C. *Approaching Death.* Washington, DC: Institute of Medicine; 1997.

6. Gibson R. The Robert Wood Johnson grantmaking strategies to improve care at the end of life. *J Palliat Med.* 1998; 1:415–417.

7. Addington-Hall J, MacDonald LD, Anderson HR, Freeling P. Dying from cancer: the views of bereaved family and friends about experiences of terminally ill patients. *Palliat Med.* 1991; 5:207–214.

8. Seale C. Communication and awareness about death. *Soc Sci Med.* 1991; 32:943–952.

9. Seale C, Addington-Hall J. Dying at the best time. *Soc Sci Med.* 1995; 40:589–595.

10. Schmidt T, Harrahill R. Family response to out-of-hospital death. *Acad Emerg Med.* 1995; 2:513–518.

11. Hendrick C, Borden R, Geisen M, Murray J, Seyfried B. Effectiveness of integration tactics in a cover letter on mail questionnaire response. *Psychon Sci.* 1972; 26:349–351.

12. Childers T, Ferrell O. Response rates and perceived questionnaire length in mail surveys. *J Market Res.* 1979; 16:429–431.

13. Steinhauser K, Clipp E, McNeilly M, Christakis N, McIntyre L, Tulsky J. In search of a good death: observations of patients, families, and health care providers. *Ann Intern Med.* 2000; 132:825–832.

14. Singer P, Martin D, Merrijoy K. Quality end-of-life care. *JAMA.* 1999; 281:163–168.

15. Solomon M. The enormity of the task: the SUPPORT study and changing practice. *Hastings Cent Rep.* 1995; 25:S28–S32.

16. Hanson L, Danis M, Garrett J. What is wrong with end-of-life care? opinions of bereaved family members. *J Am Geriatr Soc.* 1997; 45:1339–1344.

17. Emanuel E, Emanuel L. The promise of a good death. *Lancet.* 1998; 251:21–29.

18. Martin DK, Theil EC, Singer PA. A new model of advance care planning. *Arch Intern Med.* 1999; 159: 86–92.

19. Christakis N. *Death Foretold: Prophecy and Prognosis in Medical Care.* Chicago, Ill: University of Chicago Press; 2000.

20. Christakis N, Iwashyna T. Attitude of self-reported practice regarding prognostication in a national sample of internists. *Arch Intern Med.* 1998; 158:2389–2395.

21. Erikson E. *The Life Cycle Completed: A Review.* New York, NY: WW Norton; 1982.

22. Tulsky J, Cassileth B, Bennett C. The effect of ethnicity on ICU use and DNR orders in hospitalized AIDS patients. *J Clin Ethics.* 1997; 126:381–388.

23. Garrett J, Harris R, Norburn J, Patrick D, Danis M. Life-sustaining treatments during terminal illness: who wants what? *J Gen Intern Med.* 1993; 8:361–368.

24. O'Brien L, Grisso J, Maislin G, et al. Nursing home residents' preferences for life-sustaining treatments. *JAMA.* 1995; 274:1775–1779.

25. National Hospice Organization. *New Findings Address Escalating End-of-Life Debate.* Arlington, Va: National Hospice Organization; 1996.

26. Fried T, van Doorn C, O'Leary J, Tinetti M, Drickamer M. Older persons' preference for site of terminal care. *Ann Intern Med.* 1999; 131:109–112.

27. King D. Beliefs and attitudes of hospital inpatients about faith healing and prayer. *J Fam Pract.* 1994; 39:349–352.

FUNDING/SUPPORT

This work was supported by VA Health Services Research and Development Grant IIR 96–066. Dr. Tulsky is supported by a VA Health Services Research Career Development Award and a Robert Wood Johnson Generalist Physician Faculty Scholars Award. Drs. Tulsky and Christakis are Project on Death in America Soros Faculty Scholars.

DISCLAIMER

The views expressed in this article are those of the authors and do not necessarily represent the views of the Department of Veterans Affairs.

ACKNOWLEDGMENT

We are grateful to Steven C. Grambow, Ph.D., for his expert and thorough consultation on statistical analyses.

12

USE OF HOSPITALS, PHYSICIAN VISITS, AND HOSPICE CARE DURING LAST SIX MONTHS OF LIFE AMONG COHORTS LOYAL TO HIGHLY RESPECTED HOSPITALS IN THE UNITED STATES

JOHN E. WENNBERG, ELLIOTT S. FISHER, THÉRÈSE A. STUKEL, JONATHAN S. SKINNER, SANDRA M. SHARP, AND KRISTEN K. BRONNER

EDITORS' INTRODUCTION

John E. Wennberg and his colleagues have linked their observations about the variability in medical care practices in different regions of the United States to quality, though it is difficult to define what the "right" level of care should be. This article identifies striking variation in intensity of hospital and specialist care for seriously ill patients cared for at *U.S. News & World Report* "best hospitals."

■ ■ ■

INTRODUCTION

The frequency of use of hospitals, intensive care units, and physician visits among patients with chronic illness varies extensively across hospital regions in the United States, including regions served by well-known academic medical centres. The variations are unrelated to population-based measures of need but are closely associated with the per capita supply of hospital beds and physicians.[1-4] The variations in frequency of use of these "supply sensitive" services during the last six months of life are particularly striking.[1] These variations are of concern because they do not seem to reflect patients' preferences or rates of illness. Moreover, patients with chronic illnesses who live in regions with high rates of use do not seem to have better health outcomes.[5-7] For these reasons, we have argued that the research agenda for academic medical centres should give high priority to comparative studies of their own patterns of practice with the goal of rationalizing the management of chronically ill patients and answering questions about how many hospital beds and physicians are needed to provide optimal care.[5,8] An important first step is to obtain population-based performance measures specific to academic medical centres. In this paper, we document extensive variations in end-of-life care among cohorts of patients enrolled in Medicare who receive most of their inpatient care at well-known academic medical centres in the United States.

METHODS

Selection of Cohorts

Hospital-specific utilisation measures are feasible because patients, particularly those with chronic illness, tend to receive most of their inpatient care from a given hospital.[4] For this study, we identified those patients who received most of their inpatient care during the last two years of their lives from a hospital that appeared on the 2001 *U.S. News & World Report* list of "America's best hospitals" for geriatric care and for the treatment of three common chronic illnesses: heart disease, cancer, and pulmonary disease.[9] By using Medicare's hospital admission files for all Medicare patients who died in 1999–2000, we assigned decedents to the hospital used most often during the last two years of life. In the case of a tie, assignment was to the last hospital used before death. We included only decedents who had been continuously enrolled in traditional Medicare during that period. We generated utilisation measures for the cohorts assigned to the selected hospitals. The databases used to generate performance measures included a 100 percent sample of hospital admissions and hospice enrolments and a 20 percent sample of claims from physicians and laboratories.

Outcome Measures

The measures of utilisation during the last six months of life included the number of days spent in hospital ("hospital days"), the number of days spent in intensive care units ("ICU days"), the number of physician visits, the percentage of patients seeing ten or more physicians, and the percentage of patients enrolled in a hospice. Measures of intensity of terminal care included the percentage of deaths occurring in hospital and the percentage of deaths involving a stay in an intensive care unit.

Statistical Analysis

We used Iezzoni's approach to coding chronic conditions.[10] On the basis of diagnoses that appeared on the record of the last hospital admission, we determined the presence of up to eleven chronic conditions and used these conditions to adjust for differences among cohorts in underlying rates of disease. The denominator for calculating utilisation rates in the last six months of life was the full six months of observation before death. We calculated crude hospital-specific rates by using the number of cohort members assigned to the hospital as the denominator.

In this paper, we have adjusted the hospital and visit rates directly for age, sex, race, and illness by using overdispersed Poisson regression models.[11] In the regression models, the dependent variable was the total event count per decedent and the independent variables were indicator variables for the study hospitals and for age (five categories), sex, race (nonblack, black), and chronic condition (eleven dichotomous variables). We centred all covariates about the population mean so that the rates reflect an average member of the study population. As patients were nested within hospitals, we used the overdispersion parameter to adjust the confidence intervals for correlations among outcomes of patients within the same cohort. We used overdispersed logistic regression to analyse events that could occur only once (for example, enrolment in a hospice). To transform the hospital-specific regression coefficients into a directly standardized rate on the original scale, we exponentiated and calibrated them so that they had the same overall mean as the crude hospital-specific rates.

We evaluated relations between hospital-specific rates by using product-moment correlation. We used the coefficient of variation and interquartile and extremal range ratios to compare the degree of variation among utilisation measures. We also compared variation graphically by displaying the directly standardised rate for each hospital, expressed as a ratio to the mean rate among the seventy-seven hospital cohorts.

Final Sample of Hospital Specific Cohorts

Ninety-two acute general hospitals appeared one or more times on the *U.S. News & World Report* list for 2001. We excluded hospitals with fewer than one hundred decedents with data for physician claims, leaving seventy-seven hospital cohorts. In keeping with the principles of population-based epidemiology, performance measures reflect the total amount of care received, regardless of where or by whom care was provided. However, as patient loyalty (defined as percentage of all days in hospital that occurred in the assigned hospital) tended to be strong, the measures primarily reflect services undertaken by providers affiliated with the medical centre to which the patients were assigned. Among the seventy-seven hospital-specific cohorts, patient loyalty, measured over the two years before death, ranged from 64.6 percent to 91.9 percent, with a median of 82.5 percent and a mean of 81.4 percent.

Results

Table 12.1 shows the characteristics of the study population. Of the 115,089 patients, 98,415 (85 percent) were chronically ill, many with two or more conditions. The intensity of care during the last six months of life and at the time of death varied substantially. The figure shows the standardised utilisation ratios and statistical measures of variation among the seventy-seven hospital cohorts. Among the seventy-seven hospital cohorts, the average number of days spent in hospital during the last six months of life was more than 27 days—almost a month—in the highest-ranked cohort and fewer than 10 days in the lowest-ranked cohort. Average ICU days varied by a factor of six, from 1.6 to 9.5 days per person; physician visits varied by a factor of four, from less than eighteen to more than seventy-six visits per decedent. The propensity to use multiple physicians varied from less than 17 percent of patients seeing ten or more physicians in the last six months of life to more than 58 percent of patients. The percentage of deaths occurring in hospital ranged from less than 16 percent to more than 55 percent; deaths associated with a stay in an intensive care unit varied from less than 9 percent to more than 36 percent. Enrolment in a hospice varied among the cohorts from less than 11 percent of decedents to more than 43 percent.

Table 12.2 examines the intensity of care during the last six months for cohorts loyal to major teaching hospitals located in metropolitan regions with two or more major teaching hospitals. They are ranked according to the (unweighted) average number of patient days per decedent. By this measure, the hospitals located in Manhattan provided the most care. Other regions with high hospital day rates included Los Angeles, Philadelphia, and Washington, D.C. Patient cohorts loyal to the teaching hospitals in these regions also tended to have a higher frequency of physician visits, and a higher proportion saw ten or more physicians. However, the use of intensive care units varied: the rates were high among the listed teaching hospital cohorts in

TABLE 12.1. **Illness and Demographic Characteristics Among Patients Assigned to 77 Hospital Cohorts.**[a]

Characteristic	Patients (*n* = 115,089)
Chronic conditions	
Cancer: solid tumours	31,764 (27.6)
Lymphomas and leukaemias	6,279 (5.5)
AIDS	103 (0.1)
Chronic pulmonary disease	25,864 (22.5)
Coronary artery disease	9,931 (8.6)
Congestive heart failure	37,584 (32.7)
Peripheral vascular disease	5,958 (5.2)
Severe chronic liver disease	2,317 (2.0)
Diabetes with end organ damage	2,902 (2.5)
Chronic renal failure	6,809 (5.9)
Nutritional deficiencies	12,068 (10.5)
Dementia	17,062 (14.8)
Functional impairment	3,040 (2.6)
No. of chronic conditions:	
None	17,674 (15.4)
1 only	49,568 (43.1)
2 only	33,914 (29.5)
3 only	11,656 (10.1)
≥4	2,277 (2.0)
Demographic characteristics:	
Age 65–69	12,912 (11.2)
Age 70–74	19,811 (17.2)
Age 75–79	23,545 (20.5)
Age 80–84	22,995 (20.0)
Age ≥85	35,826 (31.1)
Male	52,313 (45.5)
Female	62,776 (54.5)
Non-black	97,740 (84.9)
Black	17,349 (15.1)

[a]Values are numbers (percentages).

TABLE 12.2. Age, Sex, Race, and Illness Adjusted Rates (95% Confidence Intervals) for Hospital Days, Days in Intensive Care, and Physician Visits and Percentage Seeing 10 or More Physicians During Last Six Months of Life Among Patient Cohorts Loyal to Selected Academic Medical Centres by Region of Location

Hospital by Region[a]	Hospital Days per Decedent	ICU[b] Days per Decedent	Physician Visits per Decedent	% Seeing ≥10 Physicians
New York (23.8)				
Mount Sinai Hospital	22.8 (22.1 to 23.5)	2.8 (2.6 to 3.0)	53.9 (50.6 to 57.4)	58.5 (51.8 to 66.0)
New York Presbyterian Hospital	21.6 (21.0 to 22.2)	4.5 (4.2 to 4.7)	40.3 (37.9 to 42.8)	37.7 (33.2 to 42.7)
NYU Medical Center-University Hospital	27.1 (26.1 to 28.1)	6.7 (6.4 to 7.2)	76.2 (71.3 to 81.3)	57.1 (49.0 to 66.4)
Los Angeles (18.7)				
UCLA Medical Center	16.1 (15.2 to 17.1)	9.2 (8.6 to 9.8)	43.9 (39.7 to 48.5)	50.9 (42.2 to 61.4)
Cedars-Sinai Medical Center	21.3 (20.6 to 22.0)	7.0 (6.7 to 7.4)	66.2 (62.7 to 69.9)	48.2 (42.5 to 54.8)
Washington, DC (18.4)				
Georgetown University Hospital	18.5 (17.3 to 19.8)	3.6 (3.1 to 4.1)	43.0 (37.2 to 49.7)	55.1 (42.6 to 71.3)
Washington Hospital Center	18.2 (17.4 to 19.0)	3.0 (2.7 to 3.2)	37.0 (33.5 to 40.9)	39.4 (32.5 to 47.9)
Philadelphia (18.3)				
Hospital of the University of Pennsylvania	17.2 (16.2 to 18.2)	3.8 (3.4 to 4.2)	40.3 (35.7 to 45.5)	44.7 (35.4 to 56.4)
Thomas Jefferson University Hospital	19.4 (18.6 to 20.2)	9.5 (9.1 to 10.0)	55.0 (50.8 to 59.4)	53.7 (45.8 to 62.8)
Baltimore (16.3)				
Johns Hopkins Hospital	16.1 (15.2 to 17.0)	3.2 (2.9 to 3.5)	28.1 (24.9 to 31.7)	36.7 (29.6 to 45.4)
Francis Scott Key Medical Center	16.5 (15.7 to 17.5)	5.7 (5.3 to 6.1)	23.0 (20.0 to 26.5)	29.4 (22.9 to 37.9)
Chicago (16.1)				
University of Chicago Hospital	13.4 (12.6 to 14.3)	3.5 (3.2 to 3.9)	30.2 (26.6 to 34.3)	41.7 (33.5 to 51.9)
Rush-Presbyterian-St Luke's Medical Center	17.9 (16.9 to 19.0)	4.5 (4.1 to 4.9)	48.9 (44.1 to 54.3)	35.1 (27.4 to 44.9)
Northwestern Memorial Hospital	17.1 (16.3 to 17.9)	3.5 (3.2 to 3.8)	34.9 (31.7 to 38.4)	40.4 (33.8 to 48.3)

Hospital by Region[a]	Hospital Days per Decedent	ICU[b] Days per Decedent	Physician Visits per Decedent	% Seeing ≥10 Physicians
Boston (14.5)				
Boston Medical Center	15.6 (14.5 to 16.8)	3.9 (3.5 to 4.4)	31.5 (27.0 to 36.6)	47.8 (37.2 to 61.4)
Massachusetts General Hospital	16.5 (15.8 to 17.1)	2.5 (2.3 to 2.7)	38.8 (35.8 to 41.9)	46.2 (40.0 to 53.3)
Beth Israel Deaconess Medical Center	12.2 (11.6 to 12.8)	2.4 (2.2 to 2.6)	29.2 (26.5 to 32.2)	34.3 (28.7 to 41.1)
Brigham and Women's Hospital	13.9 (13.1 to 14.7)	3.2 (2.9 to 3.6)	31.9 (28.3 to 36.0)	43.7 (35.6 to 53.6)
St. Louis (14.5)				
Barnes-Jewish Hospital	16.1 (15.6 to 16.7)	4.4 (4.2 to 4.7)	29.5 (27.3 to 31.9)	30.9 (26.5 to 36.0)
St Louis University Hospital	12.9 (12.0 to 13.9)	6.1 (5.6 to 6.7)	31.5 (27.0 to 36.7)	38.1 (28.7 to 50.4)
Cleveland (13.0)				
University Hospitals of Cleveland	12.5 (11.9 to 13.2)	2.4 (2.2 to 2.6)	26.0 (23.3 to 29.0)	30.5 (25.0 to 37.4)
Cleveland Clinic	13.4 (12.8 to 14.1)	3.0 (2.8 to 3.3)	30.9 (28.2 to 33.9)	45.9 (39.5 to 53.4)
Minneapolis (11.4)				
Hennepin County Medical Center	9.6 (8.7 to 10.6)	4.0 (3.6 to 4.5)	18.1 (14.7 to 22.4)	28.3 (20.1 to 39.8)
Fairview-University Medical Center	13.3 (12.3 to 14.4)	2.3 (1.9 to 2.6)	23.9 (20.0 to 28.6)	34.8 (25.8 to 46.9)
San Francisco/Bay Area (10.8)				
University of CA San Francisco Medical Center	11.5 (10.6 to 12.4)	2.6 (2.3 to 3.0)	27.2 (23.0 to 32.2)	30.3 (22.0 to 41.9)
Stanford University Hospital	10.1 (9.4 to 10.9)	4.3 (4.0 to 4.7)	22.6 (19.4 to 26.3)	23.1 (17.1 to 31.3)

[a]Regions ranked by unweighted average for patient days among listed hospital cohorts; average given in parentheses.
[b]ICU: intensive care unit.

Los Angeles, low in Washington, D.C., and varied substantially according to specific hospital cohorts in Philadelphia and New York. Cohorts in Boston and St. Louis exhibited considerable within-area variation in hospital days and ICU days. By contrast, those in Minneapolis and San Francisco had low rates on all four measures of intensity of care in the last six months of life.

The observed variation could have been generated by substitution between hospital use, physician visits, and hospice care. Enrolment in a hospice was inversely correlated with hospital days in the last six months of life (r = −0.41; P < 0.0002), the chance of dying in a hospital (r = −0.51; P < 0.0001), and the percentage of deaths occurring in association with a stay in the intensive care unit (r = −0.28; P = 0.012). However, the percentage enrolled in a hospice was not correlated significantly (P > 0.05) with fewer physician visits, seeing ten or more physicians, or ICU days in the last six months of life. We found a strong positive correlation between the number of days spent in hospital and the number of physician visits within the last six months of life (r = 0.77; P < 0.0001).

FIGURE 12.1. *Distribution of rates and statistical measures of variation for end of life care among 77 cohorts assigned to hospitals with national reputations for high quality ICU-intensive care unit.*

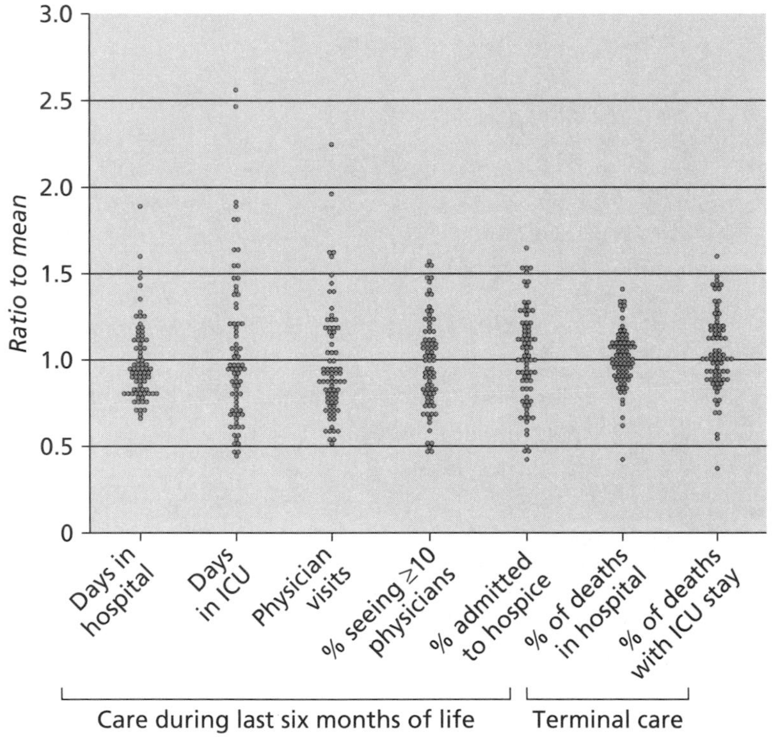

	Care during last six months of life				Terminal care		
Mean	14.5	3.72	34.1	37.3	26.9	39.6	23.1
Interquartile ratio	1.38	1.72	1.55	1.47	1.46	1.22	1.34
Extremal ratio	2.89	5.85	4.33	3.46	4.05	3.50	4.38
Coefficient of variation	0.23	0.42	0.34	0.28	0.28	0.17	0.23

DISCUSSION

Academic medical centres in the United States with reputations for excellence differed dramatically in the care they provided to patients during the last six months of life. For example, patient cohorts loyal to the University of California Medical Center in San Francisco had, on average, twenty-seven physician visits, with 30 percent seeing ten or more physicians and spending an average of 11.5 days in hospital. For the New York University hospital cohort, average physician visits were seventy-six, nearly triple the frequency in San Francisco, with 57 percent seeing ten or more physicians and spending an average of 27.1 days in hospital. The context of terminal care also varied. For example, the chance that death was associated with a stay in an intensive care unit was 1.84 times greater for patients loyal to Cedars-Sinai Hospital in Los Angeles (36.8 percent) than for patients loyal to New York's Mt. Sinai Hospital (21.1 percent).

What Explains Such Variation?

Among regions, a direct relation exists between supply and utilization of services. The frequency of use of physician services is strongly associated with the local workforce supply,[1,12,13] and bed supply "explains" more than half of the variation in hospital admission rates for medical conditions.[1] The effect of bed supply is to influence the threshold for admitting patients with chronic illnesses such as congestive heart failure, chronic pulmonary obstructive disease, and cancer.[2-4,14] Finally, physicians have been shown to adapt their decisions about admission and discharge to the availability of intensive care unit beds, admitting more patients with lower severity of illness and extending their length of stay when more beds are available.[15,16] In the light of this evidence, the likely explanation for the variations in acute hospital care and physician visits is variation in bed and workforce capacity relative to the size of population loyal to the seventy-seven hospitals.

The key question is whether greater frequency of physician visits and hospital care for chronically ill patients (many of whom are in the sample of decedents) results in better health outcomes. Using a variety of measures, two randomised trials of elderly patients from the U.S. Veterans Affairs health care system found that more frequent office visits and more intensive primary care were associated with increased use of the hospital but no improvement in health or function.[17,18] Both studies found that more frequent office-based visits were associated with a nonsignificant increase in mortality. Recently, we compared practice patterns and health outcomes across regions of the United States that were similar in baseline health status but that differed by 60 percent in overall utilisation of services.[6] Greater frequency of use was associated with worse outcomes: quality and access to care were slightly worse in higher-spending regions, and mortality was between 2 percent and 5 percent higher, suggesting that overuse of supply-sensitive services was leading to harm, possibly because greater use of hospital and specialist care exposes populations to greater risks of medical errors.[7]

Limitations of the Study

Our study has limitations. Firstly, the focus was on acute hospital care and frequency of physician visits. With the exception of hospice care, we were unable to evaluate the contribution of community care services such as home health agencies or nursing homes. Interestingly, whereas hospice enrolment varied substantially among the seventy-seven cohorts, we did not find that increased use of hospice led to less use of intensive care units or physician visits during the last six months of life. It was, however, associated with fewer deaths in hospital and, to a lesser degree, with a decrease in the chance that death was associated with a stay in an intensive care unit. We had no information on patients' or caregivers' preferences for end-of-life care or on their satisfaction with the services provided, the effectiveness of pain control, or the degree of emotional or physical support provided by each health care system. However, the SUPPORT study documented deficiencies in these aspects of care across five major medical centres (two of which were included in our study) and showed that the differences in hospital care were due neither to case mix nor to patients' preferences.[19] Indeed, patients' stated preferences to avoid deaths in hospital were commonly unfulfilled, whereas the local bed supply was correlated with probability of dying in hospital.

Secondly, the "follow back" design means that we excluded patients who did not experience at least one hospital admission during their last two years of life. Among the 306 hospital referral regions in the *Dartmouth Atlas of Health Care*, the percentage of deaths in 1999–2000 without any hospital admission within two years of death (and hence unassigned to any hospital) ranged from 8 percent to 30 percent. Thus, we based end-of-life hospital admission rates on a denominator that is too small. Assuming that the unassigned deaths in the region are assigned in proportion to the total number of deaths at each hospital would suggest adjustment of each end-of-life variable by $1/(1 - x)$, where x is the fraction of "unassigned" deaths. Adjusting our variables in this way had little impact on our results, and if anything tended to increase rather than decrease dispersion across hospitals. Thirdly, we have underestimated loyalty for medical centres that use affiliated hospitals, because information on affiliation was not available.

Generalisability

Variations in end-of-life care among the best hospitals in the United States raise questions about the appropriate role for acute hospital care in the management of chronically ill patients. Patterns of practice during this period of care are highly correlated with variation at other stages in the progression of chronic illness. Thus end-of-life measures provide a good indicator of how hospitals are treating all patients with chronic illness, not just those near death.[6] Typically, hospital-level comparisons are confounded by differences in case mix across communities. However, all patients in the last six months of life are quite similar with regard to at least one critical case-mix adjuster—they are all dead within six months. This allows comparisons of use of hospitals during this period of life, with confidence that regional differences in illness are not an important cause of the variations seen. Although we have found

What Is Already Known on This Topic

Population-based rates of use of hospitals, intensive care units, and physician visits vary extensively across U.S. regions, particularly during the last six months of life.

Population-based rates are uncorrelated with illness and patients' preferences but are closely associated with the supply of hospital beds and physicians.

The outcomes of care are no better among the cohorts of patients with chronic illness who receive care in regions with higher rates of use of services.

What This Study Adds

Population-based rates of use of hospitals and physician services can be measured among populations loyal to specific hospitals.

End-of-life care varies extensively among patient cohorts who receive most of their care from well-known academic medical centres, even among those located in the same region.

Hospital-specific information opens the opportunity for academic medical centres to participate in studies to improve the quality and efficiency of care.

that regions allocating the least resources to patients at the end of life tend to have lower mortality and do better on other measures of quality for all of their patients,[7] this association needs to be tested in countries where the frequency of acute hospital care and physician visits is less than in the United States. We hope the international research community will focus on learning how to manage chronic illness better and how to provide end-of-life care determined by the needs and wants of patients and not the capacity of the acute care system.[20]

REFERENCES

1. Wennberg JE, Cooper MM, eds. The quality of medical care in the United States: a report on the Medicare program. *The Dartmouth atlas of health care 1999*. Chicago, IL: American Hospital Association Press, 1999.

2. Wennberg JE, Freeman JL, Culp WJ. Are hospital services rationed in New Haven or over-utilized in Boston? *Lancet*. 1987; i: 1185–8.

3. Wennberg JE, Freeman JL, Shelton RM, Bubolz TA. Hospital use and mortality among Medicare beneficiaries in Boston and New Haven. *N Engl J Med*. 1989; 321:1168–73.

4. Fisher ES, Wennberg JE, Stukel TA, Sharp SM. Hospital readmission rates for cohorts of Medicare beneficiaries in Boston and New Haven. *N Engl Med*. 1994; 331: 989–95.

5. Wennberg JE, Fisher ES, Skinner JS. Geography and the debate over Medicare reform. 2002. http://content.healthaffairs.org/cgi/content/full/hlthaff.w2.96v1/DC1 (accessed 4 Mar 2004).

6. Fisher ES, Wennberg DE, Stukel DA, Gottlieb D, Lucas FL, Pinder E. The implications of regional variations in Medicare spending: part 1, utilization of services and the quality of care. *Ann Intern Med*. 2003; 138:273–87.

7. Fisher ES, Wennberg DE, Stukel DA, Gottlieb D, Lucas FL, Pinder E. The implications of regional variations in Medicare spending: part 2, health outcomes and satisfaction with care. *Ann Intern Med*. 2003; 138: 288–98.

8. Wennberg, JE. Unwarranted variations in healthcare delivery: implications for academic medical centres. *BMJ*. 2002; 325: 961–4.

9. America's best hospitals. *U.S. News & World Report.* 2001; 131(3).

10. Iezzoni LI, Heeren T, Foley SM, Daley J, Hughes J, Coffman GA. Chronic conditions and risk of in-hospital death. *Health Serv Res.* 1994; 29: 435–60.

11. McCullagh P, Nelder JA. *Generalized linear models.* 2nd ed. New York: Chapman and Hall, 1989.

12. Wennberg J, Gittelsohn A. Small area variations in health care delivery: a population-based health information system can guide planning and regulatory decision-making. *Science.* 1973; 182: 1102–8.

13. Welch WP, Miller ME, Welch HG, Fisher ES, Wennberg JE. Geographic variation in expenditures for physicians' services in the United States. *N Engl J Med.* 1993; 328:621–7.

14. Fisher ES, Wennberg JE, Stukel TA, Skinner JS, Sharp SM, Freeman JL, et al. Associations among hospital capacity, utilization, and mortality of U.S. Medicare beneficiaries, controlling for sociodemographic factors. *Health Serv Res.* 2000; 34:1351–62.

15. Singer DE, Carr PL, Mulley AG, Thibault GE. Rationing intensive care—physician responses to a resource shortage. *N Engl J Med.* 1983; 309: 1155–60.

16. Strauss MJ, LoGerfo JP, Yeltatzie JA, Temkin N, Hudson LD. Rationing of intensive care unit services: an everyday occurrence. *JAMA.* 1986; 255: 1143–6.

17. Wasson JH, Gaudette C, Whaley F, Sauvigne A, Baribeau P, Welch HG. Telephone care as a substitute for routine clinic follow-up. *JAMA.* 1992; 267: 1788–93.

18. Weinberger M, Oddone EZ, Henderson WG, for the Veterans Affairs Cooperative Study Group on Primary Care and Hospital Readmission. Does increased access to primary care reduce hospital readmissions? *N Engl J Med.* 1996; 334: 1441–7.

19. Pritchard RS, Fisher ES, Teno JM, Sharp SM, Reding DJ, Knaus WA, et al. Influence of patient preferences and local health system characteristics on the place of death: study to understand prognoses and preferences for risks and outcomes of treatment. *J Am Geriatr Soc.* 1998; 46:1242–50.

20. Schneiderman LJ, Gilmer T, Teetzel HD, Dugan DO, Blustein J, Cranford R, et al. Effect of ethics consultations on nonbeneficial life-sustaining treatments in the intensive care setting: a randomized controlled trial. *JAMA.* 2003; 290:1166–72.

ETHICAL APPROVAL

Not needed.

CONTRIBUTORS

All authors were involved in developing the methods for measuring hospital specific performance. TAS and SMS did the statistical analyses. JEW wrote many drafts of the paper, and all authors contributed to the final draft. JEW is the guarantor.

FUNDING

Grant support by the Robert Wood Johnson Foundation and the National Institute of Aging (1PO1AG19783-01).

COMPETING INTERESTS

None declared.

13

FAMILY PERSPECTIVES ON END-OF-LIFE CARE AT THE LAST PLACE OF CARE

JOAN M. TENO, M.D., M.S., BRIAN R. CLARRIDGE, PH.D.,
VIRGINIA CASEY, PH.D., M.P.H., LISA C. WELCH, M.A., TERRIE WETLE, PH.D.,
RENEE SHIELD, PH.D., AND VINCENT MOR, PH.D.

This article originally appeared as Teno JM, Clarridge BR, Casey V, Welch LC, Wetle T, Shield R, Mor V. Family perspectives on end-of-life care at the last place of care. *JAMA.* 2004; 291(1):88–93. Copyright © 2004, American Medical Association. All rights reserved. Reprinted with permission.

EDITORS' INTRODUCTION

Joan M. Teno's body of research focuses on the experiences of seriously ill and dying patients and their families. This indictment of end-of-life care in the United States identified major quality problems with end-of-life care in hospitals, nursing homes, and home care agencies. In contrast, families rated highly the care received from hospice programs.

■ ■ ■

Over the past century, dying has become increasingly institutionalized. In the early 1900s most people died at home, but by the middle of the twentieth century the majority of deaths in industrialized nations occurred in health care institutions. With recent changes in health care, society is struggling with the role that governmental and non-governmental regulatory structures should play in ensuring that the health care system provides competent, coordinated, and compassionate care at life's end.[1]

Early efforts to define a "good death" were based on expert opinion.[2-4] Recent attempts have used focus groups and in-depth interviews to capture patient and family perspectives.[5-7] Several authors of the current study developed a conceptual model of quality of end-of-life care[7] with input from dying patients, their families, structured review of professional guidelines, and experts. This research indicates that high-quality end-of-life care results when health care professionals (1) ensure desired physical comfort and emotional support, (2) promote shared decision making, (3) treat the dying person with respect, (4) provide information and emotional support to family members, and (5) coordinate care across settings. Outcome measures based on each of these domains have been developed and validated.[8] The goal of this study was to use these measures to provide national estimates of the dying experience and to examine whether family members' perceptions of the quality of end-of-life care differed by the last place of care.

METHODS

We conducted a mortality follow-back survey of deaths in 2000. We contacted the informant listed on the death certificate, usually a close family member, to ask whether she or he knew how and where the decedent was treated in the last few weeks of life. If not, the informant was asked to identify another person who would know about the circumstances of the decedent's death and dying experience. Decedents dying as a result of trauma (for example, homicide, motor vehicle crashes) and decedents under the age of eighteen were excluded. The majority (72 percent) of the interviews were conducted between nine and fifteen months after the patient died.

A two-stage probability sample[9-10] (designed to select states, then individuals within states) was used to generate national estimates of the dying experience. Detailed information on the sampling and calculation of the weights is available at http://www.chcr.brown.edu/dying/factsondying.htm. Based on 1998 U.S. mortality data, two strata were created: eight states accounting for nearly one-half of the deaths in the United States were selected with certainty, and seventeen of the forty-two remaining states were randomly selected (because South Dakota law precludes release of death certificate data, it was not part of the frame). Wisconsin and New Mexico refused to participate, citing privacy concerns, and Georgia delayed data transfer too long for the data to be useable. Deaths in the twenty-two identified states accounted for 70.4 percent of all annual deaths in the United States. Restrictions placed by the New York City branch of the state vital statistics made inclusion untenable. The study design and informed consent procedures were reviewed by institutional review boards at Brown University, the University of Massachusetts, and within each participating state.

With this strategy we sampled 3,275 death certificates. For 549 (16.7 percent), an informant could not be located. Of the remaining 2,727 cases, 1,578 (57.9 percent) resulted in completed interviews, 3 were ineligible, 66 had no informant listed on the death certificate, 688 listed that informants refused to participate, 40 contacts reached households in which English was not spoken, and 12 informants were too ill to be interviewed. At the end of the field period, 335 cases were still active. Our assumption that an eligible respondent could have been found for about half the cases remaining in the field resulted in a conservative cooperation rate of 65 percent. To calculate national estimates, data were weighted to account for the sampling design and differential nonresponse among states. A total of 1,578 interviews represent 1.97 million deaths in the year 2000.

In comparing the available demographic information on death certificates resulting in interviews and those without interviews, there were no differences by sex ($P = .32$), but respondents representing decedents sixty-four years and younger were less likely to be interviewed (completion rate: 39.3 percent versus 50.6 percent; $P < .001$), as were Hispanic and African American respondents (35.6 percent versus 49.4 percent; $P < .001$).

Respondents were asked about quality of care at the last place the patient spent at least forty-eight hours. The main outcome measures were based on a conceptual model of patient-focused, family-centered medical care.[7] The first domain (that is, providing the desired level of physical comfort and emotional support)[8] was measured by unmet needs regarding pain, shortness of breath, or emotional distress. We calculated the rate of unmet needs for each symptom. A need was defined as unmet when the respondent reported that the patient did not receive any or not enough help with that symptom. The second domain (that is, promoting shared decision making) was considered unmet when the respondent reported that the patient had no contact with physicians but desired such contact, or when the informant expressed concerns with physician communication about shared decision making. We inquired whether the dying person was treated with respect by asking the respondent, "While [the patient] was at [the last place of care], how often was [he or she] treated with respect by those who were taking care of him/her—always, usually, sometimes, or never?" We report the rate of family respondents indicating that patients were not always treated with respect. We summarized each of the three remaining domains (that is, attending to family needs for information and emotional support, and coordinating care) as a count of the number of reported quality-of-care concerns as perceived by the informant. For these analyses, we compared those who expressed "no concern" with those who expressed "1 or more concerns." The actual survey tool, calculation of scores, and information on the psychometrics of the measures are available at http://www.chcr.brown.edu/dying/factsondying.htm.

All analyses were performed using SUDAAN version 8.0 (RTI International, Research Triangle Park, NC) to account for the complex sampling design. We used the χ^2 test to examine associations between reported perceptions of care and site of care. In the case of ordered responses, the Mantel-Haenzel χ^2 test was used. Multivariate logistic regression analyses were conducted to examine whether the association of last place of care and reported perceptions of care persisted after adjusting for the decedent's age, years of education, sex, race, the underlying cause of death, respondent perceptions of whether death was unexpected, and whether the decedent had difficulty rising from a chair or bed ninety days prior to death.

RESULTS

Characteristics of Decedents and Respondents

Table 13.1 describes decedents by their last place of care, defined as where they spent forty-eight hours prior to death. The site of death and last place of care were the same for 92.1 percent of cases. For the majority (68.9 percent), the last place of care was an institutional setting, either a hospital or nursing home. Home was the last place of care for 31.1 percent; of those, 36.1 percent died without any nursing services, 12.4 percent had home nursing services, and 51.5 percent had home hospice services. Older women and those currently unmarried were more likely to reside in a nursing home. Persons who died with home hospice services were more likely to have had cancer, while those who died at home without formal services were more likely to have died from heart disease. Thirty-seven percent of those persons who died at home without formal services were functionally impaired, defined as having difficulty rising from a bed or chair. A written advance directive (either a living will or a durable power of attorney for health care) was reported for 70.7 percent of decedents. Characteristics of respondents are shown in Table 13.2. Most were family members who were in close contact with the dying person; 72.1 percent either saw or spoke with the patient for all seven days prior to death.

Family Perceptions of the Quality of End-of-Life Care

Family perceptions of quality of care differed by the last place of care in which the decedent received formal services. Table 13.3 shows the unadjusted and adjusted results for the last place of care where the decedent received formal services. Nearly one fourth of all respondents reported that the patient did not receive any or enough help with pain (24.2 percent) or dyspnea (22.4 percent). Family members of persons whose last place of care was a nursing home or home with home health nursing services had a higher

TABLE 13.1. Characteristics of Decedents by Last Place of Care[a]

Characteristic	1993 Comparison Data[d]	Last Place of Care, % (95% CI)[b][c]					
		Total	Home Without Nursing Services	Home With Home Care Nursing Services	Home With Hospice Services	Nursing Home	Hospital
Sample size, No.							
Actual	10,122	1,578	198	65	256	487	572
Weighted	1,980,388	1,966,705	221,071	76,231	315,165	600,802	753,436
Age, mean (95% CI), y	73.9	74.8 (73.5-76.1)	71.4 (69.0-73.6)	79.2 (74.9-83.5)	72.9 (70.8-75.0)	83.8 (82.1-85.5)	74.8 (73.5-76.1)
Women	50.1	53.4 (50.2-56.6)	42.7 (34.1-51.2)	56.3 (40.8-71.8)	49.7 (42.2-57.1)	67.0 (60.8-73.1)	47.0 (42.6-51.4)
Race/ethnicity							
White, non-Hispanic	83.2	86.8 (82.8-90.8)	88.4 (81.7-95.0)	78.3 (65.6-91.0)	81.3 (71.8-90.8)	92.5 (89.4-95.7)	84.8 (79.7-89.9)
Black, non-Hispanic	11.6	7.8 (5.0-10.5)	7.8 (2.0-13.7)	12.8 (3.6-21.9)	7.4 (3.0-11.7)	5.1 (2.3-7.9)	9.6 (5.3-13.8)
Hispanic	3.2	4.8 (2.5-7.2)	3.8 (1.2-6.5)	8.9 (0.0-18.5)	10.0 (3.2-16.7)	1.8 (0.6-3.1)	5.1 (1.6-8.5)
Education less than high school degree	46.7	36.5 (31.8-41.2)	29.7 (19.2-40.2)	34.0 (18.2-49.9)	30.6 (23.9-37.2)	41.9 (35.9-47.9)	36.8 (30.0-43.7)
Married	42.5	28.0 (25.4-30.6)	46.0 (38.8-53.2)	32.4 (17.6-47.3)	54.7 (45.1-64.4)	22.4 (17.6-27.3)	48.4 (42.7-54.0)
Cause of death							
Cancer	25.8	40.7 (37.0-44.3)	7.9 (1.7-14.1)	29.2 (12.8-45.5)	68.3 (61.0-75.6)	15.9 (12.8-19.0)	26.6 (22.2-31.0)
Heart disease	36.2	41.9 (39.2-44.7)	77.2 (68.5-85.8)	40.7 (27.5-54.0)	11.5 (7.1-16.0)	47.1 (42.4-51.8)	40.3 (35.9-44.7)
Stroke syndrome	7.6	9.4 (7.7-11.0)	7.3 (2.4-12.3)	5.5 (0.0-12.0)	0.6 (0.0-1.2)	14.0 (10.4-17.7)	10.4 (7.8-12.9)
Dementia		6.0 (4.6-7.5)	1.0 (0.0-2.5)	1.0 (0.0-2.8)	3.2 (0.0-6.9)	16.0 (12.3-19.8)	1.3 (0.3-2.3)
Difficulty rising from bed/chair in last year of life	NA	65.3 (62.6-67.9)	37.1 (28.3-45.9)	65.8 (51.1-80.5)	70.8 (64.6-76.9)	80.4 (77.0-83.8)	59.1 (53.6-64.6)
Written advance directives	NA	70.7 (67.5-73.9)	55.6 (47.4-63.9)	70.8 (52.6-89.1)	81.6 (75.5-87.6)	80.8 (77.2-84.4)	62.5 (57.3-67.8)

[a] P<.001 for comparison of all characteristics except education less than high school degree (P = .33).

[b] Abbreviations: CI, confidence interval; NA, not available.

[c] All percentages are weighted. "Last place of care" indicates the last location where the decedent spent more than forty-eight hours prior to death. For 125 out of the 1,578 cases, the site of death was not the last place of care. Of these 125 cases, 96 were persons who were transferred to a hospital emergency department or who died soon after hospital admission.

[d] Comparison data from the 1993 US Mortality Follow-back Survey.[11]

TABLE 13.2. Characteristics of Survey Respondents by Decedents' Last Place of Care[a]

Characteristic	Total	Home Without Nursing Services	Home With Home Care Nursing Services	Home With Hospice Services	Nursing Home	Hospital
Sample size, No.						
Actual	1,578	198	65	256	487	572
Weighted	1,966,705	221,071	76,231	315,165	600,802	753,436
Women	71.0 (68.2-73.7)	67.8 (57.5-78.1)	78.1 (65.4-90.8)	69.0 (61.3-76.8)	70.5 (65.9-75.0)	72.4 (67.4-77.3)
Less than high school degree	10.4 (7.8-12.9)	12.7 (7.9-17.5)	12.4 (1.0-23.7)	11.0 (5.6-16.3)	9.8 (6.0-13.7)	9.7 (6.4-13.0)
Relationship to decedent						
Spouse	30.1 (26.7-33.4)	34.9 (26.5-43.4)	25.9 (12.0-39.7)	42.3 (32.5-52.0)	14.6 (11.3-17.9)	36.3 (30.3-42.2)
Child	40.5 (37.0-44.1)	32.0 (24.3-39.7)	50.3 (34.3-66.2)	39.2 (29.0-49.4)	48.3 (43.8-52.8)	36.4 (30.9-42.0)
Friend/other	3.2 (2.3-4.2)	2.3 (0.0-4.5)	4.2 (0.0-10.7)	1.4 (0.0-2.9)	5.3 (3.1-7.6)	2.6 (1.3-3.8)
Contact with patient all 7 days in last week of lifep	72.1 (68.7-75.4)	67.4 (59.8-75.1)	73.3 (58.2-88.3)	91.2 (86.7-95.8)	57.4 (51.1-63.7)	76.2 (71.8-80.6)
Dying was "extremely" unexpected	22.6 (19.7-25.4)	65.0 (58.0-72.1)	33.6 (17.8-49.5)	7.1 (2.1-12.0)	12.0 (8.2-15.7)	23.8 (19.6-28.1)

Abbreviation: CI, confidence interval.
*P<.001 for comparison of all characteristics except sex (P = .74).
†All percentages are weighted.

[a] P<.001 for comparison of all characteristics except sex (P = .74).
[b] CI: confidence interval.
[c] All percentages are weighted.

TABLE 13.3. Patient- and Family-Centered Outcomes at the Last Place of Care[a]

Outcome	Total, Unadjusted % (95% CI[c])	Last Place of Care[b] Home With Home Care Nursing Services Unadjusted %	Adjusted OR (95% CI)[d]	Home With Hospice Care Unadjusted %	Adjusted OR (95% CI)[d]	Nursing Home Unadjusted %	Adjusted OR (95% CI)[d]	Hospital Unadjusted %	Adjusted OR (95% CI)[d]
Provided Desired Physical Comfort and Emotional Support to Patient									
Patient did not receive any or enough help with									
Pain	24.2 (21.2-27.3)	42.6	1.6 (1.1-2.0)	18.3	Reference	31.8	1.6 (1.0-2.2)	19.3	1.2 (0.3-1.9)
Dyspnea	22.4 (18.7-26.0)	38.0	1.4 (0.5-2.2)	25.6	Reference	23.7	1.0 (0.6-1.7)	18.9	0.7 (0.3-1.2)
Emotional support	50.2 (44.4-56.0)	70.0	2.7 (1.7-3.1)	34.6	Reference	56.2	1.3 (1.1-1.5)	51.7	1.3 (1.0-1.6)
Supported Shared Decision Making									
Respondent wanted but did not have contact with physician	30.1 (24.1-36.1)	22.5	1.6 (0.5-3.3)	14.0	Reference	31.3	2.0 (1.4-2.5)	51.3	1.8 (1.5-1.9)
Respondents with contact had concern(s) about physician communication	23.9 (20.1-26.4)	26.6	1.1 (0.4-2.1)	17.6	Reference	17.7	1.2 (0.5-2.1)	27.0	1.3 (0.8-1.9)
Treated Patient With Respect									
Not always treating patient with respect	21.1 (18.3-23.9)	15.5	2.9 (1.5-4.3)	3.8	Reference	31.8	2.6 (2.3-2.9)	20.4	3.0 (2.2-3.8)
Attended to Needs of the Family									
Concern(s) about emotional support	34.6 (31.5-37.8)	45.4	1.6 (1.0-1.9)	21.1	Reference	36.4	1.6 (1.3-1.9)	38.4	1.5 (1.3-1.8)
Concern(s) about information regarding what to expect while patient was dying	29.2 (22.3-36.1)	31.5	0.9 (0.4-1.8)	29.2	Reference	44.3	1.5 (1.2-1.7)	50.0	1.4 (1.1-1.6)
Coordinated Care									
Staff did not know enough about patient's medical history to provide best care	15.2 (12.7-17.7)	7.5	0.7 (0.2-2.3)	7.9	Reference	19.6	2.0 (1.2-2.9)	15.4	1.5 (0.9-2.4)
Overall Assessment of Quality of Care									
Excellent	49.4 (45.9-52.9)	46.5	0.4 (0.2-0.8)	70.7	Reference	41.6	0.4 (0.3-0.6)	46.8	0.6 (0.3-0.7)

[a]Results are presented only for the 1,380 decedents who had contact with health care institutions. Questions regarding the quality of care were not asked of the 198 persons who died at home without nursing services.

[b]All percentages are weighted.

[c]CI: confidence interval; OR: odds ratio.

[d]Adjusted OR from a multivariate logistic regression model adjusting for age, sex, underlying cause of death, education, race/ethnicity, respondents' perceptions of whether the death was expected, and whether the patient had difficulty rising from a chair three months prior to death. In addition, ORs are adjusted to approximate the relative risk according to the method of Zhang and Yu.[12]

rate of reported unmet needs for pain (nursing home: adjusted odds ratio [OR], 1.6; 95 percent confidence interval [CI], 1.0–2.2; home with nursing services: adjusted OR, 1.6; 95 percent CI, 1.1–2.0), compared with those persons with home hospice services. Unmet needs for dyspnea did not differ by setting of care. Overall, half of family members reported that the patient did not receive enough emotional support. Recipients of home hospice care had lower rates of unmet needs (34.6 percent), compared with the other settings of care. About one in four families reported concerns with physician communication regarding medical decision making, although there was no difference by setting of care. Families reported more concerns with whether the patient was always treated with respect when the last place of care was a nursing home (adjusted OR, 2.6; 95 percent CI, 2.3–2.9), hospital (adjusted OR, 3.0; 95 percent CI, 2.2–3.8), or home with home health services (adjusted OR, 2.9; 95 percent CI, 1.5–4.3), compared with persons who died at home with hospice services. Similarly, in contrast to other settings of care, family members of those dying at home with hospice services reported fewer concerns with the amount of emotional support provided to them. Overall satisfaction was better for those who received home hospice services: 70.7 percent rated care as "excellent" versus less than 50 percent for the other settings of care (P < .001).

COMMENT

No national study has adequately characterized the U.S. experience of dying.[13] Key findings of our study are that bereaved family members reported high rates of unmet needs for symptom management, concerns with physician communication about medical decision making, a lack of emotional support for themselves, and a belief that their dying family member was not always treated with respect. A higher rate of concerns with the quality of end-of-life care was reported for persons whose last place of care was a nursing home or hospital. Increasingly, nursing homes are replacing hospitals as the last place of care.[14] With the "baby boom generation" starting to reach retirement, there is an urgent need for improving the end-of-life care in the United States.

Our finding that bereaved family members of patients with home hospice services (in contrast to the other settings of care) reported higher satisfaction, fewer concerns with care, and fewer unmet needs is consistent with smaller and less generalizable studies that have examined the effect of hospice or palliative-care services.[15] However, there are important opportunities to improve hospice care, with more than one in four respondents reporting unmet needs in the management of dyspnea and in the emotional support provided. An overly simplistic reaction would be to place blame with the nursing home or hospital industry. Yet, in the past decade, each has been faced with substantial limitations in federal funding and with challenges in care management. For example, nursing homes are now caring for sicker patients despite shortages of nursing staff and high rates of staff turnover.[16] These factors influence not only the quality of end-of-life care but also the incidence of decubitus ulcers, inadequacy of feeding assistance, and potentially preventable hospitalizations.[17] Most likely, these perceptions of bereaved family members are the result of a complex set of interactions that include our death-denying culture and existing financial incentives that reinforce invasive treatment approaches to medical care.

Important limitations should be acknowledged in the interpretation of these results. Because of the difficulty in prognosticating death and defining who should be counted in the denominator, we used a mortality follow-back approach that easily defines the denominator and uses death certificates to contact next of kin.[18–19] Family members both acted as a proxy for the decedents and reported their own perceptions of the quality of end-of-life care based on their own interactions with clinicians. They may have inaccurately perceived patients' unmet needs for symptom management; however, a recent synthesis of literature suggests that families are able to accurately report on many quality-of-care domains.[11] In addition, we interviewed only 65 percent of the persons who could be located. Younger persons, African Americans, and Hispanics were somewhat less likely to participate in this survey. Nonetheless, as reported in Table 13.1, our sample is comparable to the 1993 U.S. National Mortality Follow-back Survey.[20] Finally, interpretation of the results of last place of care and quality of end-of-life care must take into account the nonexperimental design. While we adjusted for leading cause of death, age, and other characteristics, location of death is to some extent self-selected.

Despite these limitations, this is the largest study to date using a mortality follow-back approach and new survey methods to examine family perceptions of the quality of end-of-life care. Such national information on the quality of end-of-life care in the United States has been sorely lacking. Bereaved family members voiced significant concerns with the quality of end-of-life care, regardless of whether care was provided in a nursing home or hospital. Only bereaved family members whose loved one received home hospice services reported higher satisfaction and fewer unmet needs. However, simply increasing access to hospice services may not adequately improve end-of-life care in the United States, given that qualification for the Medicare hospice benefit requires that two physicians certify a six-month prognosis, and accurately prognosticating life expectancy for persons dying of diseases other than cancer is difficult.[21] Rather, our results call for a public health approach that uses sustained and multifaceted interventions to improve end-of-life care in the United States.[1]

REFERENCES

1. Singer PA, Bowman KW. Quality care at the end of life. *BMJ*. 2002; 324:1291–1292.

2. Emanuel EJ, Emanuel LL. The promise of a good death. *Lancet*. 1998; 351(suppl 2): SII21–SII29.

3. Field MJ, ed, Cassel CK, ed, Institute of Medicine, Committee on Care at the End of Life. *Approaching Death: Improving Care at the End of Life*. Washington, DC: National Academy Press; 1997.

4. Lynn J. Measuring quality of care at the end of life: a statement of principles. *J Am Geriatr Soc*. 1997; 45:526–527.

5. Singer PA, Martin DK, Kelner M. Quality end-of-life care: patients' perspectives. *JAMA*. 1999; 281:163–168.

6. Steinhauser KE, Clipp EC, McNeilly M, Christakis NA, McIntyre LM, Tulsky JA. In search of a good death: observations of patients, families, and providers. *Ann Intern Med*. 2000; 132:825–832.

7. Teno JM, Casey VA, Welch L, Edgman-Levitan S. Patient-focused, family-centered end-of-life medical care: views of the guidelines and bereaved family members. *J Pain Symptom Manage*. 2001; 22:738–751.

8. Teno JM, Clarridge B, Casey V, Edgman-Levitan S, Fowler J. Validation of toolkit after-death bereaved family member interview. *J Pain Symptom Manage*. 2001; 22:752–758.

9. Kish L. *Survey Sampling*. New York, NY: Wiley & Sons; 1965.

10. Cochran WG. *Sampling Techniques*. New York, NY: Wiley & Sons; 1977.

11. McPherson C, Addington-Hall J. Judging the quality of care at the end of life: can proxies provide reliable information? *Soc Sci Med*. 2003; 56:95–109.

12. Zhang J, Yu KF. What's the relative risk? a method of correcting the odds ratio in cohort studies of common outcomes. *JAMA*. 1998; 280:1690–1691.

13. Council on Scientific Affairs, American Medical Association. Good care of the dying patient. *JAMA*. 1996; 275:474–478.

14. Teno JM. Facts on dying: policy relevant data on care at the end of life. 2000. Available at: http://www.chcr.brown.edu/dying/factsondying.htm. Accessibility verified October 31, 2003.

15. Higginson I, Finlay I, Goodwin D, et al. Do hospital based palliative teams improve care for patients or families at end of life? *J Pain Symptom Manage*. 2002; 23:96–106.

16. Zerzan J, Stearns S, Hanson L. Access to palliative care and hospice in nursing homes. *JAMA*. 2000; 284:2489–2494.

17. Harrington C, Kovner C, Mezey M, et al. Experts recommend minimum nurse staffing standards for nursing facilities in the United States. *Gerontologist*. 2000; 40:5–16.

18. Teno JM, Coppola KM. For every numerator, you need a denominator: a simple statement but key to measuring the quality of care of the "dying." *J Pain Symptom Manage*. 1999; 17:109–113.

19. Addington-Hall J, McPherson C. After-death interviews with surrogates/bereaved family members: some issues of validity. *J Pain Symptom Manage*. 2001; 22:784–790.

20. Weitzen S, Teno JM, Fennell M, Mor V. Factors associated with site of death: a national study of where people die. *Med Care*. 2003; 41:323–335.

21. Fox E, Landrum-McNiff K, Zhong Z, Dawson NV, Wu AW, Lynn J, SUPPORT Investigators. Evaluation of prognostic criteria for determining hospice eligibility in patients with advanced lung, heart, or liver disease. *JAMA*. 1999; 282:1638–1648.

CORRESPONDING AUTHOR AND REPRINTS

Joan M. Teno, M.D., M.S., 2 Stimson Ave., Providence, RI 02912 (e-mail: joan_teno@brown.edu).

AUTHOR CONTRIBUTIONS

Dr. Teno, as principal investigator of this study, had full access to all of the data in the study and takes responsibility for the integrity of the data and the accuracy of the data analyses.

STUDY CONCEPT AND DESIGN

Teno, Clarridge, Casey, Welch, Mor.

ACQUISITION OF DATA

Teno, Clarridge.

ANALYSIS AND INTERPRETATION OF DATA

Teno, Wetle, Shield, Mor.

DRAFTING OF THE MANUSCRIPT

Teno, Casey, Welch, Mor.

CRITICAL REVISION OF THE MANUSCRIPT FOR IMPORTANT INTELLECTUAL CONTENT

Teno, Clarridge, Casey, Welch, Wetle, Shield, Mor.

STATISTICAL EXPERTISE

Teno.

OBTAINED FUNDING

Teno.

ADMINISTRATIVE, TECHNICAL, OR MATERIAL SUPPORT

Teno, Clarridge, Wetle, Mor.

STUDY SUPERVISION

Teno, Clarridge, Mor.

FUNDING/SUPPORT

Funding for this research was provided by grant 037188 from the Robert Wood Johnson Foundation.

ROLE OF SPONSOR

The Robert Wood Johnson Foundation did not have any role in the design, conduct, interpretation, review, approval, or control of this article.

DISCLAIMER

The opinions and findings in this manuscript are those of the authors and do not necessarily represent the views of the Robert Wood Johnson Foundation.

ACKNOWLEDGMENT

We thank the survey staff at the Center for Survey Research for their tireless efforts in conducting this study. We especially thank Jack Fowler, Ph.D., and Tony Roman, M.S., for help with the sampling design and calculations of sampling weights.

AUTHOR AFFILIATIONS

Center for Gerontology and Health Care Research, Brown Medical School (Drs. Teno, Casey, Wetle, and Shield; Ms Welch) and Department of Community Health, Brown University, Providence, RI (Drs. Teno, Mor, Wetle, and Shield); and the Center for Survey Research, University of Massachusetts at Boston (Dr. Clarridge).

PALLIATIVE CARE

PAIN AND MEDICAL DECISION MAKING

Kathleen M. Foley, "The Treatment of Cancer Pain"

Timothy E. Quill and Ira R. Byock, for the ACP-ASIM End-of-Life Care Consensus Panel, "Responding to Intractable Terminal Suffering: The Role of Terminal Sedation and Voluntary Refusal of Food and Fluids"

Daniel P. Sulmasy, Wayne A. Ury, Judith C. Ahronheim, Mark Siegler, Leon Kass, John Lantos, Robert A. Burt, Kathleen Foley, Richard Payne, Carlos Gomez, Thomas J. Krizek, Edmund D. Pellegrino, and Russell K. Portenoy, "Response to Quill and Byock, 'Responding to Intractable Suffering'"

14

THE TREATMENT OF CANCER PAIN

KATHLEEN M. FOLEY, M.D.

This article originally appeared as Foley, KM. The treatment of cancer pain. *N Engl J Med.* 1985;313(2):84–95.

EDITORS' INTRODUCTION

Kathleen Foley is the nation's most prominent leader in pain research and palliative medicine. This 1985 article identifies untreated pain as a major public health problem and describes the science and the safety of appropriate pain management with narcotic analgesics. Twenty-three years later, progress in adhering to Foley's recommendations remains too slow, but this article was influential in the effort to change physicians' attitudes and behaviors towards pain management.

■ ■ ■

Advances in the diagnosis and treatment of cancer, coupled with an expanded understanding of the physiology, pharmacology, and psychology of pain perception, have led to improved care of the patient with pain from cancer.[1] Improved methods of cancer diagnosis and treatment provide the best approach to managing pain by treating its cause. Before the start of antitumor therapy, or when such therapy is unsuccessful or irreversible injury to bone, soft tissue, or nerve has occurred, however, adequate pain control is essential.

Management of pain in patients with cancer requires specific expertise that includes a knowledge of the clinical pain syndromes that are common in cancer and their pathophysiologic mechanisms, the psychological state of the patient, and the indications and limitations of the available therapeutic approaches. Clinical experience suggests that patients with cancer pain are treated most effectively with a multidisciplinary approach that includes adequate analgesic drug therapy, neurological and anesthetic procedures, behavioral methods, and supportive care.[2-5]

The goal of pain therapy for patients receiving active treatment is to provide them with sufficient relief to tolerate the diagnostic and therapeutic approaches required to treat the cancer. For patients with advanced disease, pain control should be sufficient to allow the patients to function at a level that they choose and to die relatively free of pain.[6,7] Critical to the management of cancer pain is the establishment of a trusting relationship between the patient and a physician who takes the pain seriously and assesses its nature and severity.

EPIDEMIOLOGY

Large-scale epidemiologic studies of the incidence and severity of cancer pain are lacking, but numerous studies in specialized medical care settings have demonstrated that the prevalence of pain increases with the progression of disease. Patients with cancer frequently have multiple causes of pain.[8] Some 15 percent of patients with nonmetastatic cancer have pain.[9] One-third of adults and children with metastatic cancer report pain that interferes with and reduces their activity level and requires the use of analgesics.[10] With advanced disease, 60 to 90 percent of patients report substantial pain.[3,11,12] It is postulated that 25 percent of all patients with cancer throughout the world die without relief from severe pain.[9] To remedy this situation, and as part of a broader cancer program, the Cancer Unit of the World Health Organization has formulated a pain-relief program to conduct an epidemiologic investigation of cancer pain throughout the world, to provide guidelines for pain management, particularly in patients with advanced disease, and to encourage national governments to help make therapeutic approaches available, specifically oral narcotic drug therapy.[13]

TYPES OF PAIN

Patients with cancer have two types of pain: acute and chronic. This division is based on an increased understanding of the mechanisms of pain transmission and the recognition that the central modulation of acute and chronic pain states may differ, along with their clinical management and response to treatment.[14,15] For this discussion the definition of pain proposed by the International Association for the Study of Pain is most useful: "an unpleasant sensory and emotional experience associated with actual or potential tissue damage or described in terms of such damage."[16] Because pain is a subjective experience, evaluation of it is difficult. The physician has limited objective signs to confirm the severity of reported pain. The patient and physician are best served if the physician believes the patient's report.

Acute pain is characterized by a well-defined temporal pattern of onset. It is generally associated with subjective and objective physical signs and hyperactivity of the autonomic nervous system. These signs serve as objective evidence to the physician, substantiating the patient's report of pain. In contrast, chronic pain is pain that persists longer than six months, in which adaptation of the autonomic nervous system occurs. Patients with chronic pain lack the objective signs common to acute pain. Chronic pain leads to marked changes in personality, life style, and functional ability. Such pain requires an approach that encompasses not only treatment of the cause of the pain but also treatment of its psychological and social consequences.[15,17]

Patients with chronic or acute pain from cancer can be further subdivided, providing the physician with a useful classification when considering therapeutic approaches (Table 14.1).

Group I comprises patients with acute cancer-related pain. A subgroup of this category includes patients in whom pain is the major symptom leading to the diagnosis of cancer. For this group, pain has a special meaning as the harbinger of their illness. The occurrence of pain during the course of the illness or after successful therapy has the immediate implication of recurrent disease. Determination of the cause of the pain may present a diagnostic problem, but effective treatment of the cause—for example, irradiation of bone metastases—is usually possible and is associated with dramatic pain relief in the majority of patients.

TABLE 14.1. Types of Patients with Pain from Cancer

I.   **Patients with acute cancer-related pain**

    a.   Associated with the diagnosis of cancer

    b.   Associated with cancer therapy (surgery, chemotherapy, or radiation)

II. **Patients with chronic cancer-related pain**

    a.   Associated with cancer progression

    b.   Associated with cancer therapy (surgery, chemotherapy, or radiation)

III. **Patients with preexisting chronic pain and cancer-related pain**

IV. **Patients with a history of drug addiction and cancer-related pain**

    a.   Actively involved in illicit drug use

    b.   In methadone maintenance programs

    c.   With a history of drug abuse

V.   **Dying patients with cancer-related pain**

The second subgroup includes patients who have acute pain associated with cancer therapy—for example, pain after surgery or secondary to the acute effects of chemotherapy. The cause of the pain is readily identified, and its course is predictable and self-limited. Such patients endure pain for the promise of a successful outcome.

Group II, which consists of patients with chronic cancer-related pain, represents difficult diagnostic and therapeutic problems. This group can be subdivided into patients with chronic pain from tumor progression and those with chronic pain related to cancer treatment. Both subgroups have pain that has persisted for more than six months.

In patients with chronic pain associated with the progression of disease—for example, those with carcinoma of the pancreas—the pain escalates in intensity, and combinations of antitumor therapy, analgesic drug therapy, anesthetic blocks, and behavioral approaches to pain control are all attempted with varying degrees of success.

Psychological factors play an important part in this group of patients, in whom palliative therapy may be of little value and is physically debilitating.[11,18] The sense of hopelessness and fear of impending death may add to and exaggerate the pain, which in turn contributes to the overall suffering of the patient. Identification of both the pain and the suffering component is essential to the provision of adequate therapy. Saunders has used the phrase "total pain" to describe the etiologic components other than the noxious physical stimulus, including emotional, social, bureaucratic, financial, and spiritual pain.[4] Those caring for this group of patients must be concerned with all aspects of distress and discomfort if the experience of physical pain is to be alleviated. The chronicity of the pain is associated with a series of psychological signs—for example, disturbances in sleep, reduction in appetite, impaired concentration, and irritability—and with clinical signs and symptoms mimicking a depressive disorder.[15]

Patients with chronic pain associated with cancer therapy usually require treatment directed at the symptoms, not the cause. Treatment of the pain is often limited by the lack of available methods to remove the cause of the pain—for example, a traumatic neuroma. This group of patients closely parallels those in the general population with chronic, intractable pain. Identification of this group of patients is imperative because recognition of the cause of the pain as independent of the cancer markedly alters the patient's therapy, prognosis, and psychological state. All approaches intended to maintain the functional status of the patient should be employed.[15,17] Approaches other than drug therapy provide effective alternatives for pain management. This group is increasing in size and accounts for 25 percent of patients referred to one cancer pain clinic.[10]

Group III includes patients with a history of chronic, nonmalignant pain who have cancer and associated pain. Psychological factors play an important part in these patients, whose psychological and functional status is already compromised. They are at high risk of further functional incapacity and escalating chronic pain. However, their history should not be used in a punitive way to minimize their complaints. Identification of this group of patients as a high-risk group helps to improve their psychological assessment and intervention.

Group IV includes patients with a history of drug addiction who have cancer-related pain. Three subgroups can be identified: patients actively involved in illicit drug use and drug-seeking behavior, those receiving methadone in a maintenance program, and those who have not used drugs for several years. Undertreatment with analgesic drugs occurs most commonly in this group of patients. Assessment of reported pain by physicians and nurses is colored by the fact that the pain symptoms are confused with drug-seeking behavior. Attention to the medical and psychological needs of these patients requires individualized assessment and consultation with experts in drug-related problems.[18] The first subgroup represents a major management problem, straining the most tolerant of medical care systems. Pain in the other two subgroups is readily managed, with the recognition that the psychological stresses consequent to the pain and cancer may place the patient at high risk for recidivism.

Group V includes dying patients with pain. In this group, diagnostic and therapeutic considerations should be directed at maintaining the comfort of the patient. The issues of hopelessness, death, and dying become prominent, and the suffering component of the illness must be addressed. Inadequate control of pain exacerbates the suffering and demoralizes both the family and the medical personnel, who feel that they have failed in treating the patient's pain at a time when adequate treatment may matter most. Rapid escalation of analgesic drug therapy and attempts to ameliorate the psychological symptoms should be employed. The risk-benefit ratios associated with analgesic approaches become less of an issue when the goal of pain therapy is the comfort of the patient.

These types of cancer pain point up the necessity of understanding the psychological needs of the patient and the temporal factors in order to assess the pain and manage it appropriately.

Cancer pain has also been classified according to a series of common pain syndromes and their pathophysiologic mechanisms.[12] The pain syndromes that commonly occur in patients with cancer have been divided into three major categories.

The first and most common cause of pain in patients with cancer is that associated with direct tumor involvement. This accounted for 78 percent of pain problems in a survey of the Memorial Sloan-Kettering Cancer Center inpatient population[5] and for 62 percent of problems in an outpatient survey.[9] Metastatic bone disease, nerve compression or infiltration, and hollow viscus involvement are the most common causes of pain from direct tumor involvement.

The second group of pain syndromes are those associated with cancer therapy. This group accounts for approximately 19 percent of pain problems in an inpatient population and 25 percent of problems in outpatients. It includes pain that occurs in the course of or as a result of surgery, chemotherapy, or radiation therapy.

The third category of pain syndromes includes those unrelated to the cancer or the cancer therapy. Approximately 3 percent of inpatients have pain unrelated to cancer or cancer therapy, and this figure increases to 10 percent when an outpatient population is surveyed.

The pathophysiologic mechanisms of these common pain syndromes are not well understood. It is currently thought that a series of neuropharmacologic and neurophysiologic changes occur in bone, soft tissue, lymphatics, blood vessels, nerve and viscera, activating and sensitizing nociceptors and mechanoreceptors by mechanical (tumor compression or infiltration) or chemical (metastases in bone) stimuli. Acute, intermittent, or continuous pain results. Most therapeutic approaches are partially effective in controlling this kind of pain.[19] In contrast, pain from nerve injury after nerve section or chronic tumor infiltration or compression produces partial damage of axons and nerve membranes, which become extremely sensitive to any mechanical or chemical stimuli. Chronic unremitting pain results, which is poorly controlled by the majority of therapeutic approaches. Experimental studies indicate that pain from deafferentation leads to central neuronal hyperactivity in the spinal cord and, possibly, in the thalamus.[20]

These different physiologic mechanisms account in part for the differences in the responses of various types of cancer pain to analgesic, neurosurgical, and anesthetic approaches. For example, drug therapy and neurosurgical procedures are often effective in managing pain from lumbosacral plexopathy in its early acute stage, but once deafferentation has occurred, the success of such procedures diminishes rapidly.[20]

MANAGEMENT OF CANCER PAIN

There are certain general principles that should be followed in evaluating all patients with cancer and pain.[21] Lack of attention to these principles is the major cause of misdiagnosis and inappropriate management of a specific pain syndrome. The principles include a complete assessment of the history of pain and an evaluation of the psychosocial status of the patient. A careful medical and neurologic examination must be coupled with the use of appropriate diagnostic procedures to determine the nature of the pain. Early treatment with analgesics markedly improves the patient's ability to participate in these procedures. No patient should be inadequately evaluated because of pain. Continual reassessment of the patient's response to prescribed therapy provides the best method of validating the accuracy of the initial diagnosis. If the response to therapy is less than predicted or if exacerbation of pain occurs, reassessment of the treatment approach or a search for a new cause of pain should be considered. Management of pain in patients with cancer requires continuity of care from the diagnosis to treatment.[22]

THERAPEUTIC APPROACHES

Non-narcotic, narcotic, and adjuvant analgesic drugs are the mainstay of therapy for patients with cancer pain. Effective use of these drugs requires an understanding of their clinicopharmacologic characteristics, with selection of a particular drug and dose geared to the needs of the individual patient. Neurosurgical, anesthetic, and behavioral approaches are commonly used in combination with drug therapy.

Changing attitudes toward the use of narcotic analgesics for cancer pain, coupled with the recognition of the dynamic complexity of pain modulation, have led to reassessment of the role of anesthetic and neurosurgical approaches. These approaches are most useful for managing localized pain before the development of serious nerve injury and a consequent deafferentation state. Although these procedures have been widely used, controlled studies of their effectiveness, as compared with that of other methods of pain control, are lacking. Published reports provide survey data on techniques and successful outcome in small numbers of patients.

These techniques require specific expertise, and certain guidelines apply to their use. These include a thorough evaluation of the nature of the pain and the patient's prognosis, an adequate prior trial of analgesic drug therapy and anticancer therapy, and the patient's awareness of the potential risks and benefits of the planned procedures. The types of anesthetic and neurosurgical procedures are listed in Tables 14.2 and 14.3. Historically, these procedures have been employed late in the course of a patient's illness, and full assessment of their efficacy has been limited by disease progression and diffuse as well as focal pain. Many patients prefer to defer these procedures until they complete their anticancer therapy, with the hope that such therapy will provide relief. Also, when informed about the small but potential risk of neurologic impairment associated with these procedures, many patients are not willing to accept such a risk for pain control alone.

There is a need to develop strategies for the appropriate use of these procedures. A detailed review of them is beyond the scope of this discussion. Drug therapy is stressed in the following discussion because all physicians caring for patients with pain must develop competence and confidence in the use of drugs.

Drug Therapy

Non-narcotic Agents Non-narcotic analgesics are the first-line agents for the management of mild to moderate cancer pain.[22-25] In patients with severe pain, these drugs serve to potentiate the effects of narcotic analgesics. Non-narcotic analgesics have a ceiling effect, and their long-term use is limited by gastrointestinal and hematologic side

TABLE 14.2. **Neuroablative, Neurostimulatory, and Neuropharmacologic Procedures for Relief of Pain from Cancer**

Site	Procedure		
	Neuroablative	Neurostimulatory	Pharmacologic
Peripheral nerve	Neurectomy	Transcutaneous and percutaneous electrical nerve stimulation	Local anesthetics
Nerve root	Rhizotomy		Local anesthetics Neurolytic agents
Spinal cord	Dorsal-root entry-zone lesions Cordotomy Myelotomy	Dorsal-column stimulation	Epidural and intrathecal local anesthetics and opiates
Brain stem	Mesencephalic tractotomy	Periaqueductal stimulation	Intraventricular opiates
Thalamus	Thalamotomy	Thalamic stimulation	
Cortex	Cingulumotomy Frontal lobotomy		
Pituitary	Transspenoidal hypophysectomy		Chemical hypophysectomy

effects. In contrast to narcotic analgesics, non-narcotic agents do not cause tolerance or physical dependence.

There is increasing evidence to suggest that these drugs may have a unique role in the management of certain kinds of pain from bone metastases.[26–28] Anecdotal reports indicate that both aspirin and indomethacin relieve bone pain, and in an animal tumor model, aspirin has been shown to have antitumor effects. These effects are thought to be mediated in part through inhibition of prostaglandin synthesis, specifically prostaglandin E2, which is important in the development of bone metastases in solid tumors.

The choice and use of these drugs must be individualized, with the patient receiving maximal levels of one drug before another is tried. Combinations of nonsteroidal and antiinflammatory drugs that produce additive analgesia remain controversial. If pain control is ineffective or the non-narcotic agents are poorly tolerated, the use of narcotic analgesics is indicated.

Narcotic Analgesics The narcotic analgesics are classified as agonist or antagonist drugs, depending on their ability to bind to opiate receptors and produce analgesia. The narcotic agonist drugs, such as morphine, bind to specific opiate receptors, resulting in analgesia. These drugs are commonly used in the management of cancer pain.

TABLE 14.3. **Types of Anesthetic Procedures Commonly Used for Cancer Pain**

Type of Procedure	Most Common Indications
Nerve block	
Peripheral	Pain in discrete dermatomes in chest and abdomen
Epidural	Unilateral lumbar or sacral pain Midline perineal pain Bilateral lumbosacral pain
Intrathecal	Midline perineal pain Bilateral lumbosacral pain
Autonomic	
Stellate ganglion	Reflex sympathetic dystrophy (for example, frozen shoulder) Arm pain
Lumbar sympathetic	Reflex sympathetic dystrophy Lumbosacral plexopathy Vascular insufficiency of the lower extremity
Celiac plexus	Midabdominal pain
Continuous epidural infusion with local anesthetics	Unilateral and bilateral lumbosacral pain Midline perineal pain
Chemical hypophysectomy	Diffuse bone pain
Inhalation therapy	Generalized pain Incident pain
Trigger-point injection	Focal muscle pain

The narcotic antagonist drugs block the effect of morphine at its receptor. Included in this category is a group of drugs with analgesic properties referred to as "mixed agonist-antagonist" drugs.[29] These drugs are of limited use in patients with cancer, for several reasons: they produce psychotomimetic effects with increasing doses; except for pentazocine, they are available only for parenteral administration (nalbuphine and butorphanol); oral pentazocine is available only in combination with naloxone, aspirin, or acetaminophen; and they precipitate withdrawal in narcotic-dependent patients. One of the newer drugs in this class, buprenorphine, has been shown to be clinically effective without marked psychotomimetic effects in patients with cancer and to result in less physical dependence than morphine.[29–31] Drugs in this class may offer special advantages to the management of pain from cancer.

Traditionally, the narcotic analgesics have been used to manage acute pain. Long-term use has been discouraged because of the development of tolerance, physical dependence, and psychological dependence.[21] Tolerance is a state in which escalating doses of drug are needed to maintain an analgesic effect. Physical dependence is characterized by the onset of acute symptoms and signs of withdrawal if the narcotic is suddenly stopped or a narcotic antagonist is administered. Psychological dependence, or addiction, is separate from physical dependence and tolerance and is a concomitant behavioral pattern of drug abuse characterized by a craving for the drug and overwhelming involvement in obtaining and using it.

Because of the misconception by both clinicians and patients that physical dependence and addiction (psychological dependence) are interchangeable terms, the use of narcotic analgesics in patients with acute or chronic pain remains inadequate at best. This overriding fear of addiction coupled with physicians' lack of knowledge about the clinicopharmacologic properties of narcotic agents further limits effective use of them.[33-35] However, advances in our understanding of endogenous opiates in pain modulation and the plight of the patient with pain from cancer have led to a reevaluation of the role of narcotic analgesics in the management of chronic pain.

The long-term use of narcotic analgesics, administered orally, to manage cancer pain was heralded by the English hospice movement[3,4] and has long been advocated in the care of patients dying from cancer.[32,36,37] Studies of the patterns of chronic narcotic drug use in patients with cancer and in those with other medical illnesses have demonstrated that tolerance and physical dependence occur but that psychological dependence (addiction) is rare.[38,39] This clinical experience with long-term narcotic drug use supports the concept that psychological dependence is separate from physical dependence.[10] Drug use is not the sole factor in the development of psychological dependence; psychological, social, and economic factors also play a part. This observation has been supported by studies of heroin use by U.S. military personnel in Vietnam.[40] The concept of "addiction" should be redefined in order to place the use of narcotic analgesics in perspective.[41]

Several reviews of oral and parenteral analgesics in the management of cancer pain provide guidelines for their use.[42-48] The American Medical Association[6] and the American College of Physicians[7] have outlined approaches to drug therapy in the management of severe chronic pain associated with advanced disease. Both groups have stressed the importance of providing adequate pain control and supportive care so that the patient can die relatively free of pain. They have also stressed the need to educate physicians and other health professionals in the care of patients with pain from cancer and in the use of narcotic analgesics.

Guidelines for the practical use of narcotic analgesics are presented in Table 14.4. Tables 14.5 and 14.6 list some of the important pharmacologic properties of the non-narcotic and narcotic analgesics commonly used to treat cancer pain. The guidelines are based in part on clinicopharmacologic principles and in part on the empirical use of these drugs in clinical practice. They serve as a useful reference point, but there remains a tremendous need to develop scientifically based guidelines.

Several controversies have arisen in the use of narcotic analgesics, including the best choice of an analgesic (for example, morphine, methadone, or heroin), the route and schedule of administration (fixed or as needed), and the risk of psychological dependence with long-term use.[49] Although resolution of these controversies awaits controlled repetitive dosage studies, some of the available data are briefly reviewed below.

TABLE 14.4. Guidelines for the Use of Narcotic Analgesics in Pain Management

1. Start with a specific drug for a specific type of pain.

2. Know the pharmacology of the drug prescribed.
   a. Duration of the analgesic effect.
   b. Pharmacokinetic properties of the drug.
   c. Equianalgesic doses for the drug and its route of administration (see Tables 14.5 and 14.6).

3. Adjust the route of administration to the patient's needs.

4. Administer the analgesic on a regular basis after initial titration of the dose.

5. Use drug combinations to provide additive analgesia and reduce side effects (for example, nonsteroidal antiinflammatory drugs, antihistamine [hydroxyzine], amphetamine [Dexedrine]).

6. Avoid drug combinations that increase sedation without enhancing analgesia (for example, benzodiazepine [diazepam] and phenothiazine [chlorpromazine]).

7. Anticipate and treat side effects.
   a. Sedation.
   b. Respiratory depression.
   c. Nausea and vomiting.
   d. Constipation.

8. Watch for the development of tolerance.
   a. Switch to an alternative narcotic analgesic.
   b. Start with one-half the equianalgesic dose, and titrate the dose for pain relief.

9. Prevent acute withdrawal.
   a. Taper drugs slowly.
   b. Use diluted doses of naloxone (0.4 mg in 10 ml of saline) to reverse respiratory depression in the physically dependent patient, and administer cautiously.

10. Do not use placebos to assess the nature of pain.

11. Anticipate and manage complications.
    a. Overdose.
    b. Multifocal myoclonus.
    c. Seizures.

TABLE 14.5. Oral Non-narcotic and Narcotic Analgesics for Mild to Moderate Pain

	Equianalgesic Dose (mg)[a]	Duration (hr)	Plasma Half-Life (hr)	Comments
Aspirin	650	4–6	3–5	Standard for non-narcotic comparisons; gastrointestinal and hematologic effects limit use in patients with cancer
Acetaminophen	650	4–6	1–4	Weak antiinflammatory effects; safer than aspirin
Propoxyphene	65[b]	4–6	12	Biotransformed to potentially toxic metabolite norpropoxyphene; used in combination with non-narcotic analgesics
Codeine	32[b]	4–6	3	Biotransformed to morphine; available in combination with non-narcotic analgesics
Meperidine	50	4–6	3–4	Biotransformed to active toxic metabolite normeperidine; associated with myoclonus and seizures
Pentazocine	30	4–6	2–3	Psychotomimetic effects with escalation of dose; only available in combination with naloxone, aspirin, or acetaminophen (U.S.)

[a]Relative potency of drugs, as compared with that of aspirin, for mild to moderate pain.
[b]Some investigators have reported that a much larger dose (propoxyphene, 130 mg; codeine, 60 mg) is effective in patients with mild to moderate pain.

There is no "best choice" of analgesic agent but rather a series of agents, such as those listed in Tables 14.5 and 14.6, that have been used effectively to manage cancer pain. Oral morphine is the most commonly used drug, but its availability for outpatient pain management is severely restricted in developed and developing countries. For patients who cannot tolerate morphine, there are useful alternative drugs. Choosing the drug according to the needs of the individual patient is the rule. There may be pharmacokinetic reasons to choose shorter-acting drugs, such as morphine or hydromorphone, over methadone or levorphanol, if they are given on a fixed schedule. Accumulation of a toxic active metabolite, normeperidine, limits the long-term use of meperidine. It is the knowledge of pharmacologic properties that directs the choice of a drug. Attention to these considerations will ensure effective use of drugs.

TABLE 14.6. **Oral and Parenteral Narcotic Analgesics for Severe Pain**

	Route[a]	Equianalgesic Dose (mg)[b]	Duration (hr)	Plasma Half-Life (hr)	Comments
Narcotic agonists					
Morphine	IM PO	10 60	4–6 4–7	2–3.5	Standard for comparison; also available in slow-release tablets
Codeine	IM PO	130 200[c]	4–6 4–6	3	Biotransformed to morphine; useful as initial narcotic analgesic
Oxycodone	IM PO	15 30	3–5	—	Short-acting; available alone or as 5 mg dose in combination with aspirin and acetaminophen
Heroin	IM PO	5 60	4–5 4–5	0.5	Illegal in U.S.; high solubility for parenteral administration
Levorphanol (Levo-Dromoran)	IM PO	2 4	4–6 4–7	12–16	Good oral potency, requires careful titration in initial dosing because of drug accumulation
Hydromor-phone (Dilaudid)	IM PO	1.5 7.5	4–5 4–6	2–3	Available in high-potency injectable form (10 mg/ml) for cachectic patients and as rectal suppositories; more soluble than morphine
Oxymor-phone (Numorphan)	IM PR	1 10	4–6 4–6	2–3	Available in parenteral and rectal-suppository forms only
Meperidine (Demerol)	IM PO	75 300[c]	4–5 4–6	3–4 normeperi-dine 12–16	Contraindicated in patients with renal disease; accumulation of active toxic metabolite normeperidine produces CNS excitation
Methadone (Dolophine)	IM PO	10 20		15–30	Good oral potency; requires careful titration of the initial dose to avoid drug accumulation

(continued overleaf)

TABLE 14.6. *(Continued)*

	Route[a]	Equianalgesic Dose (mg)[b]	Duration (hr)	Plasma Half-Life (hr)	Comments
Mixed agonist–antagonist drugs					
Pentazocine (Talwin)	IM PO	60 180[c]	4–6 4–7	2–3	Limited use for cancer pain; psychotomimetic effects with dose escalation; available only in combination with naloxone, aspirin, or acetaminophen; may precipitate withdrawal in physically dependent patients
Nalbuphine (Nubain)	IM PO	10 —	4–6	5	Not available orally; less severe psychotomimetic effects than pentazocine; may precipitate withdrawal in physically dependent patients
Butorphanol (Stadol)	IM PO	2 —	4–6	2.5–3.5	Not available orally; produces psychotomimetic effects; may precipitate withdrawal in physically dependent patients
Partial agonists					
Buprenor-phine (Temgesic)	IM SL	0.4 0.8	4–6 5–6	7	Not available in U.S.; no psychotomimetic effects; may precipitate withdrawal in tolerant patients

[a]IM denotes intramuscular; PO, oral; PR, rectal; and SL, sublingual.
[b]Based on single-dose studies in which an intramuscular dose of each drug listed was compared with morphine to establish the relative potency. Oral doses are those recommended when changing from a parenteral to an oral route. For patients without prior narcotic exposure, the recommended oral starting dose is 30 mg for morphine, 5 mg for methadone, 2 mg for levorphanol, and 4 mg for hydromorphone.
[c]The recommended starting doses for these drugs are listed in Table 14.6.

Lack of knowledge of the equianalgesic doses of drugs, when a switch is made from one medication to another or from one route of administration to another, is the most common cause of undermedication. Because cross-tolerance is not complete, patients who become tolerant to the analgesic effect of one narcotic can be given another narcotic to provide better analgesia.[36,45] One-half the calculated equianalgesic dose of the new drug is recommended for titrating the starting dose. This calculation is based on clinical experience and suggests that the relative potency of some of the narcotic analgesics, specifically those with long plasma half-lives, may increase with repetitive doses.

Lack of attention to the pharmacokinetic profile has also limited the effective use of certain drugs. The plasma half-lives of the narcotic analgesics vary widely and do not correlate with their analgesic time courses. Both methadone, with a half-life of fifteen to thirty hours, and levorphanol, with a half-life of twelve to sixteen hours, produce analgesia for four to six hours.[50,51] With repeated doses, these drugs accumulate in plasma and can result in excessive sedation and respiratory depression.[52,53] It is necessary to adjust the dose and schedule according to the plasma half-life of the drug when it is introduced.[54,55]

Medication should be administered on a regular basis, with the interval between doses based on the duration of the analgesic effect. The pharmacologic objective is to maintain the plasma level of the drug above a "minimal effective concentration for pain relief."[56] However, the time required to reach a steady state after repeated administration depends on the half-life of the drug, and full assessment of the analgesic efficacy of a drug regimen may thus take twenty-four hours, for a drug such as morphine, or up to five to seven days, for methadone.[54]

The use of a combination of drugs enables the physician to improve pain relief without escalation of the narcotic dose. Several combinations have been proved effective, including a narcotic plus a non-narcotic (600 mg of aspirin or acetaminophen[36] or 400 mg of ibuprofen[57]), a narcotic plus an antihistamine (100 mg of hydroxyzine given intramuscularly),[58] and a narcotic plus an amphetamine (10 mg of dextroamphetamine [Dexedrine] given intramuscularly).[59] Other drugs, which do not provide additive analgesia but are commonly employed in combination with narcotic agents, include diazepam, chlorpromazine, and cocaine.[60-62]

The Brompton Cocktail, which consists of varying doses of diacetylmorphine (heroin) or morphine, cocaine, phenothiazine, alcohol, and chloroform water, has been reported to control pain in 90 percent of patients. Studies by Twycross have demonstrated that analgesic efficacy results from the narcotic alone and that morphine can be substituted for heroin. He has therefore advocated using oral narcotic solutions in titrated doses according to the needs of the individual patient rather than using cocktails.[3,63]

The route of drug administration must also be selected according to the needs of the patient. The oral route is most practical, but the oral bioavailability of drugs varies widely. Recent studies have helped to establish a kinetic basis for the rational use of oral morphine and methadone in patients with cancer[55,64-66] and have demonstrated that oral heroin, although effective as an analgesic, is inefficient as a means of delivering morphine.[67] Several novel methods and routes of administration have been developed to maximize pharmacologic effects and to minimize undesirable effects associated with standard methods—for example, slow-release morphine tablets that are effective for eight to twelve hours. Novel routes under investigation include intranasal, transdermal, and sublingual drug administration. The advantage of these routes is that they avoid drug metabolism by the liver (presystemic clearance), which substantially reduces the oral potency of morphine and some of the other narcotics. These alternative routes offer a special advantage, particularly in the patient with gastrointestinal obstruction, limited venous access, or reduced muscle mass. To date, only one drug, buprenorphine, is produced in a sublingual form, but it is not available in the United States.

Continuous infusions of narcotics by intravenous and subcutaneous routes have been employed to meet the needs of select populations of patients with cancer.[68-71] Although the indications for these techniques, their limitations, and their efficacy have not been fully assessed and the pharmacokinetic basis for their use remains undefined, their clinical use is widespread and expanding. The inability to predict an ideal maintenance infusion rate and to accommodate differences among patients makes it difficult to use these techniques.[72] The intravenous or oral equianalgesic doses are not known for many of the drugs. When a switch is made from the intramuscular route to continuous intravenous infusions, the starting dose is calculated as the equivalent morphine dose for a twenty-four-hour period. This calculation is based on clinical experience, not controlled studies.[47]

Epidural and intrathecal administration of narcotics is based on the demonstration of opiate receptors in the dorsal horn and suppression of spinothalamictract neurons to noxious stimuli by opiates applied to the spinal cord.[73-78] Localized selective analgesia is produced without motor blockade. This approach minimizes the distribution of drugs to receptors in the brain stem and cerebral hemispheres, avoiding the side effects of systemic administration. The clinical efficacy of continuous infusions by this route, using the Infusaid pump, has been studied in patients with pain from cancer. The clinical and pharmacokinetic data demonstrate that profound analgesia can be produced with small doses of morphine. Because the dose and subsequent systemic uptake are much higher with epidural administration, the intrathecal route has been advocated. However, both epidural and intrathecal administration are associated with rostral redistribution of drug and central side effects. Also, tolerance occurs and is most problematic in the patient with progressive disease. Considerable cross-tolerance is induced by systemic narcotics, making it difficult to determine the proper timing for use of these techniques in the management of pain from cancer. Intraventricular administration of narcotics in patients with cancer has also been shown to provide profound analgesia when small doses of drug are administered through an Ommaya reservoir.[79]

As noted above, tolerance occurs with long-term administration in patients with progressive disease, but increased doses of drug continue to produce analgesia, suggesting that with the narcotic agonist drugs there is no limit to tolerance. Tolerance of each of the effects of the narcotics occurs at a different rate. Switching to an alternative narcotic, adding non-narcotic agents, and employing neurosurgical and anesthetic approaches are methods commonly used to manage pain in the patient with a tolerance to a particular narcotic agent.

These guidelines notwithstanding, the management of pain with analgesics remains difficult. Much of the difficulty encountered arises from differences in the responses of individual patients to the same dose of drug. Kaiko and colleagues have described some of the sources of variation in the responses of patients with cancer to morphine and the need for dose adjustment on the basis of age.[80,81] The efficacy of such drugs is based on an understanding of their clinicopharmacologic properties and improved methods to manage their side effects. Effective use of narcotic agents is now possible because of the development of specific and sensitive techniques to quantitate drugs in biofluids, the availability of well-defined clinical methods to measure the pain response, and the application of pharmacokinetic and pharmacodynamic models to relate plasma concentrations of narcotics to analgesic effects.[82,83] Recent studies demonstrate that equianalgesic doses of heroin are comparable to morphine in their analgesic effect, side effects, and influence on mood. These studies refute anecdotal reports of heroin's superiority.[84] Studies of repeated meperidine administration in patients with cancer have demonstrated that central nervous system hyperirritability results from accumulation of the active toxic metabolite normeperidine.[85]

Adjuvant Analgesic Drugs Adjuvant analgesic agents constitute a third group of drugs used to treat patients with pain from cancer.[86,87] This group includes several different categories of drugs, such as anticonvulsant agents,[88] phenothiazines,[89] butyrophenones,[90] tricyclic antidepressants,[91,92] antihistamines, amphetamines, and steroids,[93,94] and levodopa.[95] These drugs produce analgesia in certain painful states by mechanisms not clearly established and not directly related to the opiate receptor system. Clinical interest in their use has developed from a greater understanding of the neuropharmacologic characteristics of pain and the ability of these drugs to enhance or block neurotransmitter function. In some instances, analgesic effects have been established in controlled clinical trials, such as the use of amitriptyline in postherpetic neuralgia,[91] but for most of these drugs, anecdotal data or clinical surveys provide the rationale for their use, which is controversial at best. Although these drugs are commonly used in patients with pain from cancer, the evidence suggests that they are not as effective as narcotic analgesics in relieving pain. Adjuvant analgesic drugs have been developed and released for clinical indications other than pain relief.

Anesthetic Approaches

These approaches are most useful in treating patients with well-defined localized pain from tumor infiltration. Short-acting and long-acting anesthetics are used for temporary and diagnostic nerve blocks, whereas phenol, alcohol, and freezing (cryoanalgesia) are the common neurolytic agents used for permanent blocks.[96–99] The principal pathologic effect produced by these agents is demyelination, with secondary nerve degeneration. Local freezing causes a loss in nerve function, which reportedly lasts for several weeks only.[99] A permanent nerve block is performed if a temporary block has demonstrated efficacy. The most common indications for nerve block are listed in Table 14.3. The limitations of these procedures are that each peripheral nerve subserves sensory function over multiple levels, requiring multiple nerves to be blocked for adequate pain control. Similarly, epidural and intrathecal nerve blocks with neurolytic agents can produce motor weakness and autonomic dysfunction. The techniques, indications, and diluents and concentration of neurolytic agents vary from investigator to investigator, with satisfactory results reported in 22 to 80 percent of patients and permanent side effects, such as urinary or rectal incontinence, motor weakness, or paresthesias, in 1 to 13 percent.[96-102] However, the use of autonomic nerve blocks, such as celiac-plexus block, to manage midabdominal pain associated with carcinoma of the pancreas is very effective in 60 percent of patients and is often the procedure of choice in such patients.[101]

Intermittent or continuous epidural infusions of local anesthetics have been used for temporary management of the difficult pain syndromes involving the lumbosacral plexus and sacrum. By varying the amount and concentration of the local anesthetic delivered continuously by an infusion pump or intermittently by a subcutaneously implanted reservoir attached to a catheter placed in the epidural space, pain relief can be achieved without interruption of motor or autonomic function.[103] The advantage of this method is that it does not result in cross-tolerance with opiate analgesia, and temporary use of epidural infusions allows for a reduction in the amount of systemic opiate drugs, partially reversing tolerance. This is a useful preliminary approach to reduce tolerance when spinal opiate analgesia is under consideration as a therapeutic approach.

Two anesthetic approaches used to manage diffuse pain are chemical hypophysectomy and intermittent inhalation therapy with nitrous oxide. Chemical hypophysectomy, which involves the injection of alcohol into the sella turcica under radiologic supervision, is used to control pain in patients with widespread bony metastases. Initial studies reported dramatic pain relief in 60 percent of six hundred patients, but more recent studies report relief in 35 to 74 percent of patients.[104, 105] The mechanism of analgesia may be related in part to the tracking of alcohol up the pituitary stalk and the consequent disruption of the hypothalamic-thalamic endorphinergic pain pathway. The lack of detailed clinical data and information on the endocrine status of such patients limits critical assessment of the technique, and in many patients pain relief occurs independently of tumor regression.

Nitrous oxide is used to manage chronic pain from tumor progression or pain in the dying patient.[106] It is administered in oxygen through a nonrebreathing face mask, with concentrations ranging from 25 to 75 percent, often in combination with systemic narcotics. Patients can remain alert during its use. It is most useful in managing acute incident pain and procedure-related pain.

Lastly, trigger-point injections,[107] although considered an anesthetic procedure, are commonly used in clinical practice and require no special expertise. A focal injection of saline or local anesthetic into a painful muscle joint provides dramatic relief. However, a careful assessment of the nature of the pain should be undertaken.

Neurosurgical Approaches

At present, cordotomy and placement of epidural, intrathecal, and intraventricular catheters for narcotic drug delivery are the most common neurosurgical procedures performed for pain relief (Table 14.2).[108-115] A cordotomy involves the interruption of the anterior lateral spinothalamic tract in the cervical or thoracic region. It may be performed as a percutaneous stereotactic procedure or by an open surgical approach. It is most useful in managing unilateral pain below the waist. Initial complications include paresis in 5 percent of patients, ataxia in 20 percent, and urinary dysfunction in 10 percent, with late complications occurring in only 5 percent. Although initial pain relief from cordotomy occurs in 90 percent of patients, this figure drops to 80 percent at three months, and at the end of one year approximately 40 percent of patients report a return of pain. Another limiting factor in the success of both open and percutaneous cordotomies is that pain develops on the side opposite the cordotomy site in 7 to 10 percent of patients; even more distressing, in a comparable number of patients, pain previously unrecognized at another site becomes as intractable as the pain for which the cordotomy was performed. This is one of the most common causes for the failure of cordotomy and explains the limited usefulness of the procedure in patients with diffuse pain.

Each of the other neurosurgical procedures involves either sectioning or stimulation of the peripheral nerves, spinal cord, brain stem, or thalamus. These are specialized procedures requiring neurosurgical expertise and must often be performed at special centers.

Behavioral Approaches

Behavioral approaches, including relaxation training, biofeedback and cognitive and behavioral training, hypnosis, and music therapy, have been integrated into the management of cancer pain.[116-121] The major goal of these interventions is to promote an increased sense of control by reducing the hopelessness and helplessness that many patients with pain from cancer experience. These techniques also serve as a calming diversion of attention, breaking the pain-anxiety-tension cycle. The effectiveness of any one of these techniques, as compared with another or with standard medical or surgical therapy, is unknown, and few controlled studies have been performed. Patients are taught these techniques and then use them independently. Relaxation training can be given by all health care professionals, whereas other approaches require biophysical instrumentation or more specialized skills. Cognitive and behavioral training provides patients with a variety of strategies to divert their attention away from pain, facilitate their tolerance of pain, and increase their perceived self-control and adaptive functioning.

Music therapy has been used in hospitals and hospice settings either alone or in combination with relaxation training and hypnosis to augment the effects of these techniques.[119] Hypnosis has been studied the most extensively and has been widely used in the treatment of acute and chronic cancer pain.[120, 121] Studies report that 50 percent of patients may obtain some pain relief, yet indicate that there is no single effective hypnotic procedure.

In general, these behavioral techniques reduce pain by means of mechanisms that are in part related to their ability to modulate the affective response to painful stimuli. Studies have demonstrated that analgesia induced by hypnosis is not mediated by the endogenous opiate system, because it is not reversed by naloxone.[122]

SUPPORTIVE CARE

Numerous models of supportive care have stressed the importance of pain control for the patient at home. Inadequate control of pain in the outpatient is a common cause for readmission to the hospital. Specific guidelines for managing cancer pain at home include education of patients, their families, and health care professionals in the proper use of analgesics; twenty-four-hour availability of a physician or a nurse with expertise in pain management to adjust drug doses; adequate drug supplies for alternative routes of administration, such as the parenteral route; and education in the use of naloxone to reverse opiate-induced respiratory depression.

These approaches, coupled with psychological support for patients and their families and integration of social services, can give the patient with pain the option to remain at home.[3,4,123,124]

SUMMARY

Pain is one of the most feared consequences of cancer. Control of pain from cancer should be possible with the approaches discussed above. Changing attitudes toward the effective use of narcotic analgesics, the development of novel routes and methods of administration, and a clinical approach based on scientific principles and humane care offer the promise of improved management of pain in patients with cancer.

REFERENCES

1. Payne R, Foley KM. Advances in the management of cancer pain. *Cancer Treat Rep.* 1984; 68:173–83.

2. Bonica JJ. Importance of the problem. In: Bonica JJ, Ventafridda V, Fink RB, Jones LE, Loeser JD, eds. *Advances in pain research and therapy.* Vol. 2. New York: Raven Press, 1979:1–12.

3. Twycross RG, Lack SA. *Symptom control in far advanced cancer: pain relief.* London: Pitman, 1984.

4. Saunders CM. *The management of terminal illness.* London: Edward Arnold, 1967.

5. Foley KM. The management of pain of malignant origin. In: Tyler HR, Dawson DM, eds. *Current neurology.* Boston: Houghton Mifflin, 1979:279–302.

6. McGivney WT, Crooks GM, eds. The care of patients with severe chronic pain in terminal illness. *JAMA.* 1984; 251:1182–8.

7. Health and Public Policy Committee, American College of Physicians. Drug therapy for severe chronic pain in terminal illness. *Ann Intern Med.* 1983; 99:870–3.

8. Twycross RG, Fairfield S. Pain in far-advanced cancer. *Pain.* 1982; 14:303–10.

9. Daut RL, Cleeland CS. The prevalence and severity of pain in cancer. *Cancer.* 1982; 50:1913–8.

10. Kanner RM, Foley KM. Patterns of narcotic drug use in a cancer pain clinic. *Ann NY Acad Sci.* 1981; 362:161–72.

11. Cleeland CS. The impact of pain on patients with cancer. *Cancer.* 1984; 54:2635–41.

12. Foley KM. Pain syndromes in patients with cancer. In: Bonica JJ, Ventafridda V, Fink RB, Jones LE, Loeser JD, eds. *Advances in pain research and therapy.* Vol. 2. New York: Raven Press, 1979:59–75.

13. Swerdlow M, Stjernswärd J. *Cancer pain relief— an urgent problem. World Health Forum* 1982; 3:325–30.

14. Basbaum AI, Fields HL. Endogenous pain control mechanisms: review and hypothesis. *Ann Neurol.* 1978; 4:451–62.

15. Sternbach RA. *Pain patients: traits and treatment.* New York: Academic Press, 1974.

16. IASP Subcommittee on Taxonomy Pain Terms: a list with definitions and notes on usage. *Pain.* 1979; 6:249–52.

17. Spiegel D, Bloom JR. Pain in metastatic breast cancer. *Cancer.* 1983; 52:341–5.

18. Fultz JM, Senay EC. Guidelines for management of hospitalized narcotic addicts. *Ann Intern Med.* 1975; 82:815–8.

19. Bonica JJ. *The management of pain*. Philadelphia: Lea & Febiger, 1953.

20. Tasker RR, Tsuda T, Hawrylyshyn P. Clinical neurophysiological investigation of deafferentation pain. In: Bonica JJ, Lindblom U, Iggo A, eds. *Advances in pain research and therapy*. Vol. 5. New York: Raven Press, 1981:713–38.

21. Foley KM. Clinical assessment of cancer pain. *Acta Anesthesiol Scand* [suppl]. 1982; 74:91–6.

22. Twycross RG, Ventafridda V, eds. *The continuing care of terminal cancer patients*. Oxford: Pergamon Press, 1980.

23. Gerbershagen HU. Nonnarcotic analgesics. In: Bonica JJ, Ventafridda V, Fink RB, Jones LE, Loeser JD, eds. *Advances in pain research and therapy*. Vol. 2. New York: Raven Press, 1979:255–73.

24. Kantor TG. Control of pain by nonsteroidal anti-inflammatory drugs. *Med Clin North Am.* 1982; 66:1053–9.

25. Moertel GG. Treatment of cancer pain with orally administered medications. *JAMA.* 1980; 244:2448–50.

26. Brodie GN. Indomethacin and bone pain. *Lancet.* 1974; 2:1160.

27. Brereton HD, Halushka PV, Alexander RW, Mason DM, Keiser HR, DeVita VT Jr. Indomethacin-responsive hypercalcemia in a patient with renal-cell adenocarcinoma. *N Engl J Med.* 1974; 291:83–5.

28. Galasko CSB. Mechanisms of bone destruction in the development of skeletal metastases. *Nature.* 1976; 263:507–10.

29. Houde RW. Analgesic effectiveness of the narcotic agonist-antagonists. *Br J Clin Pharmacol.* 1979; 7:297S–308S.

30. Robbie DS. A trial of sublingual buprenorphine in cancer pain. *Br J Clin Pharmacol.* 1979; 7:315S–85S.

31. Ventafridda V, DeConno F, Guarise G, et al. Chronic analgesic study on buprenorphine action in cancer pain— comparison with pentazocine. *Drug Res.* 1983; 4:587–90.

32. Jaffe JH, Martin WR. Opioid analgesics and antagonists. In: Gilman AG, Goodman LS, Gilman A, eds. *The pharmacological basis of therapeutics*. 6th ed. New York: Macmillan, 1980:494–534.

33. Marks RM, Sachar EJ. Undertreatment of medical inpatients with narcotic analgesics. *Ann Intern Med.* 1973; 78:173–81.

34. Charap AD. The knowledge, attitudes and experience of medical personnel treating pain in the terminally ill. *Mt Sinai J Med.* 1978; 45:561–80.

35. Sriwatanakul K, Weis OF, Alloza JL, Kelvie W, Weintraub M, Lasagna L. Analysis of narcotic analgesic usage in the treatment of postoperative pain. *JAMA.* 1983; 250:926–9.

36. Houde RW, Wallenstein SL, Beaver WT. Evaluation of analgesics in patients with cancer pain. In: Lasagna L, ed. *International encyclopedia of pharmacology and therapeutics*. Section 6. Clinical pharmacology. Vol. 1. New York: Pergamon Press, 1966:59–97.

37. Paulshock BZ. William Heberden and opium— some relief to all. *N Engl J Med.* 1983; 308:53–5.

38. Angell M. The quality of mercy. *N Engl J Med.* 1982; 306:98–9.

39. Porter, J, Jick H. Addiction rare in patients treated with narcotics. *N Engl J Med.* 1980; 302:123.

40. Robins LN, David DH, Nurco DN. How permanent was Vietnam drug addiction? *Am J Public Health.* 1974; 64:38–43.

41. Newman RG. The need to redefine "addiction." *N Engl J Med.* 1983; 308:1096–8.

42. Beaver WT. Management of cancer pain with parenteral medication. *JAMA.* 1980; 244:2653–7.

43. Shimm DS, Logue GL, Maltbie AA, Dugan S. Medical management of chronic cancer pain. *JAMA.* 1979; 241:2408–12.

44. Inturrisi CE. Narcotic drugs. *Med Clin North Am.* 1982; 66:1061–71.

45. Inturrisi CE, Foley KM. Narcotic analgesics in the management of pain. In: Kuhar M, Pasternak G,

eds. *Analgesics: neurochemical, behavioral and clinical perspectives*. New York: Raven Press, 1984: 257–87.

46. Houde RW, Wallenstein SL, Beavers WT. Clinical measurement of pain. In: deStevens G, ed. *Analgesics*. New York: Academic Press, 1965:75–122.

47. Foley KM. The practical use of narcotic analgesics. *Med Clin North Am.* 1982; 66:1091–104.

48. Rane A, Säwe J, Dahlström B, Paalzow L, Kager L. Pharmacological treatment of cancer pain with special reference to the oral use of morphine. *Acta Anaesthesiol Scand* [suppl]. 1982; 74:97–103.

49. Foley KM. Current controversies in the management of cancer pain. In: *NIDA Res Monograph Series.* 1981; 36:169–81.

50. Inturrisi CE, Verebely K. Disposition of methadone in man after a single oral dose. *Clin Pharmacol Ther.* 1972; 13:923–30.

51. Dixon R, Crews T, Mohacsi C, Inturrisi C, Foley K. Levorphanol: radioimmunoassay and plasma concentration profiles in dog and man. *Res Commun Chem Pathol Pharmacol.* 1980; 29:535–47.

52. Ettinger DS, Vitale PJ, Trump DL. Important clinical pharmacologic considerations in the use of methadone in cancer patients. *Cancer Treat Rep.* 1979; 63:457–9.

53. Symonds P. Methadone and the elderly. *Br Med J.* 1977; 1:512.

54. Breivik H, Rennemo F. Clinical evaluation of combined treatment with methadone and psychotropic drugs in cancer patients. *Acta Anaesthesiol Scand* [suppl]. 1982; 74:135–40.

55. Säwe J, Hansen, J, Ginman C, et al. Patient-controlled dose regimen for methadone for chronic cancer pain. *Br Med J.* 1981; 282:771–3.

56. Paalzow LK. Pharmacokinetic aspects of optimal pain treatment. *Acta Anaesthesiol Scand* [suppl]. 1982; 74:37–43.

57. Ferrer-Brechner T, Ganz P. Combination therapy with ibuprofen and methadone for chronic cancer pain. *Am J Med.* 1984; 77:78–83.

58. Beaver WT, Feise G. Comparison of analgesic effects of morphine sulfate, hydroxyzine and their combination in patients with postoperative pain. In: Bonica JJ, Albe-Fessard D, eds. *Advances in pain research and therapy*. Vol. 1. New York: Raven Press, 1976:553–7.

59. Forrest WH Jr, Brown BW Jr, Brown CR, et al. Dextroamphetamine with morphine for the treatment of postoperative pain. *N Engl J Med.* 1977; 296:712–5.

60. Singh PN, Sharma P, Gupta PK. Chemical evaluation of diazepam for relief of postoperative pain. *Br J Anaesth.* 1981; 53:831–5.

61. Dundee JW, Moore J. The myth of phenothiazine potentiation. *Anaesthesia.* 1961; 16:95–6.

62. Twycross R. Value of cocaine in opiate-containing elixirs. *Br Med J.* 1977; 2:1348.

63. Twycross RG. Clinical experience with diamorphine in advanced malignant disease. *Int J Clin Pharmacol Ther Toxicol.* 1974; 9:184–98.

64. Säwe J, Dahlström B, Paalzow L., Rane A. Morphine kinetics in cancer patients. *Clin Pharmacol Ther.* 1981; 30:629–35.

65. Säwe J, Dahlström B, Rane A. Steady-state kinetics and analgesic effect of oral morphine in cancer patients. *Eur J Clin Pharmacol.* 1983; 24:537–42.

66. Säwe J, Svensson JO, Rane A. Morphine metabolism in cancer patients on increasing oral doses—no evidence for autoinduction or dose-dependence. *Br J Clin Pharmacol.* 1983; 16:85–93.

67. Inturrisi CE, Max MB, Foley KM, Schultz M, Shin S-U, Houde RW. The pharmacokinetics of heroin in patients with chronic pain. *N Engl J Med.* 1984; 210:1213–7.

68. DeChristoforo R, Corden BJ, Hood JC, Narang PK, Magrath IT. High-dose morphine infusion complicated by chlorobutanol-induced somnolence. *Ann Intern Med.* 1983; 98:335–6.

69. Fraser DG. Intravenous morphine infusion for chronic pain. *Ann Intern Med.* 1980; 93:781–2.

70. Miser AW, Miser JS, Clark BS. Continuous intravenous infusion of morphine sulfate for control of severe pain in children with terminal malignancy. *J Pediatr.* 1980; 96:930–2.

71. Campbell CF, Mason JB, Weiler JM. Continuous subcutaneous infusion of morphine for the pain of terminal malignancy. *Ann Intern Med.* 1983; 98:51–2.

72. Graves DA, Foster TS, Batenhorst RL, Bennett RL, Baumann TJ. Patient controlled analgesia. *Ann Intern Med.* 1983; 99:360–6.

73. Yaksh TL. Spinal opiate analgesia: characteristics and principles of action. *Pain.* 1981; 11:293–346.

74. Coombs DW, Saunders RL, Gaylor MS, Pageau MG. Epidural narcotic infusion reservoir: implantation technique and efficacy. *Anesthesiology.* 1982; 56:469–73.

75. Coombs DW, Saunders RL, Gaylor MS, et al. Relief of continuous chronic pain by intraspinal narcotics infusion via an implanted reservoir. *JAMA.* 1983; 250:2336–9.

76. Onofrio BM, Yaksh TL, Arnold PG. Continuous low-dose intrathecal morphine in the treatment of chronic pain of malignant origin. *Mayo Clin Proc.* 1981; 56:516–20.

77. Poletti CE, Cohen AM, Todd DP, Ojemann RG, Sweet WH, Zervas NT. Cancer pain relieved by long-term epidural morphine with permanent in-dwelling systems for self-administration. *J Neurosurg.* 1981; 55:581–4.

78. Greenberg HS, Taren J, Ensminger WD, Doan K. Benefit from and tolerance to continuous intrathecal infusion of morphine for intractable cancer pain. *J Neurosurg.* 1982; 57:360–4.

79. Lobato RD, Madrid JL, Fatela LV, Rivas JJ, Reig E, Lamas E. Intraventricular morphine for control of pain in terminal cancer patients. *J Neurosurg.* 1983; 59:627–33.

80. Kaiko RF. Age and morphine analgesia in cancer patients with postoperative pain. *Clin Pharmacol Ther.* 1980; 28:823–6.

81. Kaiko RF, Wallenstein SL, Rogers AG, Houde RW. Sources of variation in analgesic responses in cancer patients with chronic pain receiving morphine. *Pain.* 1983; 15:191–200.

82. Houde RW. Methods for measuring clinical pain in humans. *Acta Anaesthesiol Scand* [suppl]. 1982; 74:25–9.

83. Colburn WA. Simultaneous pharmacokinetic and pharmacodynamic modeling. *J Pharmacokinet Biopharm.* 1981; 9:367–88.

84. Kaiko RF, Wallenstein SL, Rogers AG, Grabinski PY, Houde RW. Analgesic and mood effects of heroin and morphine in cancer patients with postoperative pain. *N Engl J Med.* 1981; 304:1501–5.

85. Kaiko RF, Foley KM, Grabinski PY, et al. Central nervous system excitatory effects of meperidine in cancer patients. *Ann Neurol.* 1983; 13:180–5.

86. Halpern LW. Psychotropics, ataractics and related drugs. In: Bonica JJ, Ventafridda V, eds. *Advances in pain research and therapy.* Vol. 2. New York: Raven Press, 1979:275–83.

87. Hanks GW. Psychotropic drugs. *Clinics Oncol.* 1984; 3:135–51.

88. Swerdlow M. Anticonvulsant drugs and chronic pain. *Clin Neuropharmacol.* 1984; 7:51–82.

89. Beaver WT, Wallenstein SL, Houde RW, Rogers A. A comparison of the analgesic effect of methotrimeprazine and morphine in patients with cancer. *Clin Pharmacol Ther.* 1966; 7:436–46.

90. Hanks GW, Thomas PJ, Trueman T, Weeks E. The myth of haloperidol potentiation. *Lancet.* 1983; 2:523–4.

91. Watson CP, Evans RJ, Reed K, Merskey H, Goldsmith L, Warsh J. Amitriptyline versus placebo in postherpetic neuralgia. *Neurology* (NY). 1982; 32:671–3.

92. Walsh TD. Antidepressants and chronic pain. *Clin Neuropharmacol.* 1983; 6:271–95.

93. Schell HW. The risk of adrenal corticosteroid therapy with far-advanced cancer. *Am J Med Sci.* 1966; 252:641–9.

94. Idem. Adrenal corticosteroid therapy in far-advanced cancer. *Geriatrics.* 1972; 27:131–41.

95. Minton JP. The response of breast cancer patients with bone pain to L-dopa. *Cancer.* 1974; 33:358–63.

96. Cousins MJ, Bridenbaugh PO, eds. *Neural blockade.* Philadelphia: JB Lippincott, 1980.

97. Arnér S. The role of nerve blocks in the treatment of cancer pain. *Acta Anaesth Scand* [suppl]. 1982; 74:104–8.

98. Brechner VL, Ferrer-Brechner T, Allen GD. Anesthetic measures in management of pain associated with malignancy. *Semin Oncol.* 1977; 4:99–108.

99. Lloyd JW, Barnard JDW, Glynn CJ. Cryoanalgesia: a new approach to pain relief. *Lancet.* 1976; 2:932–4.

100. Swerdlow M. Spinal and peripheral neurolysis for managing Pancoast syndrome. In: Bonica JJ, Ventafridda V, Pagni CA, Jones LE, eds. *Advances in pain research and therapy*. Vol. 4. New York: Raven Press, 1982:135–44.

101. Moore DC. Role of nerve block in neurolytic solutions for pelvic visceral cancer pain. In: Bonica JJ, Ventafridda V, eds. *Advances in pain research and therapy*. Vol. 2. New York: Raven Press, 1979:593–6.

102. Ventafridda V, Martino G. Clinical evaluation of subarachnoid neurolytic blocks in intractable cancer pain. In: Bonica JJ, Albe-Fessard D, eds. *Advances in pain research and therapy*. Vol. 1. New York: Raven Press, 1976:699–703.

103. Pilon RN, Baker AR. Chronic pain control by means of an epidural catheter: report of a case with description of the method. *Cancer.* 1976; 37:903–5.

104. Moricca G. Chemical hypophysectomy for cancer pain. In: Bonica JJ, ed. *Advances in neurology*. Vol. 4. New York: Raven Press, 1974:707–14.

105. Miles J, Lipton S. Mode of action by which pituitary alcohol injection relieves pain. In: Bonica JJ, Albe-Fessard D, eds. *Advances in pain research and therapy*. Vol. 1. New York: Raven Press, 1976:867–9.

106. Fosburg MT, Crone RK. Nitrous oxide analgesia for refractory pain in the terminally ill. *JAMA.* 1983; 250:511–3.

107. Travell J. Myofascial trigger points: clinical review. In: Bonica JJ, Albe-Fessard D, eds. *Advances in pain research and therapy*. Vol. 1. New York: Raven Press, 1976:919–26.

108. Friedberg SR. Neurosurgical treatment of pain caused by cancer. *Med Clin North Am.* 1975; 59:481–5.

109. Ventafridda V, Sganzerla EP, Fochi C, et al. Transcutaneous nerve stimulation in cancer pain. In: Bonica JJ, Ventafridda V, eds. *Advances in pain research and therapy*. Vol. 2. New York: Raven Press, 1979:509–15.

110. Loeser JD. Dorsal column and peripheral nerve stimulation for relief of cancer pain. In: Bonica JJ, Ventafridda V, eds. *Advances in pain research and therapy*. Vol. 2. New York: Raven Press, 1979:499–507.

111. Meyerson BA. Central nervous stimulation for cancer pain: possible methods of manipulating the physiology of pain control. In: Bonica JJ, Ventafridda V, Pagni CA, Jones LE, eds. *Advances in pain research and therapy*. Vol. 4. New York: Raven Press, 1982:149–64.

112. Nathan PW. Pain in cancer: comparison of results of cordotomy and chemical rhizotomy. In: Fusek I, Kunc T, eds. *Present limits of neurosurgery*. Amsterdam: Excerpta Medica, 1972:513–6.

113. Idem. Results of antero-lateral cordotomy for pain in cancer. *J Neurol Neurosurg Psychiatry.* 1963; 26:353–62.

114. Ventafridda V, DeConno F, Fochi C. Clinical percutaneous cordotomy. In: Bonica JJ, Ventafridda V, Pagni CA, Jones LE, eds. *Advances in pain research and therapy*. Vol. 4. New York: Raven Press, 1982:185–98.

115. Nashold BS, Ostdahl, RH. Dorsal root entry zone lesions for pain relief. *J Neurosurg.* 1979; 51:59–69.

116. Turk DC, Meichenbaum DH, Berman WH. Application of biofeedback for the regulation of pain: a critical review. *Psychol Bull.* 1979; 86:1322–38.

117. Chappell MN, Stevenson TI. Group psychological training in some organic conditions. *Ment Hyg.* 1936; 20:588–97.

118. Rybstein-Blinchik E. Effects of different cognitive strategies on chronic pain experience. *J Behav Med.* 1979; 2:93–101.

119. Munro S, Mount B. Music therapy in palliative care. *Can Med Assoc J.* 1978; 119:1029–34.

120. Koerner ME. Using hypnosis to relieve pain of terminal cancer. *Hypnosis Q.* 1977; 20:39–46.

121. Barber J, Gitelson J. Cancer pain: psychological management using hypnosis. *Cancer*. 1980; 30:130–5.

122. Mayer DJ, Price DD. Central nervous system mechanisms of analgesia. *Pain*. 1976; 2:379–404.

123. Meyers AR, Master RJ, Kirk EM, et al. Integrated care for the terminally ill: variations in the utilization of formal services. *Gerontology*. 1983; 23:71–4.

124. Coyle N, Monzillo E, Loscalzo M, Farkas C, Massie MJ, Foley KM. A model of continuity of care for cancer patients with pain and neuro-oncologic complications. *Cancer Nurs*. 1985; 8:111–9.

ACKNOWLEDGMENTS

I am indebted to Dr. Raymond W. Houde for information on the equianalgesic doses of non-narcotic and narcotic analgesics and for his critical review of the manuscript, and to Mary Callaway for assistance in the preparation of the manuscript.

RESPONDING TO INTRACTABLE TERMINAL SUFFERING

The Role of Terminal Sedation and Voluntary Refusal of Food and Fluids

TIMOTHY E. QUILL, M.D., AND IRA R. BYOCK, M.D., FOR THE ACP-ASIM
END-OF-LIFE CARE CONSENSUS PANEL

This article first appeared as Quill TE, Byock IR. Responding to intractable terminal suffering: the role of terminal sedation and voluntary refusal of food and fluids. *Ann Intern Med.* 2000;132:408–414. Copyright © 2000, American College of Physicians. All rights reserved. Reprinted with permission. It was followed by letters to the editor on Quill-Byock in *Ann Intern Med.* 2000;133:560–566, one of which is reprinted in Chapter 16.

EDITORS' INTRODUCTION

The co-authors are prominent leaders in the field, and though they represent differing opinions on the ethics of physician-assisted dying, they agree on a patient's right to so-called terminal options of last resort in the face of intractable suffering, including voluntary stopping of eating and drinking and sedation to unconsciousness when no other methods have adequately remedied a patient's suffering.

■ ■ ■

Palliative care, which addresses the multiple physical, psychosocial, and spiritual dimensions of suffering, should be the standard of care for the dying.[1-5] Such care is usually effective,[6-12] but some patients develop intolerable suffering despite excellent care.[13-17] This paper discusses terminal sedation and voluntary refusal of hydration and nutrition as potential last-resort responses to severe, unrelievable end-of-life suffering. As part of their palliative care skills and services, clinicians must have strategies for responding to the troubling problems of patients who experience such suffering. These two options provide a means of response for patients, families, and clinicians who oppose physician-assisted suicide.

CASE PRESENTATION

BG was a sixty-six-year-old retired radiologist who developed a large glioblastoma in the left parietal lobe. After extensive discussion, he elected to pursue a purely symptom-oriented approach. BG was married with two grown children. He was a proud, independent person who valued his intellectual abilities and physical integrity. He was a lifelong Unitarian. From his experience as a radiologist, he knew the natural history and potential burdens of aggressive treatment of similar brain tumors. He did not want to die but was fearful of becoming physically dependent and intellectually impaired.

The treatment goal was to manage his symptoms so that he could have quality time with his wife and children. Dexamethasone and antiseizure medications were the central symptom-relieving measures. Initially, his right-side weakness and headache improved for several weeks as he and his family worked to achieve closure in their lives together.

Unfortunately, BG abruptly developed right-side weakness and intermittent confusion secondary to focal motor seizures, and his symptoms steadily worsened despite treatment.

Sensing his physical and intellectual deterioration, BG wanted to "get on with it before I can't do anything for myself." Further mental and physical deterioration became more frightening to him than death. He hoped he could die quickly by stopping corticosteroid therapy. BG's physician urged him to continue his medications for symptom relief, but BG did not want to take anything that could in any way prolong his life. At his internist's insistence, BG agreed to a single visit with a psychiatrist, who confirmed that BG understood his treatment options and was not clinically depressed. After saying his good-byes to friends and family, BG discontinued dexamethasone therapy.

To BG's consternation, he did not become comatose or die. Instead, his right-side weakness worsened and his seizures became more frequent. BG found his situation intolerable. He did not explicitly request medication that could be taken in a lethal dose, but his desire for a hastened death was clear. "I just want to go to sleep and not wake up," he said.

All members of the team were committed to relieving his distress but had different views about explicitly assisting death. They searched for common ground while continuing to adjust his seizure management, support his family, and bring some quality to his days. None of their efforts changed BG's certainty that he did not want to continue living under his current circumstances. He began to consider refusing all food and fluids and asked his physician what it would be like and whether she would support him.

THE CLINICAL PROBLEM

Comprehensive palliative care is highly effective,[6–12] but survey data show that 5 percent to 35 percent of patients in hospice programs describe their pain as "severe" in the last week of life and that 25 percent describe their shortness of breath as "unbearable."[15] On occasion, such symptoms as delirium, bleeding, weakness, open wounds, profound weight loss, and seizures challenge the most experienced hospice teams.

In terminally ill persons, requests for physician-assisted death are infrequently triggered by unrelieved pain alone but more commonly result from a combination of physical symptoms and debility, weakness, lack of meaning, and weariness of dying.[18–21] Some of these patients are clinically depressed, and others are not.[22–25] Usually, their suffering is a complex amalgam of pain, physical symptoms, and psychosocial, existential, and spiritual issues, which are balanced by hope, love, connection, and meaning.[26–30] Understanding each patient's unique situation and responding to it in a multifaceted way is the crux of palliative medicine. Suffering can arise from a sense of impending disintegration of one's person[26] or a loss of meaning[27] that may have little to do with uncontrolled physical symptoms.

BG feared becoming a burden to his family and developing progressive loss of mental capacity more than he feared uncontrolled pain. He had no moral reservations about hastening death under his current circumstances. For him, the humaneness and effectiveness of the intervention were more important than whether it required his physician's "active" or "passive" assistance. His physician had moral and legal reservations about hastening death but was deeply committed to BG's comfort and wanted to be responsive to the dilemma that he faced.

DEFINITION OF THE PRACTICES

Terminal Sedation

Terminal sedation is the use of high doses of sedatives to relieve extremes of physical distress. It is not restricted to end-of-life care and is sometimes used as a temporizing measure in trauma, burn, postsurgical, and intensive care. Although rendering a patient unconscious to escape suffering is an extraordinary measure, withholding such treatment in certain circumstances would be inhumane. Because most of the patients who receive heavy sedation are expected to recover, careful attention is paid to maintaining adequate ventilation, hydration, and nutrition.

When applied to patients who have no substantial prospect of recovery, terminal sedation refers to a similar last-resort clinical response to extreme, unrelieved physical suffering.[14,31–36] The purpose of the medications is to render the patient unconscious to relieve suffering, not to intentionally end his or her life.[37] However, in the context of far-advanced disease and expected death, artificial nutrition, hydration, antibiotics, mechanical ventilation, and other life-prolonging interventions are not instituted and are usually withdrawn if they are already in place. These measures are withheld during terminal sedation because they could prolong the dying process without contributing to the quality of the patient's remaining life. In the context of end-of-life care, the component practices of intensive symptom management and withholding life-sustaining treatment have widespread ethical and legal support.[31,38–40] However, because death is a foreseeable, inevitable outcome of the aggregated circumstances of the patient's condition and interventions, the act can be more morally complex and ambiguous than is often acknowledged.[31,40–43]

Terminal sedation should be distinguished from the common occurrence of a dying patient gradually slipping into an obtunded state as death approaches; this occurrence is a combination of the metabolic changes of dying and the results of usual palliative treatments. Terminal sedation is also distinct from the sedation that occasionally occurs as an unintended side effect of high-dose opioid therapy, which is used to relieve severe terminal pain.[37] In contrast, terminal sedation involves an explicit decision to render the patient unconscious to prevent or respond to otherwise unrelievable physical distress. Terminal sedation is also used regularly in critical care practice to treat symptoms of suffocation in dying patients who are discontinuing mechanical ventilation.[44]

Voluntary Cessation of Eating and Drinking

In the context of far-advanced illness, a competent patient can consciously choose to refuse food and fluid.[31,45–48] When a patient who is still capable of eating and drinking makes this decision with the intention to hasten death, it can be distinguished from the natural anorexia and loss of thirst that frequently accompany the end stages of dying. Some consider such decisions to be a form of suicide.[31] However, because such patients view continued eating and drinking as measures that prolong life without value, others argue that the decision to stop eating and drinking can be categorized as a decision to forgo life-sustaining therapy.[45-48] The patient's decision to refuse food and fluids has the ethical advantage of being neither physician ordered nor directed. In practice, however, honoring the decision requires the support of the family, physician, and health care team, who must provide appropriate palliative care as the dying process unfolds.

During food and fluid fasts, any uncomfortable emerging symptoms will need palliation. In the context of advanced oncologic illnesses, hunger is rare and transient and symptoms of dry mouth and throat usually respond to assiduous mouth care.[49] Dying under these circumstances can take several days to a few weeks, depending on the patient's disease burden and nutritional and metabolic state at the outset. Doubts on the part of the family or physician may arise as the process unfolds, especially if the process is prolonged or the patient develops preterminal delirium. If in the context of a subsequent period of confusion or delirium the patient persistently calls out for a specific food or beverage, it is reasonable to offer it. If such requests persist, the overall plan should be reevaluated. If a patient becomes severely agitated as death approaches, intensive symptom management, including terminal sedation, may be indicated to ensure comfort.

MORAL AND LEGAL STATUS

Although legal precedents guiding terminal sedation and cessation of eating and drinking are less developed than those involving other end-of-life decisions, the June 1997 U.S. Supreme Court decision on assisted suicide suggested that these practices are permitted under current law.[50-52] The court unequivocally supported the patient's right to refuse treatment, even if the intention is to hasten death, on the basis of the patient's right to bodily integrity. Furthermore, Justices O'Connor and Souter each wrote a concurrence supporting the use of medication to alleviate the pain and suffering of terminally ill patients, even to the point of causing unconsciousness or hastening death.[51,52]

Public and professional discussion of these practices is now under way.[31,37-42,48,53] In Supreme Court briefs opposing physician-assisted suicide, hospice, palliative care, and geriatric groups stated that terminal sedation and cessation of eating and drinking were morally and clinically preferable last-resort alternatives because death is not directly or intentionally hastened by the physician.[54,55] In addition, in the context of advanced disease, sedation and patient refusal to eat and drink can be used to respond to a much wider range of clinical circumstances than physician-assisted suicide, even if the latter were legal. Both sedation and refusal to eat and drink can be undertaken and supported within usual health care settings.

However, several challenging moral questions remain. Are these practices fundamentally different from physician-assisted suicide? An in-depth comparison of these last-resort options has been presented elsewhere.[31,48] Some clinicians, patients, and families believe that the differences between such practices and assisted suicide are fundamental.[39,41,42,48,53] For others, all such practices, including assisted suicide, are more similar than different.[31,37,40] Many who believe that physicians should never intentionally hasten death consider terminal sedation the end of the continuum of symptom management. Because voluntary cessation of eating and drinking is by definition a patient decision, the clinician's role is one of continued care and support. Conversely, a clinician who counters a patient's decision by forcing food or artificial nutrition and hydration risks committing assault. Many clinicians may find that these options provide morally acceptable ways to respond to severe terminal suffering without violating their consciences or abandoning the patient.

When a patient stops eating and drinking to hasten death, is clinical support for the decision equivalent to assisted suicide? The moral evaluation of clinical practice in these situations depends in part on their clinical context. For a patient with anorexia nervosa, clinical depression, or mildly symptomatic illness, cessation of eating and drinking would be considered a form of suicide that should be prevented by appropriate interventions. In contrast, for a patient with severe, unrelieved suffering and advanced, incurable illness, cessation of eating and drinking might be considered part of the right to refuse treatment.[31,48,53]

Some clinicians and ethicists, however, consider any and all intentional hastening of death by a patient to constitute suicide, making physician support of such choices unacceptable. An absolute stance of this nature creates a double bind for patients who are ready for death and desire the continued help of their physician. If such patients are honest about their intention, their request for physician support cannot be granted. To maintain a therapeutic relationship and be guaranteed continued symptom management, they and their families may have to collude in a deception and conceal the decision to stop eating and drinking.

Are physicians required to support requests for these practices? All physicians should fully explore patient requests for terminal sedation or inquiries about voluntary cessation of eating and drinking to ensure that they are not emanating from unrecognized depression or symptoms that may respond to palliative measures.[56,57] However, physicians should not be required to participate in these processes if doing so violates their fundamental moral precepts.[31] If physicians cannot find common ground with a patient, they have a responsibility to obtain palliative care or ethics consultations and to transfer care to more receptive physicians.

Additional unanswered questions provide subjects for future research, description, and discussion. How frequently will sedation or refusal of food and drink be needed in the context of state-of-the-art palliative care? How acceptable will either of these possibilities be to patients, families, and health care providers? Will predictable availability of these last-resort options diminish patients' fears that their physicians will not respond to severe terminal suffering or lessen public interest in assisted suicide? Will discussion of these options make some patients feel pressured or more fearful about physician power and potential abuse? If care of this nature were predictably available, how many patients would still prefer assisted suicide and how many physicians would still covertly break the law by providing assistance? Do patients, families, and physicians see these actions as morally different from physician-assisted suicide or euthanasia? If voluntary cessation of eating and drinking is considered a variation of forgoing life-sustaining treatment, should it be made available to incurably ill and suffering patients whose conditions are not imminently terminal?

CLINICAL GUIDELINES

The published guidelines for terminal sedation and voluntary cessation of eating and drinking are summarized in Table 15.1.[31,33] Informed consent, which includes assessing the patient's capacity to comprehend the treatment and the available alternatives, is one cornerstone of these guidelines.[56,57] Clinicians should carefully screen terminally ill patients for clinical depression because it is extremely prevalent and can be difficult to diagnose.[24–28] Although full decision-making capacity is an absolute requirement for voluntary cessation of eating and drinking, terminal sedation may sometimes be needed in acute symptomatic emergencies when the dying patient cannot respond. In such severe circumstances, family members, consultants, and other members of the health care team may have to represent the patient's values.

A second cornerstone is the presence of severe suffering that cannot be relieved by other available means. The main indication for terminal sedation is usually severe, uncontrolled physical suffering, such as intractable pain, dyspnea, seizures, or delirium. Patients who have more unrelenting, persistent, unacceptable symptoms, such as extreme fatigue, weakness, or debility, may consider refusing food and fluids. If either option is being considered by clinicians, patients, or families when the suffering person is not imminently dying, assessments should always include second opinions from mental health, ethics, and palliative care specialists.

These guidelines represent the minimum requirements for these measures. Terminal sedation should be used only in the most difficult cases, which are typically marked by intense discussion of the clinical and ethical issues on the part of the physician, the clinical team, the family, and the patient. Similarly, a patient's decision to stop eating and drinking must include thorough evaluation for depression and spiritual suffering and assiduous clarification of motives and alternatives with the patient, family, and professional caregivers. The struggle experienced by the clinical team involved with these cases is a mark of the authenticity of care and contributes to the moral acceptability of the choices made.

CLINICAL PRACTICALITIES

In response to BG's decision to stop eating and drinking, his physician discussed the likely clinical course and the symptoms he would experience. She promised to use medications for sedation if his suffering became intolerable during the dying process. His physician reassured him that the process was usually comfortable and that together they would address any discomfort that arose. BG felt liberated by having made a choice that he could openly pursue at his own volition. Two weeks would probably pass between the decision to refuse food and fluids and death, but BG did not view this prospect as an excessive burden. It would allow him some time to again say good-bye to his family, but with a predictable beginning, middle, and end. BG discussed his decision with his wife, children, and minister and the psychiatric consultant.

TABLE 15.1. **General Guidelines for Terminal Sedation and Voluntary Cessation of Eating and Drinking**

Guideline Domain	Terminal Sedation	Voluntary Cessation of Eating and Drinking
Palliative care	Must be available, in place, and unable to adequately relieve current suffering.	Must be available, in place, and unable to adequately relieve current suffering.
Usual patient characteristics	Severe, immediate, or otherwise unrelievable symptoms (for example, pain, shortness of breath, nausea, vomiting, seizures, delirium) or to prevent severe suffering (for example, suffocation sensation when mechanical ventilation is discontinued).	Persistent, unrelenting, otherwise unrelievable symptoms that are unacceptable to the patient (for example, extreme fatigue, weakness, debility).
Terminal prognosis	Usually days to weeks.	Usually weeks to months.
Patient informed consent	Patient should be competent and fully informed or noncompetent with severe, otherwise irreversible suffering (clinician should use advance directive or consensus about patient wishes and best interests).	Patient should be competent and fully informed.
Family participation in decision	Clinician should strongly encourage input from and consensus of immediate family members.	Clinician should strongly encourage input from and consensus of immediate family members.
Incompetent patient	Can be used for severe, persistent suffering with the informed consent of the patient's designated proxy and family members. If no surrogate is available, team members and consultants should agree that no other acceptable palliative responses are available.	Food and drink (oral food and fluids) must not be withheld from incompetent persons who are willing and able to eat.
Second opinion(s)	Should be obtained from an expert in palliative care and a mental health expert (if uncertainty exists about patient's mental capacity).	Should be obtained from an expert in palliative care, a mental health expert, and a specialist in the patient's underlying disease (strongly advised).
Medical staff participation in decision	Input from staff involved in immediate patient care activities is encouraged; physician and staff consent are required for their own participation.	Input from staff involved in immediate patient care activities is encouraged; physician and staff consent are required for their own participation.

All severely ill patients who experience substantial suffering and have a poor prognosis should be informed about the potential of palliative care to address their symptoms.[58,59] However, it would be burdensome and inappropriate to discuss these last-resort options with all patients who have late-stage illness. Information about terminal sedation and cessation of eating and drinking becomes important when patients express fears about dying badly or explicitly request a hastened death because of unacceptable suffering.[56,57] Such information must be presented with sensitivity, however, because some patients may consider discussion of these options coercive, potentially requiring them to justify a decision to continue living. Other patients may find the prospect of spending their final days in an iatrogenic coma to be meaningless and undignified and may prefer a more decisive action, such as assisted suicide.

BG stopped eating and drinking. The initial week was physically comfortable and personally meaningful. BG's family shared stories, played cards, and listened to music. BG took antiseizure medications with sips of water but absolutely nothing else orally. Morphine by continuous subcutaneous infusion at an initial dosage of 1.0 mg/h controlled his headaches without causing sedation. His mouth was kept moist with ice chips and swabs, but he was careful not to swallow any of the liquid. After 9 days, he could be roused but spent most of the day and night sleeping.

Although the patient's refusal of food and fluids technically does not require the physician's participation, a physician should be part of the team who assesses the patient's request and provides palliative care as the process unfolds. Therefore, physicians who oppose their patient's decision from the outset must decide whether they can provide all forms of indicated palliation. If the physician feels morally unable to do so, transfer of care to another provider should be considered.

On day 10, BG became confused and agitated and began having hallucinations. The peace and comfort that he and his family had achieved began to unravel. BG was now incapable of informed consent but had previously given permission for sedation if this problem arose. After discussions with his family, BG was started on a low-dose subcutaneous infusion of midazolam for treatment of seizures and agitation. The plan of care was to use whatever dose was required to control seizures and agitation. The initial dosage was 0.5 mg/h, with bolus doses of 0.5 to 1 mg ordered up to every 15 minutes as needed. The option of transferring BG to an inpatient unit was explored, but the family preferred to keep him at home. Around-the-clock home nursing was arranged under the "continuous care" provision of the Medicare hospice benefit program. After several bolus doses and adjustment of the infusion to 2.5 mg/h during the first six hours, BG seemed to be sleeping comfortably. No attempt was made to restore consciousness, and no further increases in medication were needed to maintain sedation.

TABLE 15.2. **Medications Used for Terminal Sedation**[a]

Medication	Type	Usual Starting Dosage	Usual Maintenance Dosage	Route
Midazolam	Rapid, short-acting benzodiazepine	0.5–1.5 mg/h after bolus of 0.5 mg	30–100 mg/d	Intravenous or subcutaneous
Lorazepam	Benzodiazepine	1–4 mg every 4–6 h orally or dissolved buccally; infusion of 0.5–1.0 mg/h intravenously	4–40 mg/d	Oral, buccal, subcutaneous, or intravenous
Propofol	General anesthetic; ultrarapid onset and elimination	5–10 mg/h; bolus doses of 20–50 mg may be administered for urgent sedation, but continuous infusion is required	10–200 mg/h	Intravenous
Thiopental	Ultrashort-acting barbiturate	5–7 mg/kg of body weight to induce unconsciousness	Initial rate may range from 20 to 80 mg/h; average maintenance rates range between 70 and 180 mg/h	Intravenous
Pentobarbital	Long-acting barbiturate	2–3 mg/kg, slow infusion, to induce unconsciousness	1 mg/h, increasing as needed to maintain sedation	Intravenous
Phenobarbital	Long-acting barbiturate	200 mg loading dose, repeated every 10–15 minutes until patient is comfortable	Approximately 50 mg/h	Intravenous or subcutaneous

[a]Adapted from references 32, 33, and 60–64. Goal of treatment is to relieve suffering by inducing sedation. Dosage should be increased by approximately 30 percent every hour until sedation is achieved. Once desired level of sedation is achieved, infusion is usually maintained at that level as long as the patient seems comfortable. If symptoms return, dosages should be increased in 30 percent increments until sedation is achieved. The ranges above are representative. Individual patients may require lower or higher doses to achieve the desired goal. Previous doses of opioids and other symptom-relieving medications should be continued.

In the context of advanced illness and imminent death, sedation can be achieved with a barbiturate or benzodiazepine infusion, which should be rapidly increased until the patient is adequately sedated and seems comfortable. A level of sedation that eliminates signs of discomfort (such as stiffening or grimacing spontaneously or with routine repositioning and nursing care) is maintained until the patient dies. Table 15.2 shows potential starting dosages and strategies for increasing dosages and monitoring. Depending on the severity of the patient's physiologic condition at the onset of the procedure, the interval from initiation to death is usually hours to days. Continuous sedation usually requires a subcutaneous or intravenous infusion and intensive involvement by the health care team for observation, monitoring, and support. When a dying patient requires sedation, opioids for pain and other symptom-relieving measures should also be continued to avoid the possibility of unobservable pain or opioid withdrawal. However, opioids are generally ineffective at inducing sedation and are not the medications of choice.

CONCLUSION

BG died quietly approximately twenty-four hours later in his home, surrounded by his family. BG's family had remained resolute in their support for his decision and firmly committed to keeping him at home. However, they also continued to have emotional family discussions and at times struggled with whether they had done too little or too much to help him die peacefully. They drew comfort from recognizing that they had kept BG's values in the forefront and made the best of a potentially devastating situation.

Medicine cannot sanitize dying or provide perfect solutions for all clinical dilemmas. When unacceptable suffering persists despite standard palliative measures, terminal sedation and voluntary refusal of food and fluids are imperfect but useful last-resort options that can be openly pursued. Patients and their families who fear that physicians will not respond to extreme suffering will be reassured when such options are predictably made available.[65] Relevant professional bodies can help by adopting policy statements that attest to the ethical and professional acceptability of these components of palliative care.

REFERENCES

1. *Caring for the Dying: Identification and Promotion of Physician Competence*. American Board of Internal Medicine End-of-Life Patient Care Project Committee. Philadelphia: American Board of Internal Medicine; 1996.

2. Decisions near the end of life. Council on Ethical and Judicial Affairs, American Medical Association. *JAMA*. 1992; 267:2229–33.

3. Good care of the dying patient. Council on Scientific Affairs, American Medical Association. *JAMA*. 1996; 275:474–8.

4. Field MJ, Cassel CK, eds. *Approaching Death: Improving Care at the End of Life*. Committee on Care at the End of Life, Division of Health Care Services, Institute of Medicine. Washington, DC: National Academy Pr; 1997.

5. Quill TE, Meier DM, Block SD, Billings JA. The debate over physician-assisted suicide: empirical data and convergent views. *Ann Intern Med*. 1998; 128:552–8.

6. Seale CF. What happens in hospices: a review of research evidence. *Soc Sci Med*. 1989; 28:551–9.

7. Wallston KA, Burger C, Smith RA, Baugher RJ. Comparing the quality of death for hospice and non-hospice cancer patients. *Med Care*. 1998; 26:177–82.

8. Byock I. *Dying Well: Prospects for Growth at the End of Life*. New York: Riverhead Books; 1997.

9. Foley KM. Pain, physician-assisted suicide and euthanasia. *Pain Forum*. 1995; 4:163–78.

10. Jadad AR, Browman GP. The WHO analgesic ladder for cancer pain management. Stepping up the quality of its evaluation. *JAMA*. 1995; 274:1870–3.

11. Quality improvement guidelines for the treatment of acute pain and cancer pain. American Pain Society Quality of Care Committee. *JAMA*. 1995; 274:1874–80.

12. Rhymes J. Hospice care in America. *JAMA*. 1990; 264:369–72.

13. Kasting GA. The nonnecessity of euthanasia. In: Humber JM, Almeder RF, Kasting GA, eds. *Physician-Assisted Death*. Totawa, NJ: Humana; 1994:25–43.

14. Ventafridda V, Ripamonti C, De Conno F, Tamburini M, Cassileth BR. Symptom prevalence and control during cancer patients' last days of life. *J Palliat Care*. 1990; 6:7–11.

15. Coyle N, Adelhardt J, Foley KM, Portenoy RK. Character of terminal illness in the advanced cancer patient: pain and other symptoms during the last four weeks of life. *J Pain Symptom Manage*. 1990; 5:83–93.

16. Ingham JM, Portenoy RK. Symptom assessment. *Hematol Oncol Clin North Am*. 1996; 10:21–39.

17. Quill TE, Brody RV. "You promised me I wouldn't die like this!" A bad death as a medical emergency. *Arch Intern Med*. 1995; 155:1250–4.

18. Back AL, Wallace JI, Starks HE, Pearlman RA. Physician-assisted suicide and euthanasia in Washington State. Patient requests and physician responses. *JAMA*. 1996; 275:919–25.

19. van der Maas PJ, van Delden JJ, Pijnenborg L. *Euthanasia and other medical decisions concerning the end of life*. Vol. 2. Amsterdam: Elsevier; 1992.

20. Meier DE, Emmons CA, Wallenstein S, Quill T, Morrison RS, Cassel CK. A national survey of physician-assisted suicide and euthanasia in the United States. *N Engl J Med*. 1998; 338:1193–201.

21. van der Maas PJ, van der Wal G, Haverkate I, de Graaff CL, Kester JG, Onwuteaka-Philipsen BD, et al. Euthanasia, physician-assisted suicide, and other medical practices involving the end of life in the Netherlands, 1990–1995. *N Engl J Med*. 1996; 335:1699–705.

22. Cassel EJ. The nature of suffering and the goals of medicine. *N Engl J Med*. 1982; 306:639–45.

23. Frankel VE. *The Doctor and the Soul, from Psychotherapy to Logotherapy*. New York: Knopf; 1955.

24. Block S. Assessing and managing depression in the terminally ill patient. *Ann Intern Med*. 2000; 132:209–18.

25. Chochinov HM, Wilson KG, Enns M, Lander S. Prevalence of depression in the terminally ill: effects of diagnostic criteria and symptom threshold judgments. *Am J Psychiatry*. 1994; 151:537–40.

26. Breitbart W, Rosenfeld BD, Passik SD. Interest in physician-assisted suicide among ambulatory HIV-infected patients. *Am J Psychiatry*. 1996; 153:238–42.

27. Kathol RG, Noyes R, Williams J, Mutgi A, Carroll B, Perry P. Diagnosing depression in patients with medical illness. *Psychosomatics*. 1990; 31:434–40.

28. Byock IR. The nature of suffering and the nature of opportunity at the end of life. *Clin Geriatr Med*. 1996; 12:237–52.

29. Byock IR. When suffering persists . . . . *J Palliat Care*. 1994; 10:8–13.

30. Quill TE. *A Midwife Through the Dying Process: Stories of Healing and Hard Choices at the End of Life*. Baltimore: Johns Hopkins Univ Pr; 1996.

31. Quill TE, Lo B, Brock DW. Palliative options of last resort: a comparison of voluntarily stopping eating and drinking, terminal sedation, physician-assisted suicide, and voluntary active euthanasia. *JAMA*. 1997; 278:2099–104.

32. Troug RD, Berde CB, Mitchell C, Grier HE. Barbiturates in the care of the terminally ill. *N Engl J Med*. 1992; 327:1678–82.

33. Cherny NI, Portenoy RK. Sedation in the management of refractory symptoms: guidelines for evaluation and treatment. *J Palliat Care*. 1994; 10:31–8.

34. Enck RE. *The Medical Care of Terminally Ill Patients*. Baltimore: Johns Hopkins Univ Pr; 1994.

35. Saunders CM, Sykes N, eds. *The Management of Terminal Malignant Disease*. 3d ed. London: Edward Arnold; 1993:1–305.

36. Stone P, Phillips C, Spruyt O, Waight C. A comparison of the use of sedatives in a hospital support team and in a hospice. *Palliat Med*. 1997; 11:140–4.

37. Quill TE, Dresser R, Brock DW. The rule of double effect—a critique of its role in end-of-life decision making. *N Engl J Med*. 1997; 337:1768–71.

38. Brody H. Causing, intending, and assisting death. *J Clin Ethics*. 1993; 4:112–7.

39. Byock IR. Consciously walking the fine line: thoughts on a hospice response to assisted suicide and euthanasia. *J Palliat Care*. 1993; 9:25–8.

40. Quill TE. The ambiguity of clinical intentions. *N Engl J Med*. 1993; 329:1039–40.

41. Billings JA, Block SD. Slow euthanasia. *J Palliat Care*. 1996; 12:21–30.

42. Mount B. Morphine drips, terminal sedation, and slow euthanasia: definitions and facts, not anecdotes. *J Palliat Care*. 1996; 12:31–7.

43. Brody H. Commentary on Billings and Block's "Slow Euthanasia." *J Palliat Care*. 1996; 12:38–41.

44. Brody H, Campbell ML, Faber-Langendoen K, Ogle KS. Withdrawing intensive life-sustaining treatment— recommendations for compassionate clinical management. *N Engl J Med*. 1997; 336:652–7.

45. Bernat JL, Gert B, Mogielnicki RP. Patient refusal of hydration and nutrition. An alternative to physician-assisted suicide or voluntary active euthanasia. *Arch Intern Med*. 1993; 153:2723–8.

46. Printz LA. Terminal dehydration, a compassionate treatment. *Arch Intern Med*. 1992; 152:697–700.

47. Eddy DM. A piece of my mind. A conversation with my mother. *JAMA*. 1994; 272:179–81.

48. Miller FG, Meier DE. Voluntary death: a comparison of terminal dehydration and physician-assisted suicide. *Ann Intern Med*. 1998; 128:559–62.

49. McCann RM, Hall WJ, Groth-Juncker A. Comfort care for terminally ill patients. The appropriate use of nutrition and hydration. *JAMA*. 1994; 272:1263–6.

50. Burt RA. The Supreme Court speaks—not assisted suicide but a constitutional right to palliative care. *N Engl J Med*. 1997; 337:1234–6.

51. *Vacco* v. *Quill,* 117 S.Ct. 2293 (1997).

52. *Washington* v. *Glucksberg,* 117 S.Ct. 2258 (1997).

53. Byock I. Patient refusal of nutrition and hydration: walking the ever-finer line. *Am J Hosp Palliat Care*. 1995; 12:8–13.

54. Lynn J, Cohn F, Pickering JH, Smith J, Stoeppelwerth AM. American Geriatrics Society on physician-assisted suicide: brief to the United States Supreme Court. *J Am Geriatr Soc*. 1997; 45:489–99.

55. Brief Amicus Curiae for the National Hospice Organization in *Vacco* v. *Quill* and *Washington* v. *Glucksberg,* Supreme Court of the United States, October 1996.

56. Quill TE. Doctor, I want to die. Will you help me? *JAMA*. 1993; 270:870–3.

57. Block SD, Billings JA. Patient requests to hasten death. Evaluation and management in terminal care. *Arch Intern Med*. 1994; 154:2039–47.

58. Lo B, Quill T, Tulsky J. Discussing palliative care with patients. ACP-ASIM End-of-Life Care Consensus Panel. *Ann Intern Med*. 1999; 130:744–9.

59. Karlawish JH, Quill T, Meier DE. A consensus-based approach to providing palliative care to patients who lack decision-making capacity. ACP-ASIM End-of-Life Care Consensus Panel. *Ann Intern Med*. 1999; 130:835–40.

60. Doyle D, Hanks GW, MacDonald N, eds. *Oxford Textbook of Palliative Medicine*. 2d ed. New York: Oxford Univ Pr; 1998:945–7.

61. Enck RE. *The Medical Care of Terminally Ill Patients*. Baltimore: Johns Hopkins Univ Pr; 1994:166–72.

62. Dunlop RJ. Is terminal restlessness sometimes drug induced? *Palliat Med*. 1989; 3:65–6.

63. Greene WR, Davis WH. Titrated intravenous barbiturates in the control of symptoms in patients with terminal cancer. *South Med J*. 1991; 84:332–7.

64. Moyle J. The use of propofol in palliative medicine. *J Pain Symptom Manage*. 1995; 10:643–6.

65. Quill TE, Cassel CK. Nonabandonment: a central obligation for physicians. *Ann Intern Med*. 1995; 122:368–74.

THE AUTHORS AND MEMBERS AND STAFF OF THE ACP-ASIM END-OF-LIFE CARE CONSENSUS PANEL

This paper was written by Timothy E. Quill, M.D., and Ira R. Byock, M.D., for the American College of Physicians-American Society of Internal Medicine (ACP-ASIM) End-of-Life Care Consensus Panel. Members of the ACP-ASIM End-of-Life Care Consensus Panel were Bernard Lo, M.D. (chair); Janet Abrahm, M.D.; Susan Block, M.D.; William Breitbart, M.D.; Ira R. Byock, M.D.; Kathy Faber-Langendoen, M.D.; Lloyd W. Kitchens Jr., M.D.; Paul Lanken, M.D.; Joanne Lynn, M.D.; Diane Meier, M.D.; Timothy E. Quill, M.D.; George Thibault, M.D.; and James Tulsky, M.D.. Primary staff to the panel were Lois Snyder, J.D. (project director), and Jason Karlawish, M.D. This paper was reviewed and approved by the Ethics and Human Rights Committee, although it does not represent official ACP-ASIM policy. Members of the Ethics and Human Rights Committee were Risa Lavizzo-Mourey, M.D. (chair); Joanne Lynn, M.D.; Richard J. Carroll, M.D.; David A. Fleming, M.D.; Steven H. Miles, M.D.; Gail J. Povar, M.D.; James A. Tulsky, M.D.; Alan L. Gordon, M.D.; S.Y. Tan, M.D., JD; Vincent Herrin, M.D.; and Lee J. Dunn Jr., JD, LLM.

GRANT SUPPORT

The Greenwall Foundation provided support to the End-of-Life Care Panel.

16

RESPONSE TO QUILL AND BYOCK, "RESPONDING TO INTRACTABLE TERMINAL SUFFERING"

DANIEL P. SULMASY, O.F.M., M.D., PH.D., WAYNE A. URY, M.D.,
JUDITH C. AHRONHEIM, M.D., MARK SIEGLER, M.D.,
LEON KASS, M.D., PH.D., JOHN LANTOS, M.D., ROBERT A. BURT, J.D.,
KATHLEEN FOLEY, M.D., RICHARD PAYNE, M.D., CARLOS GOMEZ, M.D.,
THOMAS J. KRIZEK, M.D., EDMUND D. PELLEGRINO, M.D.,
AND RUSSELL K. PORTENOY, M.D.

This letter to the editor originally appeared as Sulmasy DP, Ury WA, Ahronheim JC, Siegler M, Kass L, Lantos J, Burt RA, Foley K, Payne R, Gomez C, Krizek TJ, Pellegrino, ED, Portenoy RK. Letters to the editor responding to Quill and Byock. Responding to intractable terminal suffering. *Ann Intern Med.* 2000;133(7):560–562. Copyright © 2000, American College of Physicians. All rights reserved. Reprinted with permission.

EDITORS' INTRODUCTION

In an echo of the emotionally fraught public and political debate about withholding artificial nutrition and hydration from the vegetative Terri Schiavo, these prominent authors express strong disagreement with Quill and Byock's arguments about palliative options of last resort during circumstances of intractable suffering. The reasons they advance to account for this difference of opinion are traced to their concerns about clarity of intentions (relieving suffering or hastening death) and rejection of Quill and Byock's assertion of professional consensus on these issues.

■ ■ ■

TO THE EDITOR:

We are deeply troubled by a recent pair of papers on terminal sedation and "voluntary refusal of food and fluids"[1,2] and the process by which they were accepted and published in *Annals*. These papers appear to convey the mistaken and perhaps dangerous impression of a genuine consensus among experts and official policy endorsement of these practices. At the request of the editors, we address the issues raised by the first of these papers in this letter and address related issues separately.[3,4]

It is true that terminal sedation (perhaps better called *sedation in the imminently dying*) is being discussed and evaluated by palliative care specialists as a therapy intended to relieve the refractory symptoms of patients suffering at the end of life. We do not disagree that it could potentially be appropriate therapy when performed in carefully selected cases by a well-trained internist or palliative care specialist who understands the ethical and medical issues involved. We also recognize that patients are entitled to refuse artificial hydration and nutrition. However, Quill and Byock[1] propose as standard practice the use of "terminal sedation" intended to make patients unconscious and unable to eat so that they may die more quickly, and the use of "terminal sedation" for patients who "voluntarily refuse" to eat. We do not believe that there is anything approaching a consensus among palliative care physicians, bioethicists, or the membership of the American College of Physicians–American Society of Internal Medicine that such practices are morally, legally, and clinically appropriate.

While some might even agree that sedation was appropriate in the specific case they describe, this does not mean that one should endorse the authors' general conclusions, which would justify a much wider range of "indications" for terminal sedation. "Suffering" is a very broad term, and it is unclear what sorts of suffering might represent appropriate indications for terminal sedation.

None of us, the undersigned, feel that the practices the authors recommend represent a settled approach to palliative care. It therefore seems inappropriate for them to be urging "professional bodies [to] help by adopting policy statements that attest to the ethical and professional acceptability of these components of palliative care."[1]

Daniel P. Sulmasy, O.F.M., M.D., Ph.D.
Wayne A. Ury, M.D.
Judith C. Ahronheim, M.D.
Saint Vincent's Hospital
New York, NY 10011

Mark Siegler, M.D.
Leon Kass, M.D., Ph.D.
John Lantos, M.D.
University of Chicago
Chicago, IL 60637

Robert A. Burt, J.D.
Yale University School of Law
New Haven, CT 06511

Kathleen Foley, M.D.
Richard Payne, M.D.
Memorial Sloan-Kettering Cancer Center
New York, NY 10021

Carlos Gomez, M.D.
University of Virginia
Charlottesville, VA 22908
Thomas J. Krizek, M.D.
University of South Florida
Tampa, FL 33620

Edmund D. Pellegrino, M.D.
Georgetown University Medical Center
Washington, DC 20007

Russell K. Portenoy, M.D.
Beth Israel Hospital
New York, NY 10003

REFERENCES

1. Quill TE, Byock IR. Responding to intractable terminal suffering: the role of terminal sedation and voluntary refusal of food and fluids. ACP– ASIM End-of-Life Care Consensus Panel. *Ann Intern Med.* 2000; 132:408–14.

2. Quill TE, Lee BC, Nunn S. Palliative treatments of last resort: choosing the least harmful alternative. University of Pennsylvania Center for Bioethics Assisted Suicide Consensus Panel. *Ann Intern Med.* 2000; 132:488–93.

3. Sulmasy DP, Ury WA, Ahronheim JC, Siegler M, Kass L, Lantos J, et al. Palliative treatment of last resort and assisted suicide [Letter]. *Ann Intern Med.* 2000; 133:562–3.

4. Sulmasy DP, Ury WA, Ahronheim JC, Siegler M, Kass L, Lantos J, et al. Publication of papers on assisted suicide and terminal sedation [Letter]. *Ann Intern Med.* 2000; 133:564–5.

ISSUES AND PERSPECTIVES

Balfour M. Mount, "Challenges in Palliative Care: Four Clinical Areas That Confront and Challenge Hospice Practitioners"

David E. Weissman, Bruce Ambuel, Charles F. von Gunten, Susan Block, Eric Warm, James Hallenbeck, Robert Milch, Karen Brasel, and Patricia B. Mullan, "Outcomes from a National Multispecialty Palliative Care Curriculum Development Project"

Marjorie Kagawa-Singer and Leslie J. Blackhall, "Negotiating Cross-Cultural Issues at the End of Life: 'You Got to Go Where He Lives'"

Benjamin Goldsmith, Jessica Dietrich, Qingling Du, and R. Sean Morrison, "Variability in Access to Hospital Palliative Care in the United States"

David Casarett, Amy Pickard, F. Amos Bailey, Christine Ritchie, Christian Furman, Ken Rosenfeld, Scott Shreve, Zhen Chen, Judy A. Shea, "Do Palliative Care Consultations Improve Patient Outcomes?"

Sean Morrison, Joan D. Penrod, J. Brian Cassel, Melissa Caust-Ellenbogen, Ann Litke, Lynn Spragens, Diane E. Meier, for the Palliative Care Leadership Centers' Outcomes Group, "Cost Savings Associated with U.S. Hospital Palliative Care Consultation Programs"

17

CHALLENGES IN PALLIATIVE CARE

Four Clinical Areas That Confront and Challenge Hospice Practitioners

BALFOUR M. MOUNT, M.D.

EDITORS' INTRODUCTION

Writing over twenty years ago before the exponential growth in North American hospital palliative care programs, Balfour M. Mount identifies the core barriers to universal access to quality palliative care. Every one of the concerns he describes remains as salient today as several decades ago. Among these barriers are health professionals' denial of any problem with how we care for the seriously ill; lack of professional training; inadequate government funding and associated overreliance on philanthropy to sustain the field; the centrality of expert symptom management and spiritual concerns to patients; and the equally central, but underrecognized, importance of the family and family systems to good palliative care.

■ ■ ■

Shirley du Boulay, Cicely Saunders's biographer, has pointed out, "The dying need the friendship of the heart—its qualities of care, acceptance, vulnerability; but they also need the skills of the mind—the most sophisticated treatment that medicine has to offer. On its own, neither is enough." Those are comprehensive demands. I know of no other health care field that sustains such a broad mandate with such motivation. In attempting to fulfill these goals, we are challenged on several fronts.

In 1985, we can look back on a decade of achievement. While acknowledging our advancements, I would like to examine some of the challenges that face us. I take it that we all agree that this field needs a firmer foundation of careful clinical research on which to test our assumptions. While the research challenges that confront us are diverse and complex, I wish to focus this morning on the challenges in four clinical areas: (1) challenges related to our communities; (2) challenges related to patients; (3) family-related challenges; (4) caregiver-related challenges. I will briefly consider three challenges in each of these four areas.

CHALLENGE I: COMMUNITY-RELATED CHALLENGES

1. Definition of Need and Integration of Resources

North American studies of terminal care suggest both an intrinsic deficiency and a general lack of perception of that deficiency by the caregivers involved. Both aspects of the problem are significant, since change will only be evoked and improvements in care promoted when those responsible for health care are convinced that there is a serious need that demands attention. Thus, the first challenge facing a community needing to upgrade its services for the terminally ill is to foster an increased awareness of terminal care deficiencies. Why has inadequate care not been more clearly recognized by those responsible? There are at least four reasons.

The first has to do with the discrepancy in perspective between the sharply focused, disease-oriented preoccupation of the health care team with investigating, diagnosing, prolonging life, curing, and the diffuse or global whole-person needs of the terminally ill and their families embracing psychosocial, financial, spiritual, and physical concerns. The caregiver has been trained to see his mandate as "the fight for life" and the enemy as pathophysiology. He is pressured by the technologic information explosion to focus all energies on developing life-prolonging and curative diagnostic skills. Suffering, existential concerns, financial problems, and a host of other psychosocial issues that crowd in on the terminally ill patient and family lie outside his professional visual field.

The second factor preventing the caregiver from recognizing his contributions to deficient care is his assumption of personal sensitivity. Each of us feels that we personally are sensitive individuals. Each remembers ego-supporting examples of times when we have met the needs of others. Usually we have failed to recognize the needs we don't respond to. In any event, the memory of numberless personal hurts confirms for us our own sensitivity and we are likely to see ourselves as sensitive and responsive in our relationships with patients. Our research at the Royal Victoria Hospital has shown that each professional group thinks of itself as being sensitive to the patient's emotional needs. Furthermore, each caregiver tends to see himself as being more sensitive than his colleagues, a point of view that diminishes the probability of recognizing personal insensitivity.

Thirdly, a hospital is simply a microcosm of the surrounding society. It embodies the beliefs and attitudes of that society. Feifel has studied North American attitudes toward death in the latter half of the twentieth century and has put forward a convincing argument that we are a society uniquely ill equipped to deal with death. In his Pulitzer Prize–winning book, *The Denial of Death,* Becker suggests that our underlying fear of death is ever present and underrides the majority of the thoughts and actions of Western man. It is hardly surprising that caregivers so conditioned find personal dis-ease in confronting terminal illness in their patients.

Finally, the caregivers' view of inadequate care is clouded by the patient's need to patronize, flatter, and humor the caregiver. As Belloc put it, "When going out, stick close to nurse for fear of meeting something worse." An understanding of the above factors can assist us in educating both professional colleagues and the public. There *is* a problem! The evidence is clear:

- At least 70 percent of North Americans die in institutions. All significant studies evaluating traditional terminal care have documented unacceptable deficiencies;

- Bonica and others have documented disastrously inadequate pain control in spite of the availability of effective strategies and medications;

- The bereaved represent a high-risk population with higher incidence of suicide, cardiovascular death, functional disorders, G.I. complaints, and visits to family physicians;

- A recent Columbia Presbyterian study has demonstrated two to three times the incidence of significant early loss in populations of psychiatric patients as compared to control groups. Isn't that sobering? It brings to mind Bowlby's thesis that much of adult psychopathology is probably related to unresolved grief reactions.

I would suggest that one solution to the lack of knowledge about the need in your community is to do local studies. The thing that convinced the Royal Victoria Hospital to do something about it was the study that demonstrated that *we* had a problem in *our* hospital; that it wasn't theoretical; that it wouldn't do to say it would be nice to do more if only we had the dollars, but a clear matter of having an unacceptable problem here and a moral obligation to do something about it.

Now that the need has been identified, let us turn our attention to integrating the communities' resources. To do this, we will be forced to clarify another whole series of questions. We must first clearly define the patient populations whose needs we wish to address. Who do we include: Only the cancer patients? What of the others? What of patients with Alzheimer's or AIDS? Shall we include only those with six months or less to live? Who in the world wrote the selection criteria saying that hospice patients should have six months or less to live? I don't know anyone with the gift of prophecy. Who was the person who suggested that a patient must have a "primary caregiver" to be accepted for hospice care? I don't know about your community, but I can tell you that in Montreal, a city of 3.5 million people, many of those we care for live alone or with loved ones who must work or go to school. They're among our most needy, grateful, and rewarding patients.

How are we going to get the support we need for new hospice services? How are we going to integrate existing resources when we are the new kid on the block; when resources are scarce and the competition for inadequate funding is fierce; when there is a competition for beds, for patients; and when each special interest group jealously guards its own empire? These challenges demand strong leadership, clear-minded leadership, skilled diplomacy, and a minimum of personal insecurity on the part of everyone concerned. As long as we are guarding our individual empires, the sort of liaison that is needed won't happen.

2. The Need for Training

The second community-related challenge is that of training. I include this as a "community challenge" because at a state or national level we have a vested interest in having available hospice training in this country; good hospice training, so that we are not all flying by the seat of our pants; so that we are not all, in each little service, reinventing the wheel. If there have been valuable lessons learned in the last decade, then let's learn from each other. Let's not think we all have to know as much as the next guy and we all have to do it on our own. These are reasons why meetings like this one [The First Annual American Conference on Hospice Care] are so vital and so important. We must remember Potter's admonition to us in his important *New England Journal* article, "A Challenge to the Hospice Movement," when he said, "A high order of clinical competence is essential if abuse of the hospice is to be avoided."

In hospice programs in this country and Canada, too frequently there has been documented inadequate physician participation, inadequate charting, inadequate history taking, inadequate physical examination, and inadequate clinical skills on the part of a highly motivated team. Nobody faults the motivation, but motivation alone isn't enough. Too often there is inadequate knowledge of pharmacology and pharmacokinetics; inadequate knowledge of neurology and medical oncology; inadequate knowledge of internal medicine. In hospice, one thing we don't need is another way to do it badly. Medical incompetence by any other name is still medical incompetence, and it just won't do.

3. Funding

The third community-related need that we have in hospice today is the need for funding. It is an important need. There is an especially urgent need for new mechanisms for funding physician participation so that it is possible for a doctor to make a living giving this kind of care. This is one of the major problems facing hospice in this country and in the majority of Canadian provinces. In Quebec, the reason we can have an adequately staffed service at our hospital is because there is a provincial mechanism for placing palliative care physicians on salary.

We need to make the funding of hospice a political issue. Those of us in other countries of the world can take our hats off to the way you have been able to do that in this country. We have politicized the issue in a positive way that just hasn't been done in any other country. While that is true, I think you must see that in some other countries, with different kinds of health care systems, they've been able to move forward faster. I have just returned from Norway, where they have a more socialized health care system in their country, so they have been able to set in motion nationwide plans for symptom-control teams in all major hospitals and trial palliative care wards in two cities. That sort of sweeping change isn't possible in Canada or the United States, and the need to politicize the issue remains.

Kathy Foley of Memorial Sloan-Kettering Cancer Center points out in commenting on the recent heroin bill that the cost involved in simply operationalizing its proposals would be $3 million per year for each of the four years of the bill. That is in a country that spends $1 million a year on research and patient care. What do these figures say to us about our priorities? We need to secure a sounder funding basis for our programs. I'm sure that for many of us in this room this is the greatest cause of personal stress. We need the funding to put together the teams to do the job. If President Reagan really thinks hospice is all the things he said in his welcoming letter, and if we really have all that support, we must also have the money. As Churchill said during the Second World War, "Give us the tools and we'll finish the job."

CHALLENGE II. PATIENT-RELATED CHALLENGES

1. Symptom Control

In hospice we are concerned with the whole person. Problems in pathophysiology, the biology of disease, pharmacology, and cellular kinetics are seen in relation to psychodynamic issues, social issues, and spiritual issues. While hospice recognizes and attempts to address each dimension of human concern, the foundation of whole-person medical care is excellence in *physical* care. All the psychodynamic and psychosocial issues go by the board unless there is excellence in symptom control. Thus our first challenge is to provide good symptom control.

Once hospice turned its attention to improving symptom control for its long-neglected patient population, progress was rapid. The management of pain and malignant bowel obstruction are two outstanding examples.

The control of intractable pain in the cancer patient has been revolutionized by the work of Dame Cicely Saunders, who introduced individually optimized doses of narcotics given at intervals dependent on the kinetics of the drug in question, in conjunction with carefully chosen coanalgesics, and stressed the need for attention to the psychosocial and spiritual needs of the patient. Helpful suggestions for improved pain control are now coming from many centers. One study from Italy has reminded us of the effectiveness of both the rectal and sublingual roots of morphine administration.

Similarly, refinements in the medical management of malignant bowel obstruction now find patients who previously would have been treated by colostomy, or prolonged suck-and-drip therapy, being managed medically without surgery, I.V. fluids, or nasogastric tube.

Such progress brings with it some excellent new reference manuals in symptom control. There are two I would recommend: Saunders's *The Management of Terminal Malignant Disease,* second edition, 1984 (Edward Arnold Press), and Twycross and Lack's *Therapeutics in Terminal Cancer,* 1984 (Pittman Press).

General principles of improved symptom control include:

- Attention of one symptom improves control of all symptoms,
- Clarify who is bothered by the symptom (patient, family, or caregiver),
- Determine what was helpful in the past,
- Determine whether treatment was correctly given as prescribed.

Residual symptoms should be carefully reviewed. An attitude of quiet confidence and cautious optimism on the part of the doctors and nurses is extremely reassuring to both patient and family. There is a need to take the time to sit down at the bedside; to listen; to admit the problem; to explain what is happening; to convey to the patient your continuing involvement.

Careful history taking will disclose the patient's current priorities, dreams, and frustrations. Ingenuity is needed to ensure maximum independence for a disabled patient. Modified activities of daily living may enhance the quality of life. Care must be taken to inform and involve the patient's family and social network, while staff and volunteers should be kept abreast of current thinking regarding the patient's residual symptoms. The key to success lies in attention to detail, intensive physician involvement, skilled nursing care, the regular review of residual symptoms, and close and frequent communication on the team.

2. Meaningful Attention to Spiritual Concerns

The second patient-related challenge I wish to touch on is that of pastoral care. Even as we are ill prepared to deal with death in this secular age, we are also ill prepared to deal with the spiritual dimension of our lives. Cicely Saunders has suggested that "the special needs of a mortally ill patient and his family make the question of religious and philosophical belief a central issue." When he was dying, the poet Ted Rosenthal commented, "It's the time when the mind's own camera is forever turned on self." It is the time when previously abstract existential questions take on a deep urgent personal significance. What does it mean to be dead? Where will I be? What does it really mean? How does one reconcile the concept of a good all-powerful God on one hand and unmerited suffering on the other? As Archibald MacLeish put it, "If God is God he is not good, If God is good he is not God." There is something screwy somewhere! Maybe there are answers to these questions; maybe there aren't. One thing is certain in this setting: whatever my faith or absence of it, I shall re-ask the questions.

What indeed constitutes good pastoral care in our secular age? We are so worried that we will infringe on each other's religious rights or privacy that we tend to produce environments in our schools, hospitals, and hospices which suggest that man exists without a transcended dimension. Too often pastoral care is reduced to one of two extremes—either a highly sectarian approach that forcefully proclaims the speaker's personal beliefs, on the one hand, or watered-down counseling pap, completely devoid of spiritual fiber and substance, on the other. Is that all there is? How do we administer effective pastoral care to those of other beliefs; to atheists or agnostics? These are important questions. Surely a preliminary goal is to create an atmosphere that proclaims through attitudes, rather than simply words, that these are significant issues. Care must be taken to observe the holidays, holy days, rituals, and symbols of the faiths represented by the patients under our care.

One experiment in pastoral care at the Royal Victoria Hospital, Palliative Care Ward, has been "Partage." Held every Monday afternoon, it is a time for patients, family members, and staff to come together in order to examine a specific theme, such as community, fear, or hope. Through readings, music, shared quiet, symbols, and actions, we learn something of both our shared vulnerability and our potential strength. Partage is coordinated by the music therapist, pastoral care leader, and occupational therapist, but all contribute and all leave feeling they have received more than they have given.

Pastoral care involves not "foisting on" or "giving to" but a "listening to." It is meeting people where they are, not where we think they should be. There can be no formula. It must always be uniquely personal.

3. Nurturing and Supporting Independence

M.M. was in her late fifties. She had always been independent, productive, a self-starter. She had always enjoyed running her own show. Some would describe her as autocratic.

Now, over a period of weeks, her world shrank from that of successful career woman to that of totally dependent parasite. That was how she felt. Serious illness does not constitute a loss—it is a series of losses; the most important being the loss of the sense of personal control. To restore, even in part, this sense of control can challenge the most inventive and sensitive of caregivers. The dysphasic quadriplegic patient may find a renewed sense of control if given the opportunity to decide her daily routines—for example, to have a bath or not today, and if so, at what time.

To support independence is to nurture personhood, which presupposes having taken the time to get to know the person we are trying to help. "When my time comes, I want to die with dignity," claims Russell Myers's cartoon character Broom Hilda. "Terrific!" exclaims her friend, "It would make such an attractive contrast to the way you lived!" If we are going to meet Broom Hilda's needs, we'd better have realistic goals. We'd better recognize that if she's had warts all her life, she is going to die with warts. One of the reasons we have problems in meeting people where they are is our tendency to frame people. We frame each other. We think we know who the other person is. We jump to conclusions based on physical appearance, culture, socioeconomic status, and other superficial clues. You think you know me because of what I communicate verbally and nonverbally, yet what do you know of my fears and insecurities and secret thoughts?

This is a particular problem in the hospital setting. In home care, the caregiver has a tremendous advantage; you get a thousand clues immediately—you enter the neighborhood, walk down the street, climb the front stairs. Already you know more about the patient than you can learn from long in-hospital discussions. You walk in the door, you sit down, you smell the place, feel and listen to it, and you instinctively know who they are. In the hospital ward—even in the hospice ward, with all its preoccupations concerning personhood—all these clues are lost.

This was driven home to me one day when I observed an old woman and an old man on our ward. The old lady was one of Canada's superb artists, a lady of enormous creative power. The man had been an axe murderer who had spent most of his life in prison. On our ward, they were simply an old lady and an old man. It wasn't that I particularly wanted them to be respectively praised or penalized for all that had gone before. It was simply a recognition that, by and large, our treatment of them failed to take into consideration the texture of their previous lives, their self-images, and sense of worth. How can we hope to foster their sense of personhood and independence when our knowledge is so fragmentary? The solution starts with recognizing the problem and employing carefully thought-out specific strategies, such as primary nursing. Most of all, it depends on profound respect for the otherness and uniqueness of the one we are attempting to help.

One final thought about another kind of problem having to do with framing each other. During one of my early visits to St. Christopher's Hospice, I met a patient named Frances. She had advanced ovarian carcinoma with an incomplete large bowel obstruction. Her time in the hospice had been difficult for all concerned. Talking to the nursing staff, it became clear, in spite of their efforts to carefully word their reactions, that Frances was an irritant. They had given enormously over a long period of time. She had been demanding, irritable, and self-centered. I was puzzled. Could this be the same person I had met and learned so much from? It wasn't until some time later that we recognized that the discrepancy in our views arose from the fact that this highly experienced team was still reacting to the Frances that had been present on their ward a week or two earlier. One of the magical, marvelous things about this period in a person's life is that it is a time which is filled with potential for growth. As we grow, we change, and the change can happen very rapidly. Families may also evolve. So may caregivers. As we repeatedly confront death, the probability is that we are evolving and changing. We'd better be careful not to frame each other on the team. Maybe I'm not the same guy you were having trouble working with last year. Maybe I have grown—a little bit.

CHALLENGE III. FAMILY-RELATED CHALLENGES

1. Setting Realistic Goals

So often our goals in hospice are not realistic. We say that the family is the unit of care. The reality too often on our service is that the family is neglected. This discrepancy between expectation and reality is seen in other aspects of our work. We say the patient is number one, but we are always in meetings. We say we work as a team, but there is often poor communication. We say that listening is important, but there isn't time even for listening to each other. We say that psychosocial and spiritual concerns are important. Quite often it is lip service.

To have realistic family-related goals, we must first know who is in "the family." It isn't just the legal family. It may not be just his wife. It may also be his mistress, and we as a society may be uncomfortable with that.

One of the most memorable stories of imaginative personalized hospice care I have heard concerned a young man with advanced malignant disease admitted to a caring hospice ward. He was surrounded by color-coded walls, a television set, flowers, and a concerned team. He was miserable. Finally, in a team meeting, one of the home care nurses commented, "You know, I think we are ignoring who this man is. This young guy is a homosexual. I was in his home, and there is nothing about this place that resembles his apartment." What followed was a long discussion and a great deal of soul searching. They decided that if they were really going to meet his needs, they would have to make some significant changes. They took out all the furniture, the pictures, and the bed, and placed the mattress on the floor—the bare mattress, no bedding. Then they went and got the erotic pictures from his apartment and hung them on the walls of his remodeled hospice room. They invited his friends. Many on the hospice team were very uncomfortable and had serious questions about what they were doing. But the quality of life for that young man changed remarkably. He was now at peace, happy and able to relate to people. He had been met on his terms, where he was.

2. The Splitting Family

The splitting family is the family under stress: filled with fear, insecurity, anger, guilt, ambivalence, and charged relationships. These highly volatile families are dynamite in our services because they are skilled beyond belief at separating us as caregivers. While latching on to one person whom they emotionally drain yet fill with feelings of competence, they talk about other persons on the team in derogatory ways. It's not intentional, but it is extraordinarily destructive. The needs of this kind of family can never be met, but the unbridled motivation of the hospice team sucks everyone in.

There are three things to do. The first is to make the diagnosis that this is happening. The second thing is to share the care. The involvement of a second primary care person ensures the ability to spell each other off and promotes objectivity. Finally, it is important to openly discuss the potential divisiveness of such families in team meetings.

In helping such troubled families, indeed in working effectively with any family, we will be assisted if we familiarize ourselves with the evolving body of knowledge relating to family systems developed by Minuchin, Virginia Satir, and others.

Basic principles of family systems include the following:

First, the family is the unit of care. While that has long been a part of hospice philosophy, what strikes me is how often we say it but don't really do an effective family assessment.

A second key concept in family systems pictures the family as a mobile. This underscores the fact that the removal of even the least significant-appearing family member produces a significant shift in the position of all other persons in the mobile. Even a relatively minor change in the role or position of any one person dramatically affects the position of all others.

A third concept suggests that the system is greater than the sum of its parts. A simple family of four, for example, involves a complex series of relationships—that between the two parents, between each parent and each child, between the two children.

Fourthly, the personal tasks facing each person sustaining a loss include:

a. the need to do their own grief work

b. the need to adjust to the new role of each other person in the family system

c. the need to adapt to new routines, both personal and involving each of the others

Basic concepts in family systems! Exciting stuff! If we had more time, we could look in depth at how we assess families. Eight different areas we look into that have to do with cultural backgrounds—identification of who is really in the family; who are the support systems; how did they handle losses in the past; are they going through transition times or times of special vulnerability; what are their values and beliefs about death; their individual responses to the current illness; what resources are available to them; what immediate and long-range family needs are there? The rich material one needs to gather in carrying out a family assessment.

3. Bereavement Follow-up

A number of important questions remain with us as we try to define appropriate bereavement follow-up. Who should it be for? How do you select the high-risk people? Who should be doing it? What kind of training should they receive? How do you make it cost-effective, in that there aren't endless dollars to spend and yet we must avoid tokenism.

Last week, I made a home visit to interview the family of a woman who had died on our service a year ago. As circumstances would have it, significant bereavement follow-up by our service had come to an end, and my visit was precipitated by unrelated research that I was doing. It was chilling to recognize during that visit that each of the three children was headed for a pathologic grief reaction. The danger signals were there for all to see. We had dropped the ball. How often does it happen? These are important issues. The bereaved are a high-risk population. It looks like we can learn to identify the high risk person, and it looks like intervention programs, even simple ones, can make a difference. That doesn't imply unstructured amateurism. While we may use trained volunteers, they must be skilled, informed, and supervised, and systems for the referral of problem cases must be clearly established.

CHALLENGE IV. CAREGIVER-RELATED CHALLENGES

1. Uncertainty Regarding the Appropriateness of More Aggressive Treatment

The physicians on our hospice team held a meeting yesterday to discuss the treatment decisions involved in several recent cases. These are troubling questions for many teams—"We know he's confused. Do we investigate or not? How far do we go?" "He has a bowel obstruction. Is surgery appropriate or not? How far do we go?" "He has a painful femur with known metastatic disease. It probably signals an impending pathologic fracture. Should we pin prophylactically or not?" How we answer these questions in each of our individual hospice programs has important ramifications for the role that hospice will play in that community, for the answers we give will define how our referring colleagues will use our services. If hospices simply represent custodial care, our oncologist colleagues will be more likely to press on, seeing no alternative to the continuation of useless antitumor therapy. The nature of hospice practice, with its minimum reliance on laboratory investigation, gives rise to innumerable questions. Are we doing enough? Should we be doing more? Should we be referring? Should we be investigating? Conversely, if we do "more," we run the risk of experiencing the nagging questions facing the physicians on our team last week, when two of our patients died in the postoperative period following the pinning of a femoral fracture and the oversewing of a perforated ulcer, respectively. In looking back, we wondered if we had forgotten what hospice is all about.

I would say that it is important that such questions remain agonizing for us. This is one problem we had better keep with us because if we lose this as a problem, we have lost the ability to stay with the medical issues at hand and to recognize the uncertainty in these situations. Once we start applying easy formulas to difficult situations, we will have accepted mediocrity, and patient care will have suffered as a result.

2. Team Roles in Whole-Person Care

The second team-related problem is that of team roles in whole-person care. What in the world happened to our traditional roles when we mixed them into hospice? We can look at each professional role in turn.

Let us start with nursing, since this is the core of hospice care. Too often, hospice nurses find that they have responsibility without power. Primary nursing care has helped us change this. Hospice nursing involves heavy physical care. It is draining, and there may be little time for the psychosocial and spiritual issues that the idealized hospice manuals claim to be part of a nurse's role. One excellent nurse on our service commented, "Volunteers get all the goodies, and we get all the shit." The nurse spends long periods at the bedside. She is subjected to repeated intense interactions, repeated losses, repeated feelings of impotence, particularly when nursing patients to whom she closely relates. Her stress will depend on her setting. If she is on a home care service, professional isolation may be a factor. On a hospice ward, lack of autonomy may be stressful. If she is on a consultation or symptom-control team in an active-care institution, she'll find that she is always at the buffer zone between the traditional health care system and the direction of the hospice, and she will experience her own kind of isolation in being repeatedly subject to misinterpretation and suspicion.

What about the doctor? Yaeger and Hubert examined the stresses experienced by physicians in psychiatric residency training programs. The stressors they identified are revealingly similar to those experienced by hospice physicians. These include:

a. Boundary problems. ("What is my role compared to other mental health professionals, such as pastoral care people, counselors, family physicians, and neurologists? Will I continue to be a physician?");
b. Redefinition of self as M.D. The hospice physician is stripped of many of the diagnostic tools he/she has come to rely on, leaving diagnoses less clear and the potential for anxiety heightened. Furthermore, the holistic orientation of hospice care forces the physician to adopt a more egalitarian role. There is a shift from the active authoritarianism that has traditionally characterized the physician's role to the more passive stance of "member-of-the-team";
c. An increase in intrapsychic and interpersonal awareness;
d. The assimilation of a new body of knowledge foreign to the traditional physician role.

What about the social worker? Dame Cicely was visiting our service on one occasion when our social worker, T.N., was coming apart at the seams. Recognizing Dame Cicely's insight and experience as an "almoner" herself, we arranged a meeting. I was greatly impressed by the obvious lessening of tensions as T.N. surfaced after a good conversation and a cup of tea. When pressed to know what Dame Cicely had said,

T.N. simply replied, "We came in and sat down, and she turned to me and said, 'I know your problem. You work on a team of amateur social workers!'" T.N. had promptly burst into tears because that was exactly her problem. The reason Cicely knew was because she had been a social worker herself. In hospice, we all believe we have the answers to the questions that social workers spend a great deal of time training to handle.

What about the chaplain? What in the world is pastoral care? How do you administer to those of other beliefs? These are sensitive issues in our secular society. Like the physician and the nurse, the pastoral caregiver is often poorly equipped, poorly trained, to deal with death. Furthermore, they're often subconsciously assigned, by all of us, a lower role in the pecking order. A shrewd nun who worked on our service pointed out to me, "I'll tell you how you can see that. Just watch what happens at a hospice patient's bedside. If the pastoral caregiver comes to the door and looks in and there is a nurse or doctor sitting at the bedside, he or she will usually say, 'Oh, I'll come back later.' But if the pastoral caregiver is the one sitting at the bedside and the nurse or doctor comes into the room, it is unlikely that they will hesitate to interrupt. After all, what they had come to do is important. I am the doctor, for crying out loud!"

The physical and occupational therapists are stressed because of the difference that exists between the rehabilitation-medicine role, for which they were trained, and this new job, where their mandate is to maximize patients' ability to use their decreasing potential. Traditionally, the therapist gets her rewards from her patients being able to do more this week than last. In hospice, the patients are able to do less this week than last week. Inevitably, physical and occupational therapists will get depressed until they recognize the tremendous relevance they have in this setting. It isn't to help patients do more. It's to help patients to do as much as they can today. No one is better equipped for this task than the therapist, but to be effective, he/she must understand this change in roles.

Other members of the team also experience job-related stress—the music therapist, for instance. It is little wonder she is stressed. No one in the world knows what she actually does. The administrator is called on to respond to the demands of the whole team rather than those of a hierarchy. The researcher in this field is particularly stressed. My friend Ron Melzack, and any studies we have done, remind me of the difficulties involved in carrying out studies with the patient population. It seems that all the significant variables are always soft. How do you measure them? The brief life span of the patients, with their depleted resources and inability to fill out questionnaires, which always seem to be three hundred items long; the resentment expressed by the team if we attempt to carry out research. ("Why are we doing research? I thought we were supposed to be a hospice. I thought we were concerned with the quality of life of these people.")

Finally, the stress of the director. The problem is that it doesn't seem to matter who the director is or what his/her training has been. The training is always inadequate. The director invariably has limited knowledge and an insufficient number of arms to keep all the balls in the air at once. From an organizational point of view, services that involve all health care disciplines—focusing not only on physical but psychological, social, and spiritual care for patients that are both at home and in the hospice, as well as bereavement follow-up programs, teaching, and research—provide complex challenges, problems related to decision making and norms of functioning. Too often, team members see decision making in hospice as being autocratic or dictatorial, while the director may feel that there has to be a referendum on every topic to keep the team happy.

3. Finding Our Personal Center

Caregivers burn out, to use the vernacular. Dr. Merv Vincent reminds us that the person who is experiencing burnout is moving from caring to apathy, from involvement to distancing, from openness to self-protection, from trust to suspicion, from enthusiasm to disillusionment and often on to cynicism, from self-esteem to personal devaluation.

I would suggest that the primary task of adult life is to recognize, understand, and accept our own personhood, our own feet of clay, our own woundedness. I must come to understand my defense, my insecurities, and come to terms with what Roger Waters called our "wall," that is, the psychodynamic baggage that we drag from childhood into adult life that prevents us from functioning to our potential, that prevents us from the freedom that could be ours, that leaves us acting out and reacting.

The poet Ted Rosenthal experienced the arena of death as a teacher. In facing a terminal illness, he came to see life differently. He talked enthusiastically about living "in the moment" rather than living "for the moment." He said, "You know, I'm happier for what I've been through." He was a poet. He didn't mince words. It is striking that he didn't say, "I'm better" or "I'm wiser." He said, "I'm *happier.*"

Viktor Frankl, in his book *Man's Search for Meaning,* which he wrote in the remarkably short period of eight days after being freed from Auschwitz, pointed out that the arena of death left him with a deeper sense of commitment to life.

Those of us working as caregivers in hospice may be given a gift by being faced day by day with the transcience and preciousness of life. We can use this gift as an invitation to deal with our own personal walls so that we may come to more completely live in the moment and celebrate life more effectively. While for each of us coming to terms with our own wall is a highly personal thing, and for each of us the path will be different, whatever the path toward wholeness, it is likely to involve things like slowing down and giving up things, simplifying and opening rather than striving, accumulating, competing, and attaining. I wish each of you well in your quest for personal centeredness, for such growth lies at the heart of our sustained effectiveness, both personal and professional.

Thank you very much.

OUTCOMES FROM A NATIONAL MULTISPECIALTY PALLIATIVE CARE CURRICULUM DEVELOPMENT PROJECT

DAVID E. WEISSMAN, M.D. , BRUCE AMBUEL, PH.D. , CHARLES F. VON GUNTEN, M.D., PH.D. , SUSAN BLOCK, M.D., ERIC WARM, M.D., JAMES HALLENBECK, M.D., ROBERT MILCH, M.D., KAREN BRASEL, M.D., AND PATRICIA B. MULLAN, PH.D.

This article originally appeared as Weissman DE, Ambuel B, Von Gunten CF, Block S, Warm E, Hallenbeck J, Milch R, Brasel K, Mullan PB. Outcomes from a national multispecialty palliative care curriculum development project. *J Palliat Med*. 2007;10:408–19. Copyright © 2008, American Academy of Hospice and Palliative Medicine. All rights reserved. Reprinted with permission.

EDITORS' INTRODUCTION

Change is really possible. This successful effort demonstrated the feasibility of integrating palliative medicine teaching into 358 internal medicine, family medicine, neurology, and general surgery residency programs (27 percent of all eligible training programs). Using a two-day intervention of focused short-term instruction of residency program directors, more than 50 percent of participating programs were able to incorporate palliative medicine teaching, and more than 70 percent of the internal and family medicine residencies involved their trainees in direct bedside exposure to hospital palliative care and hospice clinical programs.

■   ■   ■

INTRODUCTION

Efforts to improve palliative care training for physicians in training has been a priority in United States medical education for only the past ten years.[1] Although palliative care topics, particularly the ethics of end-of-life care, have been widely instituted in undergraduate preclinical education, little has been instituted in the graduate training programs in which physicians learn the skills they will use in practice.[2-4] A major step forward was the first graduate training requirements specific to palliative care by a major medical specialty, internal medicine, in 1997. Since then, palliative care requirements have been added to a small number of other residency and fellowship programs.[5]

Many palliative care curriculum projects have been reported in the past ten years, largely restricted to single residency programs.[6-16] However, large-scale efforts, providing coherent and comprehensive training across medical specialties, are clearly needed. In 1998 we initiated a pilot project to stimulate curriculum development among thirty-two internal medicine residency programs recruited from the midwestern section of the United States, promoting the best available educational methods for palliative care training. After one year, 78 percent of these programs were still engaged in curriculum development and reported progress in seven key outcomes: pain assessment, pain management, nonpain symptom management, communication skills, clinical training experiences, teaching conference integration, and faculty development.[17,18] Based on these encouraging results, the project was expanded to a national cohort of internal medicine residency programs starting in 1999. Over the next five years, in response to demand and new training requirements, enrollment was expanded to include family medicine, neurology, and general surgery residency programs, as these specialties adopted their own palliative care training requirements.[19]

The goal of the expanded national project was to recruit 350 to 400 residency programs to:

- Start/expand teaching in pain and symptom management;
- Start/expand interactive palliative care communication skills training;
- Start/expand clinical care training opportunities in palliative care/hospice to reinforce didactic training and afford opportunities for clinical practice;
- Integrate palliative care content into routine educational conferences;
- Start/expand palliative care faculty development initiatives;
- Use quality improvement principles to encourage new educational initiatives.

This report provides outcomes from the residency programs that participated in this curriculum development project. We describe the extent of curriculum change achieved across and within four different specialties. The study questions include:

1. What is the feasibility and impact of a focused educational intervention on subsequent palliative care teaching practices;

2. To what extent do the strategies and findings from one medical specialty apply to other specialty-focused residency programs;

3. What is the distribution of reforms achieved among palliative care educational domains?

METHODS

This project was conducted as a prospective, multispecialty, interinstitutional study designed to assist residency directors in enhancing palliative care teaching within their residency program. The project was structured around the following steps: recruitment, needs assessment, two-day conference, one-day follow-up conference, and mentoring (Table 18.1). The project was reviewed and approved by the Medical College of Wisconsin Institutional Review Board.

Recruitment

Recruitment efforts included eliciting the support of medical specialty leadership as well as recruitment directed to residency programs within the specialties. The four oversight specialty associations (American Board of Internal Medicine, American Academy of Neurology, American College of Surgeons, and the Society of Teachers of Family Medicine) were contacted and agreed to assist in recruitment by mailing recruitment packages to program directors with a cover letter of support and/or advertising the project through organizational communication vehicles. Residencies were recruited into twelve sequential cohorts over the five years of the project; all cohorts except one had a target enrollment of thirty residencies. Cohorts 1 and 2 were exclusively for internal medicine; both internal medicine and family medicine were recruited for cohorts 3 to 6. Cohort 7 was exclusively for neurology programs, and cohort 8 was a pilot cohort for

TABLE 18.1. Project Steps and Rationale

Recruitment process
Obtain support from national residency organizations to participate in recruitment process.
  Rationale: increase the potential for project buy-in from residency program directors.

Needs assessment
  (a) Program director and senior resident complete independent curriculum review.
       Rationale: Increase validity of curriculum review process and bring resident "voice" into the project.
  (b) Invite all residents and teaching faculty to complete 36-item knowledge and self-comfort-confidence surveys.
       Rationale: Increase tension for change by demonstrating knowledge deficits.

Two-day conference
  (a) Participation by senior residents with their program directors.
       Rationale: Increase resident buy-in to curriculum reform process and awareness of career opportunities in palliative care.
  (b) Private feedback of needs assessment and knowledge test data to individual program directors.
       Rationale: Increase tension for change for residencies—demonstrate areas of strength and weakness that are program specific.
  (c) Exclusive use of small group interactive teaching.
       Rationale: Opportunity for palliative care educators to role model optimal teaching techniques.
  (d) Teaching modules: Pain, Giving Bad News, and Goal Setting communication skills.
       Rationale: These are the most basic elements of improving clinical care in palliative care.
  (e) Teaching module: Clinical experiential opportunities in palliative care.
       Rationale: Increase awareness of opportunities to utilize clinical teaching as an essential adjunct to didactic and small group teaching.
  (f) Teaching module: Basics of instructional design.
       Rationale: Acquaint attendees with alternative teaching formats besides lecture, especially for attitude-based content domains.
  (g) Teaching module: Faculty development
       Rationale: Encourage faculty development as key aspect of palliative care curriculum reform.
  (h) Scavenger hunt for educational resource material
       Rationale: Provide opportunity for attendees to review all of the educational material provided as take-home resource material.

Follow-up conference
Presentation of residency progress reports with opportunity for publication.
  Rationale: Reinforce enthusiasm for continuing curriculum reform; opportunity for program directors to obtain academic credit for curriculum reform.

Mentoring
Contact between faculty mentor and program director following two-day conference.
  Rationale: Provide support and encouragement to program directors; discuss barriers to implementation and seek alternative approaches; encourage participation in the one-day conference; encourage completion of progress report.

surgery residencies, with only eight programs recruited to test new materials developed for a surgical audience. Cohorts 9 to 12 contained programs from all four specialties.

Required conditions for participation included a signed commitment letter from the department chair, and agreement to complete baseline assessments, to send a team to participate in a two-day training workshop, and to complete a twelve-month progress report. The residency programs were responsible for travel costs and a conference registration fee.

Needs Assessment

Residency directors and a chief resident independently completed a written review of current curriculum offerings in palliative care. All residents and faculty were asked to complete a thirty-six-item knowledge assessment and a self-confidence and comfort survey regarding their palliative care skills and attitudes.[20-22]

Two-Day Conference

A team from each residency program, comprised of the program director or designee, one or two additional faculty, and a senior resident, attended a two-day workshop with other residency teams from their assigned cohort. Each program received extensive education resource material for use in curriculum development (Table 18.2). During the conference, to enhance awareness of the variety of educational resources provided to the residency teams, a scavenger hunt was conducted; attendees were asked to locate sixteen different educational products within the resource material. One residency program, from those that submitted correct scavenger hunt answers, was selected at random to receive a $1,000 financial stipend for a two-day visiting preceptorship to one of three palliative care programs directed by program faculty.

The conference format consisted of six small-group training sessions attended in rotation by all faculty participants (Table 18.3). The focus of the six sessions included the following topics: Pain Management; Communication Skills I: Giving Bad News; Communication Skills II: Goal Setting and Do-Not-Resuscitate (DNR) discussion; Clinical Experiences; Instructional Design; and Faculty Development. Each session included learning objectives, review of best-practice educational strategies, and demonstration of educational techniques. An additional training session was attended solely by residents to allow discussion of resident-specific issues in palliative care while their faculty attended the faculty development session. Within the most appropriate session, attendees were introduced to one of four educational quality improvement projects. Each project was designed for a chief resident to collect data from five to ten charts, data that could be used to demonstrate the need for changes in palliative care practice behavior: (1) pain assessment documentation; (2) analgesic prescribing; (3) advance care planning; and (4) hospice referrals. The teaching faculty for the two-day conference were consistent across the twelve cohorts except for one faculty change starting with cohort 5.

TABLE 18.2. **Educational Resource Material Provided to Residency Programs**

Conference Syllabus. Teaching resource material used during the 2-day conference containing examples of teaching objectives, lesson plans, content outlines, pegagogical methods, palliative care educational and clinical resources, and four quality improvement projects.

Improving End of Life Care: A resource guide for physician education. Weissman DE, Ambuel B and Hallenbeck J. Medical College of Wisconsin, 2001. Contains learning objectives, content outlines, pre-tests, role-playing scenarios, small group exercises, and educational references. www.mcw.edupallmed

Improving End of Life Care: A Faculty Development Resource Book. Weissman DE. Medical College of Wisconsin, 2000.

Communication Skills for the End-of-Life Educator. Weissman DE and Biernat K. Medical College of Wisconsin, 1998. Package contains a trigger video of common palliative care encounters, lesson plans, content outlines, slide sets, learner evaluation materials. www.mcw.edu/pallmed

Medical Guidelines for Determining Prognosis in Selected Non-Cancer Diseases, 2nd ed. Alexandria, VA: National Hospice and Palliative Care Organization, 1996.

Fast Facts and Concepts provided by weekly email; available at www.eperc.mcw.edu. Fast Facts were originally designed by Dr. Eric Warm during his work as a residency project participant during the pilot phase of this project.[23]

One-Day Follow-Up Conference

Six to nine months after the two-day conference, an optional one-day meeting was held for programs to review their progress, discuss barriers, and review additional requested educational methods obtained through a preconference needs assessment sent to all programs. At the end of the conference, participants had an opportunity to review and update their initial action plan. Participants were invited to draft a structured progress report, using a suggested template, suitable for presentation at the conference and for publication.[24-26]

Structured Mentoring

A set of strategies was incorporated into the training program to provide a structured mentoring experience. At the end of each of the six training sessions during the two-day conference, residency teams worked to identify strengths and gaps in their current training, and plan new curriculum initiatives. An additional sixty minutes of scheduled time was included for curriculum planning at the end of each day. To support the planning process, each residency program director met privately with the project evaluation specialist to receive a customized report detailing results from

TABLE 18.3. Two-Day Conference Learning Objectives

Pain Management

Review common house-staff barriers to providing good pain management.
Learn three educational methods for teaching and evaluating pain assessment and treatment.
Learn different educational methods for teaching (a) analgesic pharmacology and (b) assessing addiction—differentiating from pain.
Review educational resource material for pain education.

Communication Skills I

Learn three teaching strategies for giving bad news.
Learn how to incorporate personal reflection into communication skills teaching.
Plan a *Giving Bad News* simulated teaching exercise.
Review educational resources for communication skills.

Communication Skills II

Learn steps in initiating a discussion of goal setting and treatment withdrawal.
Learn how to structure a teaching program focused on goal setting and DNR[a] orders.
Learn how to incorporate personal reflection into communication skills teaching.
Plan a simulated teaching session on goal setting and DNR orders.

Clinical Experiences

Learn options for supervised clinical experiences in end-of-life care.
Learn how to utilize traditional educational formats to include greater EOL[b] emphasis (for example, grand rounds, tumor board, morning report).
Learn supervision and resident evaluation strategies for EOL clinical opportunities.
Plan one new EOL-focused clinical experience.

Instructional Design

Demonstrate how to construct teaching objectives for attitudes, knowledge and skill-based objectives.
Review the concept of "teaching scripts" used in clinical teaching.
Demonstrate how to develop teaching scripts for three common clinical topics.
Review opportunities for introducing palliative care teaching into different educational settings.

Faculty Development

Understand the barriers to and opportunities for faculty education.
Learn how to design a faculty development course.
Plan a faculty development program.
Know at least three ways to build tension for curriculum change.
Understand the two common paths to curriculum change within academic medicine.

[a]DNR: do not resuscitate
[b]EOL: end of life

their previously submitted needs assessment, including results of the knowledge and confidence surveys. Following the last conference session, residency teams developed a final action plan including specific curriculum goals and a one-year timeline of specific tasks and responsibilities. To further support the planning process, each residency was assigned to one project faculty member who met with the residency team at the end of each conference day to review and discuss the residency's evolving strategic plan.

Three months following the conference, the assigned project faculty member telephoned the residency contact and completed a ten-minute structured telephone interview. The project and program faculty reviewed progress toward action plan completion and discussed strategies to overcome institutional barriers. Participants were encouraged to contact project faculty mentors or other project faculty at any time to discuss the implementation of their strategic plans. All conference attendees were placed on an e-mail distribution list to receive announcements describing professional palliative care development opportunities, teaching tips, and pertinent palliative care education references. In addition, the project disseminated fast facts, an educational intervention developed by a physician participant in the project's pilot, presenting short focused palliative care–based questions and answers.[23]

Project Outcome Evaluation

To assess progress at twelve months, program directors were asked to complete a structured report identifying new educational initiatives arising from both the direct training at the workshops and from the educational resource material provided to each residency program. The following domains were sampled in the twelve-month progress report: new curriculum content in pain management and nonpain symptom management; new teaching in seven specific palliative care communication domains; integration of palliative care into one of three regularly scheduled conferences (grand rounds, morbidity and mortality, or morning report); development of new required or elective palliative care or hospice clinical experiences; use of the educational quality improvement projects; and new efforts directed at improving the palliative care knowledge or skills among faculty. Program directors were also asked if they had used any of the five educational resources provided to them and to rate their estimated progress towards completion of their action plan goals. Finally, recognizing that this project was occurring at a time of other palliative care educational and system change initiatives, program directors were asked to rate the percentage of new palliative care educational work that they attributed directly to their participation in this project. The survey was mailed and followed by e-mail reminders and a second mailing if there was no response; telephone calls were made to nonresponders encouraging completion.

Some residency programs did not complete the structured twelve-month report but did submit structured progress reports for the one-day follow-up conference that were subsequently published. The published reports from residency programs that did not complete the structured twelve-month report were reviewed for documentation of new curricular, faculty development, and clinical experiences consistent with the questions from the twelve-month report. Additional data from mentoring phone calls and ad hoc communication were available for review but not included in the final outcome analysis as the data were not elicited with methods comparable to the structured twelve-month progress reports or published progress reports.

Project cost was calculated by totaling the project grant funding and estimating residency program expenses for conference attendance. An average airfare of $300 per attendee was used plus $50 in round-trip taxi fare per program. The sole hotel used for conferences offered a package rate for room and all meals of $229 per day. No attempt was made to develop a cost analysis for the number of hours spent on new curriculum integration once programs returned to their home institution.

RESULTS

Three hundred seventy-eight programs filed an initial commitment letter; 20 withdrew prior to the two-day conference and are not included in the analysis. The 358 evaluable programs included internal medicine (n = 169), family medicine (n = 106), neurology (n = 39) and surgery (n = 44), representing, respectively, 47 percent, 22 percent, 33 percent, and 17 percent of all U.S. residency programs in each specialty, or 27 percent of all potential programs from the four residencies combined. Residency programs from forty-nine states and Puerto Rico were represented. The average number of residents from all training years combined, per program, was 33 (range, 6–177); 983 faculty and residents attended the twelve two-day conferences (2.7 participants per residency); 219 attendees from 157 programs participated in the one-day follow-up conferences.

Results of the attendee evaluation of the training conferences indicated that participants perceived that the educational sessions met their objectives and engaged the participants in curriculum planning; these findings were consistent across the cohorts, replicating the experience that participants reported in the pilot project.[17,18]

Twelve-month reports were completed by 188 programs (53 percent); another 36 (10 percent) submitted progress reports for publication but did not submit a twelve-month report. Interim reports from mentoring calls were available from another 26 programs (7 percent) but were not included in the analysis. A lower percentage of residency programs provided follow-up reports or progress reports in neurology (38 percent) and surgery programs (45 percent) than internal medicine (67 percent) or family practice (72 percent).

The breakdown of integration in four curriculum domains—pain, nonpain symptoms, communication skills and clinical experiences—by specialty is shown in Figure 18.1. Over 75 percent of all programs reported new curriculum features in pain management and communication skills. In particular, family practice and internal medicine reported the greatest curriculum change; 94 percent of internal medicine and 90 percent of family practice programs added new content in pain, while 83 percent of internal medicine and 92 percent of family practice added new training in communication skills. Sixty percent or more of internal medicine, family practice, and surgery programs reported new training in nonpain symptoms. Seventy percent or more of internal medicine or family practice programs began new experiential training opportunities, while 40 percent of neurology and 10 percent of surgical programs developed such opportunities.

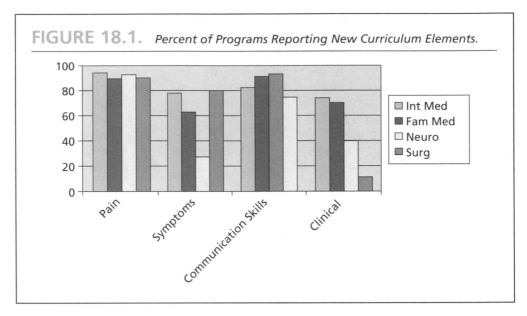

FIGURE 18.1. *Percent of Programs Reporting New Curriculum Elements.*

Data from 224 programs submitting 12-month follow-up data or a published progress report. Pain, pain assessment and management education. Symptoms, non-pain symptom assessment and management education. Communications skills, at least one of the following: giving bad news, discussing prognosis or do-not-resuscitate (DNR) orders, running a family conference, discussing hospice referral, or completing a spiritual assessment. Clinical, at least one of the following: palliative care elective or required outpatient or inpatient experience, or required or elective hospice home visits.

Figure 18.2 shows a breakdown of specific communication skills teaching by specialty. Over 50 percent of internal medicine and family practice programs started educational training dealing with giving bad news, prognosis, and DNR discussions, goals of care/family conferencing, and hospice referrals. More than 40 percent of internal medicine and family practice programs began training in spiritual assessment and provided opportunities for trainee personal reflection. Over 50 percent of neurology and surgery programs started new training programs for giving bad news and DNR discussions, with lesser penetration of the other communication topics.

Figure 18.3 provides a breakdown of new required or elective experiential training opportunities. Over 70 percent of internal medicine and family medicine programs began required or elective palliative care or hospice-based clinical experiences for residents, while only 40 percent of neurology and 10 percent of surgery programs began such offerings. The breakdown of adjunctive curriculum features is shown in Figure 18.4. Palliative care content was integrated into existing conferences (grand rounds, morbidity and mortality, or morning report) in 67 to 83 percent of programs. Faculty development was initiated in 10 to 42 percent of programs, while 20 to 41 percent of programs used at least one quality improvement project to spur educational change. Among the quality improvement projects, pain and advance care planning

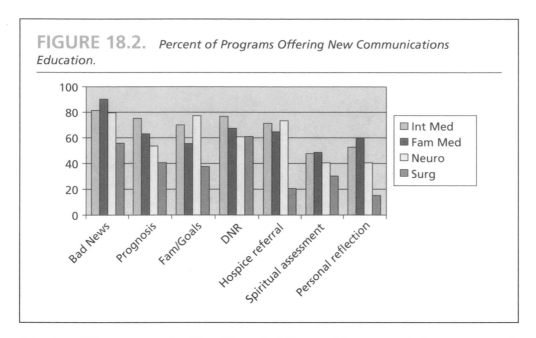

FIGURE 18.2. *Percent of Programs Offering New Communications Education.*

Data from 224 programs submitting 12-month follow-up data or published progress report. Communication skills training included any element of lecture, small group, or skills training (e.g., objective structured clinical examination [OSCE]).

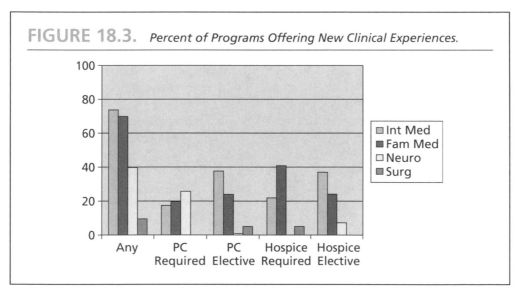

FIGURE 18.3. *Percent of Programs Offering New Clinical Experiences.*

Data from 224 programs submitting 12-month follow-up data or published progress report. Any one of the following clinical experiences: PC required, any required outpatient or inpatient palliative care experience; PC elective, any elective outpatient or inpatient palliative care experience; Hospice required, any required hospice home or inpatient hospice experience; Hospice elective, any elective hospice home or inpatient hospice experience.

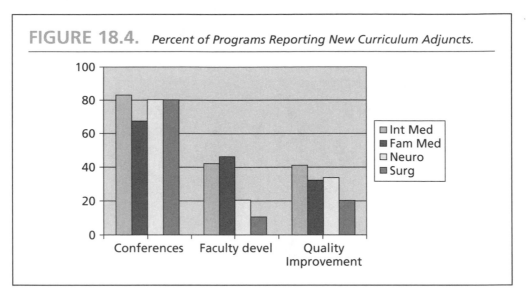

FIGURE 18.4. *Percent of Programs Reporting New Curriculum Adjuncts.*

Data from 224 programs submitting 12-month follow-up data or published progress report. Conferences, new inclusion of palliative care content in at least one of the following: grand rounds, morning report, morbidity/mortality conferences. Faculty development, any report of faculty training via lecture, workshop or small group work. QI, any use of one of four quality improvement projects: pain assessment, pain management, advance care planning, or hospice referral.

projects were used more than the hospice referral project. The educational materials provided to programs were well utilized following the teaching conference, especially the conference syllabus, the resource guide for physician education, and Fast Facts (Figure 18.5).

Programs felt they made good progress toward completion of their action plan goals with a mean rating of 3.5 ± 74 (1 = no progress, 5 = extensive progress). Residencies reported that, on average, they attributed 70 percent $\pm$ 26 percent of their progress directly to their participation in this program (internal medicine, 67 percent; family medicine, 70 percent; neurology, 92 percent; surgery, 78 percent).

The total grant support for this project was $1,353,690. The estimated total direct costs for each residency to attend the conferences was $988,015, making a total project expenditure of $2,341,705 or $6,541 per residency, or $198 per resident.

DISCUSSION

The new medical specialty of palliative medicine is rapidly growing and becoming part of the fabric of medical care and medical education. The past ten years have seen a flurry of physician education activities, including new resource material, large-scale physician-education projects, faculty development initiatives, textbook revision projects, and individual medical school and residency curriculum change projects. A national conference on palliative care physician education was held in 1999, from which a series

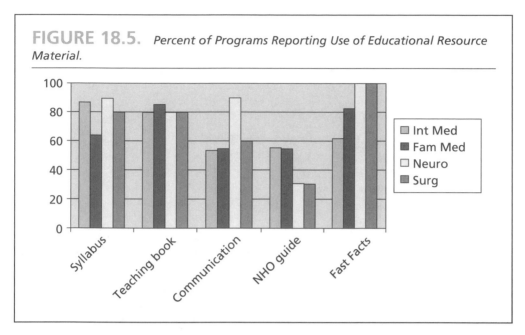

FIGURE 18.5. *Percent of Programs Reporting Use of Educational Resource Material.*

Data from 224 programs submitting 12-month follow-up data. See Table 18.2 for description of teaching resource material.

of consensus documents were developed, outlining optimal pedagogical approaches within specific educational settings.[28–30]

The aim of this project was to help a diverse group of residency programs apply existing knowledge about best educational practice in palliative care and develop and implement new curriculum elements in their training programs. The decision to initiate this project in internal medicine, and then extend it to family medicine, neurology, and general surgery programs, was based solely on new palliative care training requirements developed by the specialty's residency review committee or by their parent specialty organization. Thus the development of a new training requirement was the leverage point, the point of educational tension, for curriculum change.

The project intervention and endpoints were designed to move residency programs to adopt a comprehensive approach to curriculum development that would move beyond simply a new palliative care lecture series. First, we wanted programs to adopt new didactic or small-group education in the key educational domains where well-documented knowledge deficits exist—namely, pain and symptom management. Second, we believed that the attitude, knowledge, and skill deficiencies related to doctor-patient communication needed special attention, given the central role of and challenging and time-consuming learning process for mastering communication competencies in palliative care. Thus we devoted one-third of the educational contact time in the two-day workshop to demonstration and discussion of communication skills teaching. Third, we hoped that incorporation of palliative care into routine conferences such as grand rounds, morbidity and mortality conferences, and morning report would enhance the overall palliative care curriculum and demonstrate that palliative care was an appropriate content area, similar to traditional educational content taught in other parts of residency. Fourth, we believed that faculty development was vital for sustainability of palliative care education. Fifth, we believed that clinical palliative care experiences were an essential curriculum component to reinforce didactic and small-group teaching and to permit development of clinical skills. Sixth, we hoped that quality improvement techniques could be used as leverage for curriculum change. Finally, we were cognizant that few program directors or resident teaching faculty, especially in the early years of this project, would have the time or expertise to develop new educational materials. To meet this need, we amassed a coherent set of teaching materials that could be directly applied to resident education, including learning objectives, lesson plans, a communication-trigger videotape and communications teaching workbook, pocket reference cards, content outlines, and key educational and clinical references.

Project results indicate considerable success in all areas of curriculum development. The easiest curriculum features to incorporate—namely, didactic or small-group teaching of pain and nonpain symptom management and integration of palliative care into routine large-venue conferences—were added to most training programs. This finding tells us that, contrary to popular belief, residency program directors were able to find curricular time for new content when presented with both a rationale for making changes, new training requirement, and with ready-to-use educational resources.

Second, communication skills training, a more teacher-intensive and attitude/skill-based educational domain, received more attention than we anticipated. We believe that the combination of two workshops at the two-day conference, in which exemplar educators provided demonstrations of pedagogical techniques combined with ready-to-use teaching resources for the program directors, were essential elements of success.

Two of the more labor-intensive curriculum features were found in less than 50 percent of programs: faculty development and use of quality improvement projects. The fact that any programs began such efforts is encouraging, but much more work than we could provide within the limitations of this project is needed to fully support these ambitious goals. We strongly encouraged participating programs to send one or more faculty to participate in the Harvard Medical School program in Palliative Care Education and Practice (PCEP), a national faculty-development program in palliative care, and Education on Palliative and End-of-Life Care (EPEC) courses to help drive their local faculty-development efforts.

The disparity across specialties in providing follow-up reports was striking, with neurology and surgical programs lagging behind internal medicine and family practice. Observations from the project faculty at the training conferences indicated no major differences among different specialties in project engagement. Although there were small differences between specialties regarding which new curriculum features were adopted, in general there was more similarity than difference. The two areas of greatest difference were in starting new clinical experiences and faculty development. It is not surprising that internal medicine and family medicine began more clinical experiential training, as clinical experiences in palliative care/hospice are well aligned with primary care physician training. The lack of faculty development in neurology and surgery was disappointing and worrisome for long-term sustainability of their new educational programs.

There is little return-on-investment data for complex educational interventions. This project had an estimated cost of approximately $6,500 per residency program, of which the residency programs themselves contributed 42 percent of the cost, another potential motivating force for making curriculum change. When viewed at the level of the resident, the cost was only $198 per resident, or roughly equivalent to the price of two to three specialty textbooks. If the reported curriculum changes are sustained beyond one residency cohort and/or lead to other positive changes in institutional culture of caring for seriously ill patients, then the return on investment becomes greatly magnified.

This project did not utilize a control group to assess curriculum changes for nonparticipating residencies; thus we do not know to what degree such programs began similar educational initiatives. We tried to assess this information indirectly by asking program directors how much of the new curriculum work was directly attributable to this program; the average attribution of 70 percent is an indication that most, but not all, changes resulted from this project. A second limitation was the use of self-report forms for assessing curriculum change. Without some method of externally validating program reporting, there is certainly a possibility that program directors underreported or overreported their accomplishments. Of note, the anecdotal experiences of the project faculty were that many programs underreported their progress during mentoring and ad hoc communication. It was common for program directors to verbally indicate that they had not progressed as rapidly as they felt the project faculty were expecting, even when they were making marked progress. This phenomenon, also noted in the pilot project, seems indicative of a positive project faculty-attendee relationship in which the attendee felt a responsibility to meet faculty expectations. A third limitation was the lack of outcome data from 37 percent of residencies. In the pilot project, 22 percent of programs were lost to follow-up. We anticipated a higher dropout rate following the pilot, as a natural evolution of a long-term project where there is likely to be less enthusiasm for change among late adopters. Since we have no data on programs lost to follow-up, from a reporting standpoint we can assume only one of two things: either the program did no work or it did some work that, for whatever reason, it chose not to report. We do know, based on our experience in the pilot project, that institutional and staffing changes in residency programs commonly occurred that interfered with project work. Some of the confounding problems reported to the faculty included change of program director, change in departmental leadership, or change in hospital finances that impacted faculty responsibilities. Another suspected reason for lack of curriculum change or reporting was a lack of commitment to curriculum change and/or lack of leadership skills by the project team. Finally, a limitation of this project was the one-year follow-up window; we have no knowledge about the sustainability, expansion, or retrenchment of these new initiatives beyond twelve months.

In summary, this five-year project represents a first significant attempt to bring the principles of palliative care into a national sample of residency programs. The short-term (twelve-month) results indicate significant new curriculum work that we hope will be used as a starting point for further curricular development. Other national initiatives—in particular, the growth of hospital-based palliative care programs and the move to formal specialty status—will only serve to further enhance residency education in palliative care.

REFERENCES

1. Field MJ, Cassel CK (eds). *Approaching Death: Improving Care at the End of Life*. Report from the Institute of Medicine Committee on Care at the End of Life. Washington, D.C.: National Academy Press, 1997.

2. Block SD, Sullivan AM. Attitudes about end-of-life care: a national cross-sectional study. *J Palliat Med*. 1998; 1:347–55.

3. Sullivan AM, Lakoma MD, Block SD. The status of medical education in end-of-life care: A national report. *J Gen Intern Med*. 2003; 18:685–695.

4. Billings JA, Block S. Palliative care in undergraduate medical education. Status report and future directions. *JAMA*. 1997; 278:733–738.

5. Weissman DE, Block SD. ACGME requirements of end-of-life training in selected residency and fellowship programs: A status report. *Acad Med*. 2002; 77:299–304.

6. Ogle KS, Mavis B, Thomason C. Learning to provide end-of-life care: Postgraduate medical training programs in Michigan. *J Palliat Med*. 2005; 8:987–997.

7. Egnew TR, Mauksch LB, Greet T, Farber SJ. Integrating communication training into a required Family Medicine Clerkship. *Acad Med*. 2004; 79:737–743.

8. DeVita MA, Arnold RM, Barnard D. Teaching palliative care to critical care medicine trainees. *Crit Care Med*. 2003; 31:1257–1262.

9. Fins JF, Nilson EG. An approach to educating residents about palliative care and clinical ethics. *Acad Med*. 2000; 75:662–665.

10. Serwint JR, Rutherford LE, Hutton N, Rowe PC, Barker S, Adamo G. "I learned that no death is routine": Description of a death and bereavement seminar for pediatrics residents. *Acad Med*. 2002; 77:278–284.

11. Liao S, Amin A, Rucker L. An innovative longitudinal program to teach residents about end-of-life care. *Acad Med*. 2004; 79:752–757.

12. Hallenbeck JL, Bergen MR. A medical resident inpatient hospice rotation: experiences with dying and subsequent changes in attitudes and knowledge. *J Palliat Med*. 1999; 2:197–208.

13. Fischer SM, Gozansky WS, Kutner JS, Chomiak A, Kramer A. Palliative care education: An intervention to improve medical residents' knowledge and attitudes. *J Palliat Med*. 2003; 6:391–399.

14. von Gunten CF, Mullan PB, Harrity S, Daimant J, Heffernan E, Ikeda T, Roberts WL, and Faculty, Center for Palliative Study. Residents from five training programs report improvements in knowledge, attitudes and skills after a rotation with a hospice program. *J Cancer Educ*. 2003; 18:68–72.

15. Ross DD, Shpritz D, Alexander CS, Carter K, Edelman MJ, Friedley N, Hemani A, Keay TJ, Roy SC, Silverman H, Tasker DJ, Timmel D, Schwartz J, Wolfsthal SD. Development of required post graduate palliative care training for internal medicine residents and medical oncology fellows. *J Cancer Educ*. 2004; 19:81–87.

16. Han PKJ, Keranen LB, Lescisin DA, Arnold RM. The palliative care clinical evaluation exercise (CEX): An experience-based intervention for teaching end-of-life communication skills. *Acad Med*. 2005; 80:669–676.

17. Mullan PB, Weissman DE, Ambuel B, von Gunten CF. End-of-life care education in internal medicine residency programs: an inter-institutional study. *J Palliat Med*. 2002; 5:487–496.

18. Weissman DE, Mullan PB, Ambuel B, von Gunten CF. End-of-life curriculum reform: Outcomes and impact in a follow-up study of Internal Medicine residency programs. *J Palliat Med*. 2002; 5:497–505.

19. American Medical Association, Graduate Medical Education Directory. www.ama-assn.org/ama/pub/category/3991.html#1 (last accessed February 16, 2007).

20. Weissman DE, Ambuel B, Norton A, Wang-Cheng R, Schiedermayer D. A survey of competencies and concerns in end-of-life care for physician trainees. *J Pain Symptom Manage*. 1998; 15:82–90.

21. Von Gunten CF: Interventions to manage symptoms at the end of life. *J Palliat Med*. 2005; 8(suppl 1):S88–94.

22. Mullan PB, Weissman D, von Gunten C, Ambuel B, Hallenbeck J. Coping with certainty: Perceived competency vs. training and knowledge in end of life care. *J Gen Intern Med*. 2000; 15: 40(suppl):40.

23. Warm E. Fast Facts and Concepts: An educational tool. *J Palliat Med*. 2000; 3:332–333.

24. Weissman DE, Mullan P, Ambuel B, et al. Improving end-of-life care: Internal medicine curriculum project: Project abstracts/Progress report. *J Palliat Med*. 2001; 4:75–102.

25. Weissman DE, Mullan P, Ambuel B, von Gunten CF, Block S. Improving end-of-life care: Internal medicine curriculum project: Project abstracts/progress report. *J Palliat Med*. 2002; 5:579–606.

26. Weissman DE, Mullan P, Ambuel B, et al. Improving end-of-life care: Internal medicine curriculum project: Project abstracts/progress report. *J Palliat Med*. 2003; 6:941–964.

27. Weissman DE, Mullan P, Ambuel B, et al. Improving end-of-life care: Internal medicine curriculum project: Project abstracts/progress report. *J Palliat Med*. 2005; 8:646–664.

28. Block S. National consensus conference on medical education for care near the end of life: Executive summary. *J Palliat Med*. 2000; 3:88–92.

29. Weissman DE, Block SD, Blank L, Cain J, Cassem N, Danoff D, Foley K, Meier D, Schyve P, Theige D, Wheeler HB. Incorporating palliative care education into the acute care hospital setting. *Acad Med*. 1999; 74:871–877.

30. Block SD, Bernier GM, Crawley LM, Farber S, Kuhl D, Nelson W, O'Donnell J, Sandy L, Ury W. Incorporating palliative care into primary care education. *J Gen Intern Med*. 1998; 13:768–773.

ACKNOWLEDGMENTS

The authors would like to thank staff from the American Board of Internal Medicine, the American Academy of Neurology, the American College of Surgeons, and the Society of Teachers of Family Medicine for their help in residency program recruitment. Lisa-Pelzek Braun, Rose Hackbarth, and Barb Boutot served as project managers coordinating conference logistics and data management. Special thanks to Alan Carver, M.D., and Wendy Peltier, M.D., for help in designing the neurology curriculum. Finally, thanks to Rosemary Gibson and the Robert Wood Johnson Foundation for continued support of this project.

The project was supported by grants from the Robert Wood Johnson Foundation.

19

NEGOTIATING CROSS-CULTURAL ISSUES AT THE END OF LIFE: "YOU GOT TO GO WHERE HE LIVES"

**MARJORIE KAGAWA-SINGER, PH.D., M.N., R.N.,
AND LESLIE J. BLACKHALL, M.D., M.T.S.**

This article originally appeared as Kagawa-Singer M, Blackhall LJ. Negotiating cross-cultural issues at the end of life—"You Got to Go Where He Lives." *JAMA.* 2001;286(23): 2993–3001. Copyright © 2001. American Medical Society. All rights reserved. Reprinted with permission.

EDITORS' INTRODUCTION

In a nation as diverse as the United States, the ability to provide genuinely patient- and family-centered care is critically dependent on cross-cultural literacy. The authors provide practical approaches to exploring the meaning of illness, the tolerance for truth telling, and acceptable decision-making methods with patients from different cultures.

■ ■ ■

THE PATIENTS' STORIES

Mr. and Mrs. G, an African American Couple

Mr. G is a sixty-six-year-old African American man diagnosed with stage IV squamous cell cancer of the lung in October of 1999. He has chronic obstructive pulmonary disease and has a forty pack-year smoking history. A retired factory worker, he lives at home with his wife in a large city in Alabama. After diagnosis, he received radiation therapy and a trial of chemotherapy with vinorelbine and cisplatin. In the fall of 2000, with evident progression of the disease, his pain and dyspnea increased, adding to the symptom burden of asthenia, anorexia, and delirium. On December 6, 2000, he was admitted to an inpatient palliative care unit with symptomatic hypercalcemia. He was treated with fluids and pamidronate and approximately one week later was discharged home with hospice services. He and his wife were interviewed on December 7, 2000 by Dr. C, Mr. G's European American physician.

Ms. Z, a Chinese American Woman

Ms. Z is a thirty-eight-year-old Chinese American woman who, along with her older sister, was the primary caretaker for both parents over extended illnesses. She, her older sister, and both parents were born and raised in Hawaii. Her college-educated mother was diagnosed with stage IIIB adenocarcinoma of the lung in December 1994. In the six months following her diagnosis she underwent six rounds of chemotherapy, followed by radiation. Despite treatment, the disease metastasized to the liver, brain, and bones. During a final ten-day hospital stay, she continued to undergo radiation treatment. Still hospitalized while hospice was being considered, she died in January 1996 at the age of seventy-three years. Ms. Z's father was a prominent business executive and community leader. He was diagnosed with Parkinson's disease in the early 1990s and was treated with Sinemet (levodopa and carbidopa) and other medications. He died of complications from Parkinson's disease in February 1997 at the age of seventy-eight years, following a brief admission for aspiration pneumonia. Throughout her parents' illnesses, Ms. Z lived in California and commuted to Hawaii every few months, where her parents, her forty-year-old sister, and several relatives lived. Ms. Z was interviewed by a *Perspectives* editor on January 12, 2001.

PERSPECTIVES

In the interview between Mr. G and his physician, Dr. C, for this article, Mr. G suggested how physicians could improve their relationship with patients, especially when the cultural backgrounds of the two are different.

Ms. Z related to the *Perspectives* editor her communication with her mother after the doctor indicated to them that the prognosis for survival was poor.

Mr. G: Well, you know, you got to find out the identity of a person to even get to know them. So I think that's a big "if" right there. Because if you don't know a person, you got to find out his identity, go where he lives, where he goes, where he was born, who's in his family. And he's got to open up, and tell you these things. Because the more you know about this person, his family, then that'll make you know more about you.

Ms. Z: We never discussed it [my mother's prognosis] after [the doctor told us]. . . . My father never discussed his prognosis either . . . my father knew he had Parkinson's. There was certainly [material] available for him to read if he so chose. I don't think he read it. And there does seem to be a barrier discussing it, especially about the course of treatment. I think there are two issues: one is the actual discussion about death, and one is the discussion about treatment and care up to that point. And both of my parents were resistant to discuss either issue.

CULTURE AND MEDICAL CARE

The United States is home to an increasingly diverse population, where the former dominant culture—European American (white)— is no longer a majority in some places. Encounters between patients and physicians of dissimilar ethnicities are becoming more common, yet the literature in end-of-life care has only recently begun to investigate the influence of cultural differences on the clinical encounter. The recent President's Race Initiative (1997)[1] to eliminate racial disparities in health outcomes indicates that cultural differences significantly affect the provision of health care, including at the end of life. Without concerted attention to resolve cultural differences, disparities are likely to increase.[2]

Culture is an important part of the context within which people (including health care professionals) understand their world and make decisions about how to act. Although each individual has a perspective that is influenced by many factors, such as personal psychology, gender, and life experiences, culture fundamentally shapes the way people make meaning out of illness, suffering, and dying and therefore also influences how they make use of medical services at the end of life. However, culture is not an independent, homogeneous, dichotomous variable.[3] If "culture" is simply reduced to a series of isolated acontextual beliefs or practices categorized by ethnic origin, we run the risk of stereotyping or believing we know what any one individual thinks or does because we assume we know what people of that group tend to think. In fact, there is wide variation of beliefs and behaviors within any ethnic population. The other extreme is to disregard culture's fundamental function of giving meaning to life and of providing guidelines for living.[4] Failure to take culture seriously means we elevate our own values and fail to understand the value systems held by those of different backgrounds. Dana labels this posture "culturally destructive," as compared with "culturally skilled," behavior.[5] Assuming a Chinese woman would not want to be told her diagnosis because she is Chinese is stereotyping. Insisting that she *must* be told, even at the risk of violating her rights, is a form of cultural imperialism. The challenge is to navigate between these poles.

Misperceptions caused by lack of cultural sensitivity and skills can lead to unwanted or inappropriate clinical outcomes and poor interaction with patients and their families at critical junctures as life comes to a close.[6,7] If the Chinese family mentioned in the opening scenario believes that knowing the truth is harmful to the patient, a physician who persists in telling them the direct "truth" may be perceived as cruel, uncaring, and ignorant. The result is mistrust and anger, and may even precipitate the removal of the patient from medical care altogether.[8]

Patients bring to the medical encounter different languages, explanatory models concerning the cause and treatment of illness, religious beliefs, and ways of understanding the experience of suffering and dying.[2] Styles of communication and beliefs about the role of physician, patient, and family also vary, and such differences may occur against the backdrop of experiences of societal oppression or inequities in medical care.[9] For this reason, the clinical encounter often requires a negotiation between the worldviews or cultures of the clinician and the patient and family to reach mutually acceptable goals.[2,9,10] In the end, addressing and respecting cultural differences will likely increase trust, leading to better clinical outcomes and more satisfactory care for patients and their families.[11]

Using two case studies as examples of cross-cultural encounters—an African American couple in the southern United States, and a Chinese American family in Hawaii and California—we examine six specific issues for end-of-life care (Table 19.1). These families, from two different ethnic groups, share some views more aligned with each other than with the dominant culture, such as the reluctance to accept hospice and the dynamics of extended family involvement. The issues presented, and the views of each of the interviewees, however, are by no means exhaustive or generalizable to their entire ethnic group. Cultures are not monolithic, and a range of potential responses to each issue is likely to occur in every ethnic group. Careful examination of within-group variations, such as those attributed to acculturation differences, have not yet been applied to most studies of cultural diversity at the end of life. As the science in this area moves forward, we will be able to better understand not only differences between groups but those within groups due to education, age, gender, geographic location, degree of ethnic homogeneity, social context, and individual acculturation.[12] References and the list of Web sites at the *JAMA* Web site (http://jama.amaassn.org/issues/v286n23/abs/jel10001.html) provide more nuanced variations and ranges of responses among and within different ethnic populations.

PATIENT AUTONOMY: THE DOMINANT CULTURE, THE DOMINANT MODE

In the European American model, patient autonomy is the primary focus of decision making at the end of life. Patient autonomy emphasizes the rights of patients to be informed about their condition, its possible treatments, and their ability to choose or refuse life-prolonging medical care. Advance care directives (ACDs) are meant to ensure that patients' wishes concerning end-of-life care are enforced, even when they are no longer able to speak for themselves.[13–15] This framework reflects core values of the

TABLE 19.1. **Techniques for Negotiating Issues Influenced by Culture That Are Important in End-of-Life Care**

Issue	Possible Consequences of Ignoring the Issue	Techniques and Strategies to Address the Issue
Responses to inequities in care	Lack of trust Increased desire for futile aggressive care at the end of life Lack of collaboration with patient and with the family Dissatisfaction with care by all parties involved	Address directly: "I wonder whether it's hard for you to trust a physician who is not _____ [of your same background]?" Make explicit that you and the patient and the family will work together in achieving the best care possible Work to improve access and reduce inequities Understand and accommodate desires for more aggressive care, and use respectful negotiation when this is contraindicated or medically futile
Communication/ language barriers	Bidirectional misunderstanding Unnecessary physical, emotional, and spiritual suffering	Take time to: Avoid medical or complex jargon Check for understanding: "So I can make sure I'm explaining this well for you, please tell me what your understanding is about your illness and the treatment we're considering." Hire bilingual, bicultural staff, and train in medical translation to be bridges across cultures. Translators are preferable in person, but use AT&T language line or similar services if trained staff unavailable. Avoid use of family as translators, especially minors.
Religion and spirituality	Lack of faith in the physician Lack of adherence to the treatment regimen	"Spiritual or religious strength sustains many people in times of distress. What is important for us to know about your faith or spiritual needs?" "How can we support your needs and practices?" "Where do you find your strength to make sense of this experience?"

(continued overleaf)

TABLE 19.1. *(Continued)*

Issue	Possible Consequences of Ignoring the Issue	Techniques and Strategies to Address the Issue
Truth telling	Anger, mistrust, or even removal of patient from health care system if team insists on informing the patient against the wishes of the family Hopelessness in the patient if he or she misunderstands your reason for telling him or her directly	Informed refusal: "Some patients want to know everything about their condition; others prefer that the doctors mainly talk to their families. How would you prefer to get this information?" Use a hypothetical case, for example, "Others who have conditions similar to yours have found it helpful to consider several options for care, such as nutrition, to keep them feeling as well as possible." Be cognizant of nonverbal or indirect communication when discussing serious information.
Family involvement in decision making	Disagreement and conflict between family and medical staff when the family, rather than the patient, insists on making decisions	Ascertain the key members of the family and ensure that all are included in discussions as desired by the patient: "Is there anyone else that I should talk to about your condition?" Talk with whoever accompanies the patient, and ask the patient about this individual's involvement in receiving information and decision making.
Hospice care	Reduced use of hospice services, leading to decreased quality of end-of-life care	Emphasize hospice as an adjunct or assistance to the family, but not as a replacement: "When the family is taking care of the patient at home, hospice can help them do that."

dominant culture—independence, individual rights, and even fears of receiving too much care at the end of life. While the emphasis on patient autonomy has clarified the legal status of patients to refuse therapy and increased the comfort of physicians to make these decisions, patients and families from other cultures may not share these values and concerns[16,17]

FINAL CHOICES BY AN ELDERLY AFRICAN AMERICAN COUPLE

Responses to Inequities: Social and Historical Context of Trust in the Clinical Encounter

Although Mr. G has a do-not-resuscitate (DNR) order, opted for a palliative approach to his lung cancer, and accepted home hospice, several studies in diverse regions of the country and across practice settings have shown that African American patients are more likely to want aggressive medical care at the end of life[9] and are less likely to have DNR orders or ACDs than European American patients.[18-22] For example, one study of elderly outpatients in North Carolina found that African Americans were almost three times as likely as white patients to want more treatment (42 percent versus 15 percent), a choice that did not vary with education level.[23] Similarly, African American outpatients in Miami were more likely to want life-prolonging therapy than white patients (37 percent versus 14 percent).[7] McKinley and colleagues[20] found that 37 percent of African American cancer patients wanted cardiopulmonary resuscitation when terminally ill, while only 16 percent of white patients would desire such treatment. Only 3 percent of African Americans in this study had completed an ACD, versus 34 percent of white patients. Murphy and colleagues,[21] in a study of elderly patients from four different ethnic groups in Los Angeles, reported that only 2 percent of African American elders studied had an ACD (17 percent of those with knowledge about ACDs), versus 28 percent of white subjects (40 percent of those with knowledge about ACDs). Morrison and colleagues[23] also found that Hispanic and African American patients were less likely to have appointed a health care proxy than white patients (20 percent and 31 percent versus 46 percent). In this study, however, ethnicity was not significantly associated with ACD completion after controlling for knowledge, age, availability of a health care proxy, experience with life support, and attitudes toward family involvement.[23] Although African Americans represent 12.3 percent of the U.S. population, they comprise only 8 percent of patients enrolled in hospice.[24]

Mrs. G: Because [an African American] doctor is the same nationality as myself, that causes me to want to trust him more, because he could relate better. Most of them have been there, even though they are above [it]—they've moved away from it. That helps, but like I said, as long as I know he's qualified, it would make a difference [whether he is African American or not].

Some have attributed these differences to mistrust of the medical system by African American patients, and evidence exists to support the contention that African Americans are less likely than white patients to trust the motivations of physicians who discuss end-of-life care with them. In the Miami study, Caralis and colleagues[18] found that African American patients were more likely to feel that they would be treated differently and receive lower-quality treatment if they completed an ACD. Other studies have also suggested that mistrust acts as a barrier to organ donation,[25] and as a reason not to participate in medical research.[26] In the Los Angeles study mentioned above, African American elderly persons were more likely than other groups to want life support under various conditions (for example, 27 percent wanted CPR in the event of a coma with no chance of recovery, versus 13 percent of whites, 22 percent of Mexican Americans, and 14 percent of Korean Americans).[19] Postsurvey interviews to probe the reason behind the increased desire for life support uncovered the belief that economic motivations were behind clinicians' decisions to remove life support. Several subjects cited personal experience with relatives prematurely removed from life support, or not placed on it, including one woman whose son died of acquired immunodeficiency syndrome. He was not placed on life support, and her conclusion was "They figured out, or assumed, that I didn't have money, so they weren't going to bother."

Framing this whole issue as one of mistrust, however, is problematic. McKinley and colleagues[20] found that although African American cancer patients wanted more life-sustaining treatment than white patients, 96 percent trusted the medical system, and less than 20 percent feared inadequate medical care. More importantly, as Crawley and colleagues[27] point out, framing the issue as one of mistrust implies that the main problem is the attitude of African Americans. In fact, health care institutions, both historically and in the present, have not always shown themselves to be worthy of trust.[28,29] Trust is a critical element in cross-cultural cooperation. The historical context of African Americans' experience within the dominant medical culture in the United States is the backdrop against which any discussion of trust must take place. The Tuskegee syphilis study[30,31] and segregated hospitals are in the historic memory of most older African Americans, and current treatment disparities between African American and European American patients are extensively documented.[32] Studies report less use of cardiac procedures,[33–35] fewer surgeries for lung cancer,[36] and reduced access to renal transplantation for African Americans.[36] Similar disparities exist for Hispanics, Asian Americans, and Native Americans.[37] Ultimately, until disparities in access and quality of care are eliminated or at least greatly reduced, simply encouraging African Americans and other ethnic minorities to be more "trusting" of recommendations provided by European American physicians is doomed to failure. Physicians can take steps outlined in Table 19.1 to constructively address this issue.

Communication

Although Mr. and Mrs. G appear to be blaming themselves for not understanding medical information, research has shown that African American patients have unmet needs for communication. African American patients generally want to be informed about the diagnosis and prognosis of a terminal illness and want to make decisions about medical care.[38] In the Study to Understand Prognoses and Preference for Outcomes and Risks of Treatment (SUPPORT),[22] African Americans were among those most likely to want to discuss preferences for CPR but not to have done so (odds ratio, 1.53; 95 percent confidence interval, 1.11–2.11). A 1986 telephone survey found that African American patients were more likely than European American patients to report that their physician did not sufficiently explain test results, medical conditions, and treatments.[39] A more recent study[40] found that African American patients were less likely than

Mrs. G: We have a tendency to want to treat ourselves, but we don't have enough trust . . . You know, most [doctors] use medical terms and big terminology that's beyond us, and that tends to frighten us because we don't know what [they're] talking about—we might think one thing and feel misled to a point. We hear, but experience is different . . . sometimes experience can be detrimental—you don't want to keep doing that.

Dr. C: I don't think we have the institutional racism that we had thirty years ago with the Jim Crow laws. But we have informal institutional racism, particularly here in the South. The way we decide how we're going to fund medical care and other kinds of services for people. And people are smart—they know that.

Mrs. G: We always think we know what's best for us. And because we might not understand the explanations and what's going on, we choose the easier way. I'm not saying it's the better way—but because we don't really fully understand, we just kind of stay in those same ways or traditions.

Mr. G: We're just ignorant to the facts that we don't understand.

European Americans to feel that their physicians included them in decision making. This was particularly true for those in race-discordant patient-physician relationships.

Of course, African American patients are by no means alone in their desire for better communication. Avoiding the use of medical jargon and checking for understanding are two easy ways to reduce misunderstandings with patients of any culture.[41] When the patient speaks a language not understood by the physician, adequate translation is vital. See Table 19.1 for further details and suggestions on this topic.

Religion and Spirituality

Attitudes toward end-of-life care also may be influenced by religious or spiritual concerns.[42,43] In one study,[19] African American participants revealed their beliefs that only God has knowledge about—and power over—life and death, and that physicians cannot have access to this type of knowledge. One participant said, "The doctor don't know everything. God might come into it . . . . He can do more for us than the doctor can." Participants cited this belief as a reason for trying life support. Similarly, Koenig and Gates-Williams[44] describe an African American woman with advanced pancreatic cancer who rejected hospice and DNR orders. She stated, "Only God has priority over living. That's something man can't tell you—how long you got to live." Crawley and colleagues[27] point out that the Christian religious view embraced by many in the African American community holds that suffering is redemptive. It is to be endured rather than avoided. In this setting, forgoing life support in order to avoid pain and suffering might be seen as failing a test of faith. Denial of death and a willingness to undergo potentially painful and/or futile life support may in fact be part of an "ethic of struggle."[27] This ethic of struggle can be considered part of a moral strength that ensures a better place than this one in a world in which African Americans often die younger than their white counterparts.

FINAL CHOICES BY A CHINESE AMERICAN FAMILY

Truth Telling: Prognosis and Informed Refusal

Ms. Z: The prognosis for my mother was given very gently. And given in the form of statistics. [The doctor] had a book of statistics out and said, 'This is the percentage of people who are still living after one, two, three years . . . .' So it wasn't given verbally. I think it was mentioned very delicately, and I'm not sure how much of that information he actually took in at the time . . . . We never discussed it after that.

Although informed consent is a major tenet of U.S. health care, truth telling about diagnosis, and especially about the prognosis of potentially fatal illnesses like cancer, is not the norm in much of the world.[45,46] In Italy,[47] France,[48] and Eastern Europe,[48] as well as much of Asia,[49,50] Central and South America,[18,38] and the Middle East,[43] physicians and patients often feel that withholding medical information is more humane and ethical. A report by an Italian oncologist in 1992,[49] for example, describes the decision-making style in Italy as one in which the patient is "protected" from bad news by physicians and family. In a Greek population survey,[46] only a third of the respondents believed that patients should be told of a terminal illness. Older respondents and those with less education were less likely to favor truth telling.[51] Patients who have emigrated from countries where truth telling is not common often bring that perspective to medical encounters in this country.[9,38,49]

Even in the United States, as recently as the early 1970s, physicians commonly withheld the diagnosis of cancer.[52] Not until 1979 did the first article note the practice trend of disclosing a cancer diagnosis,[53] and while open discussion of diagnosis has become the norm in this country, discussing prognosis remains difficult.[38] One study of oncologists published in 2001 found that only 37 percent would give a truthful estimate of prognosis even when asked directly by the patient.[54] The reason often given for withholding information about diagnosis or prognosis is that the truth may be cruel and is potentially harmful to the patient.[47,49] Anecdotal reports note the tendency of Chinese[7] and Ethiopian[55] families to oppose truth telling because the patient would lose hope and suffer unnecessary physical and emotional distress. In the Los Angeles study cited above,[40] 52 percent of Mexican American patients stated that patients should not be told the truth about a terminal prognosis. Within this ethnic group, older age, lower socioeconomic status, and less acculturation were associated with a desire for less truth telling.[38] Ethnographic interviews revealed the belief that the truth should never be told because it hastens death.[36] A Korean American subject from the same study reported keeping his wife's cancer diagnosis a secret, saying, "We kept it a tight secret. . . . If she knew, she would not be able to live longer because of the fear."[49] Only 35 percent of the Korean American subjects in this study believed that a patient should be told of a terminal prognosis.[28]

Ms. Z reports that prognosis was discussed only indirectly with her mother, and, as noted above, several authors have described the tendency toward nondisclosure in Chinese society.[7,56] One recent study of 1,136 Chinese persons in Hong Kong,[57] however, indicates that the patterns of preferences for patients desiring information about diagnosis (95 percent) and prognosis (97 percent) were similar to those in the United States. Such findings emphasize the importance of being specific about the group studied. For example, identifying all persons as "Chinese," whether they come from rural mainland China, Hong Kong, or Taiwan, may miss important sources of variation.

The issue of truth telling is more complex than simply whether or not to tell the truth. It also includes the problem of how to tell, and to whom. Even a patient who does not want direct disclosure may wish to know the truth through other means: indirectly, euphemistically, "delicately" (as Ms. Z puts it), or nonverbally. In far east Asian cultures, such as Korean,[36] Chinese,[58] and Japanese,[59,60] nonverbal communication is often acknowledged to be a vital means of interpersonal connection.[61] *Zhih yi* is the Chinese term that denotes nonverbal communication, "just knowing what the other thinks and feels," and the Japanese term *inshin denshin* denotes a similar concept of knowing without being told. The Korean word *nunchi* denotes understanding through social, nonverbal cues.

The purpose of indirect communication in these cultures is to preserve the "face" of the other—that is, never to put the person one is talking to into a position of embarrassment or loss of honor by directly posing potentially sensitive questions. "Face," in the Asian sense, is the preservation of family and community honor more so than individual honor. This proscription against losing face applies to all verbal communication and conduct both within and outside the family or community setting.[62,63] In these cultures, indirect or nonverbal communication may be preferable because the ambiguity saves face[64,65] and allows for the possibility of hope.[49]

In situations in which the family insists that the patient not be told, but the clinician feels that some diagnostic or prognostic information needs to be provided (for example, before radiation therapy or chemotherapy), one strategy is to make an offer of information to the patient, allowing the patient "informed refusal" (see Table 19.1).[49,66] The clinician establishes with the patient who should receive all medical information and make decisions regarding the patient's care. If the patient designates that someone else be given this responsibility, this constitutes the patient's informed refusal to be included in the discussions or decision making, and this preference should be documented.[67,68]

Another strategy is to use a hypothetical case, as described by Carrese and Rhodes[69] in their article describing decision-making styles among Navajo patients and practitioners. This technique acknowledges the patient's and/or the family's realistic fears, respects the need for indirect discussion, and implicitly invites further questions. Apparently tangential statements by the patient or family may be indirect questions and indicate the desire for more information. How the questions are answered requires sensitivity and skill to gauge the degree of information sought. Direct confrontation may frighten or offend the patient/family, and they may not pursue their inquiry. On the other hand, they may appreciate bringing the questions to light. Responses, therefore, may be indirect or couched as hypothetical, according to the capacity of the patient/family (Table 19.1). The physician should regularly seek feedback from the patient/family to assess their understanding of the progression of the disease and the treatment plan and their desire for additional information.

Family Involvement in Decision Making

The Patient Self-Determination Act, and statutes in the United States allowing patients to enact durable power of attorney for health care and other ACDs,[46] reflect a commitment to the rights of individual patients to make decisions about their care at the end of life. In other cultures, decision making may be seen primarily as a duty of the family, whose responsibility it is to protect the dying patient from the burden of making difficult choices about medical care.

Ms. Z: I think there is a lot of pressure in the Chinese culture to take care of your own and also be a part of the person's process. So I think my ethnicity expressed itself in that my sister and I went to every medical appointment with my mother and even sat in the room with the doctors.

The familial mode of decision making is clearly the ethos described by Ms. Z and is also common in many other cultures. In a study by Morrison and colleagues,[24] 67 percent of Hispanic patients believed that health care proxies were not needed when family was involved (versus 12 percent of white and 19 percent of African American subjects). Korean American (57 percent) and Mexican American (45 percent) elderly individuals were more likely than European Americans (20 percent) or African Americans (24 percent) to believe that the family should be the primary decision maker.[38] Ethnicity remained the most important predictor of decision-making style even after controlling for socioeconomic status.[28,45]

A study of Japanese nationals in Japan and of Japanese Americans (both Japanese- and English-speaking) demonstrated a preference for family-centered decision making for advance care planning in all groups (M. Shinji, D.M.S., oral and written communication, October 2, 2001). Although preference for disclosure, willingness to forgo care, and views of advance care planning shifted toward Western values as Japanese Americans acculturated, the desire for group decision making was preserved, even among the most acculturated.

It is important to note that this is a matter of relative emphasis. Family involvement in decision making occurs in all cultures. The question is: Do family members support the patient by encouraging him or her to make choices, or do they express their love by taking on the decision-making burden themselves?

Hospice Care: Filial Responsibility

Consideration of hospice care places cultural values of families into bold relief, and differences with mainstream hospice approaches become apparent when we see that although ethnic minority populations now comprise over 25 percent of the U.S. population, they represent less than 17 percent of patients enrolled in hospice.[27] Very few of these are Asian Americans. Filial piety, which is an important concept in many parts of Asia, including Korea, China, and Japan, may partly account for this.

Ms. Z: I know there's often a great resistance to the idea of hospice or placing people in hospice. A lot of the resistance comes from admitting that the patient is dying. Or it feels like a failure of the medical system. I think one of the reasons that Asians are resistant to hospice is that it feels like a failure on the part of the caretaker . . . to take care. It seems almost like giving up or admitting that the caretakers can no longer take care of their own.

Filial piety is the expectation that children will care for their parents without question, in gratitude for their parents' caring and sacrifices, and it infuses all aspects of a parent's care.[49,64,70] Hospice, which constitutes accepting care from outsiders, may dishonor the parents by sending the message within the family as well as to the community that the family is unable to provide adequate care. Although data are lacking on this point, it may be that broaching the topic of hospice, even with acculturated Asian Americans like Ms. Z and her sister, challenges the value of filial piety, and discussion must be calibrated with this in mind (Table 19.1). Asian American families will use hospice services, but usually in the home and usually with considerable oversight and control. This enables the family to feel that they are still the primary caretaker and that they are fulfilling their filial obligation. Fulfilling family obligations as primary caretaker may not appear to be different in form from any other ethnic group, since members of most cultural groups would like to be able to care for their loved ones at home. For Chinese, Japanese, and Korean groups, however, the issue of face may be present. How well they fulfill their filial obligations is open to community scrutiny and judgment and would reflect poorly on the parenting abilities of the parents and on the extended family if the children do not fulfill their obligations.[63]

EVALUATING AND ADDRESSING CULTURAL ISSUES AT THE END OF LIFE

Mr. G's perspective, noted in his opening quote, is the key to cross-cultural communication: "You got to find out the identity of a person to even get to know them . . . and he's got to open up and tell you these things." When the physician and patient are from different cultural backgrounds, the physician needs to ask questions that respectfully acknowledge these differences and build the trust necessary for the patient to confide in him or her. Physicians can use knowledge about particular cultural beliefs, values, and practices to respectfully recognize a person's identity and to assess the degree to which an individual patient or family might adhere to their cultural background. One way to begin this dialogue is by evaluating patients' and families' attitudes, beliefs, context, decision making, and environment (ABCDE) (Table 19.2). This approach is adapted from work by Koenig and Gates-Williams.[44] The purpose of this mnemonic is to help avoid the dual pitfalls of cultural stereotyping and ignoring the potential influence of culture. In this way, the risk of miscommunication may be reduced.

While understanding the patient as an individual in the context of culture does not prevent conflicts over differing values, beliefs, or practices, information gained from such an assessment serves to identify areas for negotiation of conflicts should they occur.[17] When the physician and the patient/family have some understanding of each other's perspective, such negotiations can take place in an atmosphere of mutual respect rather than frustration and misunderstanding. In the cases above, we have discussed the context for potentially divisive issues such as "informed refusal" of diagnostic or prognostic information, delegation of decision-making power to the family, and increased desire for life support. Many other important areas, including end-of-life customs or religious rituals that give meaning, security, and solace in times of need and during life transitions such as death, have been addressed in detail elsewhere.[43,71]

As the suggested lines of inquiry provided in Tables 19.1 and 19.2 indicate, timely and sensitive investigation can begin to broaden options available to the physician to explore cross-cultural differences.[3] When specific issues (such as differing desires about truth telling, or reluctance to sign "informed consent" documents) arise repeatedly, development of appropriate and respectful institutional protocols may help avoid laborious negotiations in each individual encounter.[28,72] The suggestions in Tables 19.1 and 19.2 build on the basic communication skills presented by numerous authors, with various mnemonics to promote more productive communication generally and at the end of life.[43,75-77] The reader is directed to the growing literature in cultural competency that addresses this need and the many approaches being developed.[5,78-81]

"Cultural competence" is, however, not simply a moral or ethical obligation, or a "nice thing to do." It is now the law. In December 2000, the Office of Minority Health of the U.S. Department of Health and Human Services released national standards for culturally and linguistically appropriate health services.[78] These standards are primarily directed at health care organizations, though individual providers are encouraged to use the same standards to make their practices more culturally and linguistically accessible.

Institutions such as hospitals, home care and hospice agencies, and nursing homes must take responsibility for facilitating culturally competent care. This includes knowing the groups that most frequently use the institution, seeking out and disseminating information about cultural beliefs that might affect attitudes toward illness and health care, providing adequate translation services, and identifying community resources. Hiring and training health care workers (at all levels) who are members of the ethnic group in question or knowledgeable about them, and who have credibility within these communities, may assist greatly in bridging the cultural chasm.

TABLE 19.2. Assess ABCDE to Ascertain Level of Cultural Influence[a]

	Relevant Information	Questions and Strategies
Attitudes of patients and families	What attitudes do this ethnic group in general and the patient and family in particular have toward truth telling about diagnosis and prognosis? What is their general attitude toward discussions of death and dying?	Educate yourself about attitudes common to the ethnic groups most frequently seen in your practice (see References). Determine attitudes of your patient and the family (see Table 19.1). For example, what is the symbolic meaning of the particular disease?
Beliefs	How reflective are their practices of traditional beliefs and practices? What are the patient's and family's religious and spiritual beliefs, especially those relating to the meaning of death, the afterlife, the possibility of miracles?	See Table 19.1 for strategies addressing the religious concerns of individuals and families. For general information, see list of Web resources at http://jama.ama-assn.org/issues/v286n23/abs/jel10001.html Religious and community organizations may be able to provide general information about the relevant group (see below, "Environment").
Context	Questions about the historical and political context of their lives, including place of birth, refugee or immigration status, poverty, experience with discrimination or lack of access to care, languages spoken, and degree of integration within their ethnic community	Ascertain specific information by asking the following: "Where were you born and raised?" "When did you emigrate to the United States, and what has been your experience coming to a new country? How has your life changed?" "What language would you feel most comfortable speaking to discuss your health concerns?" Life history assessment: "What were other important times in your life, and how might these experiences help us to understand your situation?"
Decision-making style	What decision-making styles are held by the group in general and by the patient and family in particular? Is the emphasis on the individual patient making his or her own decisions, or is the approach family-centered?	Learn about the dominant ethnic groups in your practice (see References): How are decisions made in this cultural group? Who is the head of the household?

	Relevant Information	Questions and Strategies
Environment	What resources are available to aid the effort to interpret the significance of cultural dimensions of a case, including translators, health care workers from the same community, community or religious leaders, and family members?	Does this family adhere to traditional cultural guidelines, or do they adhere more to the Western model (see Table 19.1)? Identify religious and community organizations associated with the ethnic groups common in your practice (hospital social worker and chaplains may be able to help you in this effort). See list of telephone translation services available at http://jama.ama-assn.org/issues/v286n23/abs/jel10001.html

^aAdapted from work by Koenig and Gates-Williams.[44]

Finally, note Mr. G's comment about physicians eliciting a complete social history from the patient: "The more you [the physician] know about this person, his family, then that'll make you know more about you."

Reflecting on the ways culture shapes the patient's worldview invites self-reflection about the physician's own biases, values, beliefs, and practices. Cross-cultural experiences may also enrich the repertoire of the physician with alternative ways to ease the dying process for patients, families, and staff. Accepting this invitation enables the growth that is the hallmark of cross-cultural communication skills.[54]

REFERENCES

1. Council of Economic Advisors. *Changing America: Indicators of Social and Economic Well-being by Race and Hispanic Origin*. Washington, DC: U.S. Government Printing Office; 1997:40–51.

2. Kleinman A. *Patients and Healers in the Context of Culture*. Berkeley: University of California Press; 1980.

3. Crawley L, Marshall P, Koeing B. *Respecting Cultural Differences at the End of Life*. Philadelphia, Pa: American College of Physicians–American Society of Internal Medicine; 2001.

4. Hallowell AI. *Culture and Experience*. Philadelphia: University of Pennsylvania Press; 1955.

5. Dana RH. *Multicultural Assessment Perspectives for Professional Psychology*. Boston, Mass: Allyn & Bacon Inc; 1993.

6. Paul B. *Health, Culture, and Community*. New York, NY: Russell Sage Foundation; 1955.

7. Muller JH, Desmond B. Ethical dilemmas in a cross-cultural context: a Chinese example. *West J Med*. 1992; 157:323–327.

8. Fadiman A. *The Spirit Catches You and You Fall Down: A Hmong Child, Her American Doctors, and the Collision of Two Cultures*. New York, NY: Farrar Straus & Giroux; 1997.

9. Crawley L. Palliative care in African American communities. *Innovations in End-of-Life-Care*. 2001. Available at http://www.edc.org/lastacts (accessibility verified November 27, 2001).

10. Kagawa-Singer M, Chung R. A paradigm for culturally based care for minority populations. *J Comm Psychol.* 1994:192–208.

11. Katon W, Kleinman A. A biopsychosocial approach to surgical evaluation and outcome. *West J Med.* 1980; 133:9–14.

12. Barker JC. Cultural diversity: changing the context of medical practice. *West J Med.* 1992; 157:248–254.

13. Fang J, Madhavan S, Alderman MH. The association between birthplace and mortality from cardiovascular causes among black and white residents of New York City. *N Engl J Med.* 1996; 335:1545–1551.

14. Emanuel LL, Emanuel EJ. Decisions at the end of life: guided by communities of patients. *Hastings Cent Rep.* 1993; 23:6–14.

15. Emanuel LL, von Gunten CF, Ferris FD. Advance care planning. *Arch Fam Med.* 2000; 9:1181–1187.

16. Annas GJ. Reconciling Quinlan and Saikewicz: decision making for the terminally ill incompetent. *Am J Law Med.* 1979; 4:367–396.

17. Braun KL, Pietsch JH, Blanchette P, eds. *Cultural Issues in End-of-Life Decision Making*. Thousand Oaks, Calif: Sage Publications Inc; 2000.

18. Veatch R, ed. *Cross-Cultural Perspectives in Medical Ethics*. Sudbury, Mass: Jones & Bartlett Publishers; 2000.

19. Caralis PV, Davis B, Wright K, Marcial E. The influence of ethnicity and race on attitudes toward advance directives, life-prolonging treatments, and euthanasia. *J Clin Ethics.* 1993; 4:155–165.

20. Blackhall LJ, Frank G, Murphy ST, Michel V, Palmer JM, Azen SP. Ethnicity and attitudes towards life sustaining technology. *Soc Sci Med.* 1999; 48:1779–1789.

21. McKinley ED, Garrett JM, Evans AT, Danis M. Differences in end-of-life decision making among black and white ambulatory cancer patients. *J Gen Intern Med.* 1996; 11:651–656.

22. Murphy ST, Palmer JM, Azen S, Frank G, Michel V, Blackhall LJ. Ethnicity and advance care directives. *J Law Med Ethics.* 1996; 24:108–117.

23. Hofmann JC, Wenger NS, Davis RB, et al., for the SUPPORT Investigators. Patient preferences for communication with physicians about end-of-life decisions. *Ann Intern Med.* 1997; 127:1–12.

24. Morrison SR, Zayas LH, Mulvihill M, Baskin A, Meier DE. Barriers to completion of health care proxies: an examination of ethnic differences. *Arch Intern Med.* 1998; 158:2493–2497.

25. NHPCO (National Hospice and Palliative Care Organization). 2001. Available at http://www.nhpco.org (acessibility verified November 27, 2001).

26. Davidson MN, Devney P. Attitudinal barriers to organ donation among black Americans. *Transplant Proc.* 1991; 23:2531–2532.

27. Corbie-Smith G, Thomas SB, Williams MV, Moody-Avers S. Attitudes and beliefs of African Americans toward participation in medical research. *J Gen Intern Med.* 1999; 14:537–546.

28. Crawley L, Payne R, Bolden J, Payne T, Washington P, Williams S. Palliative and end-of-life care in the African American community. *JAMA.* 2000; 284:25182521.

29. Devore W. The experience of death: a black perspective. In: Parry JK, ed. *Social Work Practice With the Terminally Ill: A Transcultural Perspective*. Springfield, Ill: Charles C Thomas; 1990.

30. Mouton C. Cultural and religious issues for African Americans. In: Braun K, Pietsch JH, Blaanchette P, eds. *Cultural Issues in End-of-Life Decision Making*. Thousand Oaks, Calif: Sage Publications Inc; 2000: 71–82.

31. Chadwick GL. Historical perspective: Nuremberg, Tuskegee, and the radiation experiments. *J Int Assoc Physicians AIDS Care.* 1997; 3:27–28.

32. Francis CK. The medical ethos and social responsibility in clinical medicine. *J Natl Med Assoc.* 2001; 93:157–169.

33. Council on Ethical and Judicial Affairs, American Medical Association. Black white disparities in health care. *JAMA.* 1990; 263:2344–2346.

34. Peterson ED, Shaw LK, DeLong ER, Pryor DB, Califf RM, Mark DB. Racial variation in the use of coronary-revascularization procedures: are the differences real? Do they matter? *N Engl J Med.* 1997; 336:480–486.

35. Chen J, Rathore SS, Radford MJ, Wang Y, Krumholz HM. Racial differences in the use of cardiac catheterization after acute myocardial infarction. *N Engl J Med.* 2001; 334:1443–1449.

36. Schulman KA, Berlin JA, Harless W, et al. The effect of race and sex on physicians' recommendations for cardiac catheterization [published correction appears in *N Engl J Med.* 1999; 340:1130]. *N Engl J Med.* 1999; 340:618–626.

37. Bach PB, Cramer LD, Warren JL, Begg CB. Racial differences in the treatment of early-stage lung cancer. *N Engl J Med.* 1999; 341:1198–1205.

38. Ayanian JZ, Cleary PD, Weissman JS, Epstein AM. The effect of patients' preferences on racial differences in access to renal transplantation. *N Engl J Med.* 1999; 341:1661–1669.

39. Haynes MA, Smedley BD. *The Unequal Burden of Cancer: An Assessment of NIH Research and Programs for Ethnic Minorities and the Medically Underserved*. Washington DC: Institute of Medicine; 1999.

40. Blackhall LJ, Murphy ST, Frank G, Michel V, Azen S. Ethnicity and attitudes toward patient autonomy. *JAMA.* 1995; 274:820–825.

41. Blendon R, Aiken LH, Freeman HE, Corey CR. Access to medical care for black and white Americans: a matter of continuing concern. *JAMA.* 1989; 261:278–280.

42. Cooper-Patrick L, Gallo JJ, Gonzales JJ, et al. Race, gender, and partnership in the patient-physician relationship. *JAMA.* 1999; 282:583–589.

43. Buchman R. *How to Break Bad News*. Baltimore, Md: Johns Hopkins University Press; 1992.

44. Parry JK, ed. *Social Work Practice With the Terminally Ill: A Transcultural Perspective*. Springfield, Ill: Charles C Thomas; 1990.

45. Kagawa-Singer M. Cultural diversity in death and dying. *Gerontol Geriatr Educ.* 1994; 15:101–112.

46. Koenig BA, Gates-Williams J. Understanding cultural difference in caring for dying patients. *West J Med.* 1995; 163:244–249.

47. Rothenberg L, Wenger NS, Kagawa-Singer M, et al. The relationship of clinical and legal perspectives regarding medical treatment decision-making in four cultures. *Annu Rev Law Ethics.* 1996; 4:335–379.

48. Ersek M, Kagawa-Singer M, Barnes D, Blackhall L, Koenig BA. Multicultural considerations in the use of advance directives. *Oncol Nurs Forum.* 1998; 25:16831690.

49. Surbone A. Truth telling. *Ann N Y Acad Sci.* 2000; 913:52–62.

50. Thomsen OO, Wulff HR, Martin A, Singer PA. What do gastroenterologists in Europe tell cancer patients? *Lancet.* 1993; 341:473–476.

51. Blackhall LJ, Frank G, Murphy S, Michel V. Bioethics in a different tongue: the case of truth-telling. *J Urban Health.* 2001; 78:59–71.

52. Hern HEJ, Koenig BA, Moore LJ, Marshall PA. The difference that culture can make in end-of-life decision making. *Camb Q Healthc Ethics.* 1998; 7:27–40.

53. Dalla-Vorgia P, Katsouyanni K, Garanis TN, Touloumi G, Drogarri P, Koutselinis A. Attitudes of a Mediterranean population to the truth-telling issue. *J Med Ethics.* 1992:67–74.

54. Oken D. What to tell cancer patients: a study of medical attitudes. *JAMA.* 1961; 175:1120–1128.

55. Novack DH, Plumer R, Smith RL, Ochitill H, Morrow GR, Bennett JM. Changes in physicians' attitudes toward telling the cancer patient. *JAMA.* 1979; 241:897900.

56. Lamont EB, Christakis NA. Prognostic disclosure to patients with cancer near the end of life. *Ann Intern Med.* 2001; 134:1096–1105.

57. Beyene Y. Medical disclosure and refugees: telling bad news to Ethiopian patients. *West J Med.* 1992: 328–332.

58. Kleinman A. *The Illness Narratives: Suffering, Healing and the Human Condition*. New York, NY: Basic Books; 1988.

59. Fielding R, Hung J. Preferences for information and involvement in decisions during cancer care among a Hong Kong Chinese population. *Psychooncology*. 1996: 321–329.

60. Tong K. The Chinese palliative patient and family in North America: a cultural perspective. *J Palliat Care*. 1994; 10:26–28.

61. Ishii S. Enryo-Sasshi communication: a key to understanding Japanese interpersonal relations. *Cross Currents*. 1984; 11:49–58.

62. Takayama K, Yamazaki Y, Katsumata N. Relationship between outpatients' perceptions of physicians' communication styles and patients' anxiety levels in a Japanese oncology setting. *Soc Sci Med*. 2001; 53:1335–1350.

63. Wellisch D, Kagawa-Singer M, Reid SL, Lin YJ, Nishikawa-Lee S, Wellisch M. An exploratory study of social support: a cross-cultural comparison of Chinese-, Japanese-, and Anglo-American breast cancer patients. *Psychooncology*. 1999; 8:207–219.

64. Lebra T. *Japanese Patterns of Behavior*. Honolulu: University of Hawaii Press; 1976.

65. Zane N, Yeh M. The use of culturally based variables in assessment: studies on loss of face. In: Kurasaki K, Okazaki S, Sue S, eds. *Asian American Mental Health: Assessment Theories and Methods*. Dordrecht, Netherlands: Kluwer Academic Publishers; in press.

66. Uba L. *Asian Americans: Personality Patterns, Identity, and Mental Health*. New York, NY: The Guildford Press; 1994.

67. Kim MS, Hungter JE, Miyahara A, Horvath AM, Bresnahan M, Yoon HJ. Individual versus culture-level dimensions on an individualism and collectivism: effects on preferred conversation styles. *Commun Monogr*. 1996; 63:29–49.

68. Friedman LC, Baer PE, Lewy A, Lane M, Smith FE. Predictors of psychosocial adjustment to breast cancer. *J Psychosoc Oncol*. 1988; 6:75–94.

69. Abrahm J. *A Physician's Guide to Pain and Symptom Management in Cancer Patients*. Baltimore, Md: Johns Hopkins University Press; 2000.

70. National Bioethics Advisory Commission. *Ethical and Policy Issues in Research Involving Human Participants*. Bethesda, Md: National Bioethics Advisory Commission; 2001:250.

71. Carrese JA, Rhodes LA. Western bioethics on the Navajo reservation: benefit or harm? *JAMA*. 1995; 274:826–829.

72. Yeo G, Hikoyeda N. Cultural issues in end of life decision making among Asians and Pacific islanders in the United States. In: Braun KI, Pietsch JH, Blanchette PI, eds. *Cultural Issues in End-of-Life Decision Making*. Thousand Oaks, Calif: Sage Publications Inc; 2000:356.

73. Gilbert DT, Fiske ST, Lindzey G, eds. *The Handbook of Social Psychology*. Vol 2. 4th ed. New York, NY: McGraw-Hill; 1998.

74. Irish D, Lundquist K, Nelsen V. *Ethnic Variations in Dying, Death, and Grief: Diversity in Universality*. Washington DC: Taylor & Francis Publishers; 1993.

75. National Bioethics Advisory Committee. *Ensuring Voluntary Informed Consent and Protecting Privacy and Confidentiality*. Rockville, Md: U.S. Government Printing Office; 2001:103–104.

76. Berlin EA, Fowkes WC Jr. A teaching framework for cross-cultural health care. *West J Med*. 1983; 139:934–938.

77. Stuart MR. *The Fifteen Minute Hour: Applied Psychotherapy for the Primary Care Physician*. 2nd ed. New York, NY: Praeger; 1993.

78. Like RC, Levin SJ, Gottlieb BR. Useful clinical interviewing mnemonics [appendix]. *Patient Care*. 2000;(special issue):189.

79. Carrillo JE, Green AR, Betancourt JR. Cross-cultural primary care: a patient-based approach. *Ann Intern Med.* 1999; 130:829–834.

80. Koenig BA. Cultural diversity in decision-making about care at the end of life. Paper presented at: Institute of Medicine Workshop: Dying, Decision Making and Appropriate Care; December 2– 3, 1993.

81. US Department of Health and Human Services. Assuring cultural competence in health care: recommendations for National Standards and an Outcomes-Focused Research Agenda. 65 *Federal Register* 80865 (2000).

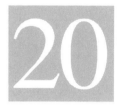

VARIABILITY IN ACCESS TO HOSPITAL PALLIATIVE CARE IN THE UNITED STATES

BENJAMIN GOLDSMITH, B.A., JESSICA DIETRICH, M.P.H.,
QINGLING DU, M.S., AND R. SEAN MORRISON, M.D.

This article originally appeared as Goldsmith B, Dietrich J, Du Q, Morrison RS. Variability in access to hospital palliative care in the United States. *J Palliat Med.* 2008;11(8):1094–1102. Copyright © 2008, American Academy of Hospice and Palliative Care, All rights reserved. Reprinted with permission.

EDITORS' INTRODUCTION

Demonstrating the same geographic variability in access to hospital palliative care services that plague virtually every aspect of our health care system, the authors identify predictors that will help drive the strategies necessary to assure reliable care during serious illness.

■ ■ ■

INTRODUCTION

Palliative care provides high-quality care for seriously ill patients and their families while making efficient use of hospital resources.[1] For patients to benefit from these services, however, hospital palliative care programs must be available locally within communities across the United States. In this report we examine the extent to which patients have access to hospital palliative care at the state level. Additionally, we examine the extent to which medical students have access to hospital palliative care programs during their clinical training. This report expands upon our prior publications in which we examined the hospital structural and demographic characteristics associated with the growth of hospital-based palliative care.[2,3]

METHODS

Data Sources

Data were obtained from four primary sources: the American Hospital Association (AHA) Annual Survey Database™ for Fiscal Year 2006 (hospital characteristics, including the presence of a palliative care program), the Association of American Medical Colleges (AAMC) (affiliated teaching hospitals for the nation's 126 public and private medical schools), the 2006 United States census (information about the hospital's community), and the *Dartmouth Atlas of Health Care 2008* (hospital admissions and deaths, ICU days and admissions, and Medicare costs by state). Supplemental data were provided through a mailed/faxed survey, telephone interviews of select medical school admission offices, and reviews of medical school Web sites as described below.

Hospital Data Data on hospital characteristics were obtained from the AHA Annual Survey Database for Fiscal Year 2006. The AHA surveys all member and nonmember hospitals in the United States and its associated areas on an annual basis. Among the over 850 elements included in the survey, data are provided on the type of authority responsible for establishing policy concerning overall operation of the hospitals (federal government, nonfederal government, nongovernment not for profit, and for profit,); clinical facilities and services offered by the hospitals (for example, general medical-surgical care, pediatric care, various types of intensive care units, physical rehabilitation, psychiatric services, cardiac programs, acquired immune deficiency disease [AIDS] care, and so on); beds and utilization; revenues and expenses; and professional staffing levels. For facilities and services, the survey also requests information on the manner in which a service is provided (that is, whether it is hospital-owned, provided by the hospital's health system or network, and/or provided through a formal contract between the hospital and another provider).

The survey also queried hospitals as to the presence of a palliative care program. The survey defines a palliative care program as "an organized program providing specialized medical care, drugs or therapies for the management of acute or chronic pain and/or the control of symptoms administered by specially trained physicians and other clinicians; and supportive care services, such as counseling on advanced directives, spiritual care, and social services, to patients with advanced disease and their families." For this study, all hospitals reporting a program, regardless of whether it was being provided by the hospital, health system, or network, or provided through a contractual arrangement or joint venture with another provider (for example, a hospice providing nonhospice palliative care to hospital patients), were coded as having an active program. The response rate for the AHA Annual Survey for Fiscal Year 2006 was 77 percent.

After publication of our last report,[3] several hospitals contacted the authors to state that the AHA had mistakenly classified them as not having hospital palliative care when indeed a program did exist at their institution (R.S. Morrison, personal communication, September 1, 2007). In order to allow hospitals to correct the data within the AHA survey, we sent a short questionnaire in January of 2007 to each hospital in the AHA Annual Survey Database for Fiscal Year 2005 that reported at least one general medical/surgical bed.

The questionnaire asked about the presence of hospital palliative care and requested details about the program if one did exist. Hospitals were also able to provide data through an online directory of hospitals via the Web site www.getpalliativecare.org. Overall, 22 percent of the surveyed hospitals responded via mailed survey or online form. Of responding hospitals, 31 percent confirmed the presence of a palliative care program, 46 percent confirmed the absence of a program, 3 percent changed their status from no program to an active program, 17 percent changed their status from an active program to no program, and 3 percent reported on data missing from the AHA survey. For hospitals that did not respond to the questionnaire, the original data provided by the AHA were used.

Medical School Data Data concerning hospital affiliation with United States allopathic medical schools were abstracted from the AAMC database of U.S. medical schools. The database records the primary teaching hospital affiliates for U.S. medical schools. After excluding those medical schools in Puerto Rico and associated with the armed forces, affiliate data were available for 100 of 121 medical schools. We reviewed Web sites and contacted the schools' offices of academic affairs by telephone to obtain data on the missing 21 schools. If the school did not report any official affiliate institutions, the primary teaching sites for the third- and fourth-year clerkship rotations were used. The AAMC also provided data concerning public and private status of the U.S. medical schools.

A medical school was considered to be affiliated with a hospital palliative care program if one or more of its main teaching hospitals reported the presence of a palliative care program. Medical school data were merged with the AHA data by hospital name and location.

Census Data Census data were obtained electronically from the United States Census Bureau Web site, http://factfinder. census.gov and reflect data current for 2006.[4] Census data were merged with primary survey data via Census Bureau county code. Census data used in this study included level of education, ethnic makeup, age distribution, and the distribution of wealth.

Health Care Utilization Data State rankings of Medicare deaths in hospital, intensive care unit/coronary care unit (ICU/CCU) admissions during terminal hospitalizations, ICU/CCU admissions per 1,000 decedents in the last six months of life, ICU/CCU days per decedent in the last six months of life, Medicare reimbursement/enrollee, and the number of Medicare hospital admissions in the last six months of life were obtained from the *Dartmouth Atlas of Health Care 2008* at www.dartmouthatlas.org/data_tools.shtm.[5]

Hospital Inclusion and Exclusion Criteria

Hospitals were included in this study if they admitted adult patients and the majority of admissions were identified as general medical-surgical, obstetrics/gynecology, cancer, or cardiac. We excluded rehabilitation hospitals, psychiatric hospitals, subacute and chronic care facilities, and eye, ear, nose, and throat hospitals. General medical-surgical and chronic disease hospitals that restricted admissions primarily to children were excluded. All hospitals falling under federal control (for example, U.S. Department of Veterans Affairs) were excluded. These hospitals are under federal mandate to reach 100 percent penetration of palliative care programs.[6] Hospitals that were located outside of the fifty states and the District of Columbia and hospitals that did not respond to the AHA survey were also excluded.

Definitions of Hospital Types

Hospitals containing 50 or more total facility beds were the primary focus of our analyses. A 50-bed cutoff was chosen because hospitals smaller than this are unlikely to be able to support a full interdisciplinary (nurse, social worker, physician) palliative care consultation team. Other subgroup analyses were completed on public hospitals, for-profit hospitals, and sole-community-provider hospitals. Public hospitals were defined as not-for-profit hospitals run by a state, county, city, joint city-county, or hospital district or authority with 50 or more total facility beds. For-profit hospitals included those institutions run by individuals, partnerships, or corporations with 50 or more total facility beds. The "sole community provider" designation is assigned to hospitals by Medicare and is defined as a hospital that is located more than thirty-five miles from other, like hospitals or that otherwise serves as the sole provider of health care services for a region, secondary to limitations in local topography or prolonged severe weather conditions. Sole-community-provider hospitals with 1 or more total facility beds were included in these analyses.

Additional analyses were done on small hospitals (less than 50 total facility beds) and large hospitals (more than 300 total facility beds).

Analyses

Multivariable logistic regression models were used to examine the association between hospital and geographic characteristics on the presence of a palliative care program, as described in our prior study.[3]Hospitals were stratified for modeling by total number of facility beds. All variables entered into the multivariable analyses appear in Table 20.1. Variables concerning age and wealth distribution by county were removed from the second model (Table 20.2) as they behaved as constants. Spearman rank correlations were used to examine the relationship between state rank of hospital palliative care penetration and state rank of the selected health care utilization measures. All analyses were performed using SAS version 9.1.3 (SAS Institute, Inc., Cary, NC). Mapping was completed using ArcGIS Desktop version 9.2. This study was exempt from Institutional Review Board (IRB) approval by the Mount Sinai School of Medicine.

RESULTS

Prevalence of Hospital Palliative Care

Adult hospital palliative care programs in facilities with 50 or more beds are displayed in Figure 20.1. States were divided into quintiles corresponding to the overall prevalence of hospital palliative care in each respective state. Nationally, state prevalence rates of hospital palliative care ranged from 10 percent in Mississippi to 100 percent in Vermont, with a cumulative national average of 52.8 percent (1,294/2,452). The lowest rates of hospital palliative care were observed in Mississippi (10 percent), Alabama (16 percent), Oklahoma (19 percent), Nevada (23 percent), and Wyoming (25 percent). The highest rates were observed in Vermont (100 percent), Montana (88 percent), New Hampshire (85 percent), the District of Columbia (80 percent), and South Dakota (78 percent).

Separate analyses were conducted on small and large hospitals. These hospitals were subject to the same exclusion criteria as the primary study population, with the exception that they contained fewer than 50 total facility beds or more than 300 total facility beds, respectively. Hospitals defined as small constituted 37 percent, and those defined as large constituted 16 percent of the nation's medical centers, respectively. The numbers of small hospitals varied widely by state: four states (Connecticut, Delaware, New Jersey, Rhode Island) and the District of Columbia did not report any hospitals in this category, whereas other states, such as Montana and South Dakota, had more than 80 percent of their hospitals in this category. State prevalence of hospital palliative care in small hospitals ranged from 0 percent in Louisiana, Maryland, Nevada, and New Mexico to 78 percent in Vermont, with a national average of 20.1 percent.

TABLE 20.1. **Prevalence of Palliative Care Programs in Sole Community Provider Hospitals**

State	# Hospitals	# HPCA^a(%)
0%–20%		
Alabama	5	0 (0)
Idaho	3	0 (0)
Indiana	1	0 (0)
Louisiana	4	0 (0)
Nevada	4	0 (0)
Oklahoma	25	1 (4)
Mississippi	16	1 (6)
Texas	56	4 (7)
Illinois	8	1 (13)
Kentucky	8	1 (13)
New Mexico	16	2 (13)
Georgia	7	1 (14)
Wyoming	22	4 (18)
21%–40%		
Utah	14	3 (21)
Pennsylvania	9	2 (22)
Colorado	18	4 (22)
Connecticut	4	1 (25)
Washington	8	2 (25)
Arkansas	19	5 (26)
Kansas	31	9 (29)
North Carolina	10	3 (30)
West Virginia	13	4 (31)
Michigan	19	6 (32)
Montana	22	7 (33)
South Carolina	9	3 (33)
Hawaii	3	1 (33)

State	# Hospitals	# HPCA[a](%)
California	27	10 (37)
Nebraska	8	3 (38)
41%–60%		
Missouri	27	11 (41)
Virginia	12	5 (42)
Oregon	14	6 (43)
North Dakota	9	4 (44)
Iowa	11	5 (45)
Massachusetts	2	1 (50)
New York	14	7 (50)
Wisconsin	12	6 (50)
Minnesota	8	4 (50)
Arizona	10	5 (50)
Alaska	8	4 (50)
South Dakota	11	6 (55)
Maine	10	6 (60)
Florida	5	3 (60)
61%–80%		
Tennessee	3	2 (67)
Vermont	7	5 (71)
81%–100%		
New Hampshire	1	1 (100)
Ohio	1	1 (100)
No sole community provider programs		
Delaware		
District of Columbia		
Maryland		
New Jersey		
Rhode Island		

[a]HPC, hospital palliative care.

TABLE 20.2. Prevalence of Palliative Care Programs in Public Hospitals with Fifty or More Beds

State	# Hospitals	# HPCA*(%)
0%–20%		
Alabama	1	0 (0)
Connecticut	1	0 (0)
Nevada	1	0 (0)
Oklahoma	8	0 (0)
Mississippi	17	1 (6)
Michigan	8	1 (13)
Kentucky	6	1 (17)
Alabama	20	4 (20)
21%–40%		
Louisiana	19	4 (21)
New York	8	2 (25)
Tennessee	8	2 (25)
South Carolina	11	3 (27)
Illinois	7	2 (29)
Texas	31	9 (29)
Washington	10	3 (30)
Colorado	3	1 (33)
Wyoming	6	2 (33)
41%–60%		
Georgia	19	8 (42)
Kansas	7	3 (43)
Indiana	19	9 (47)
Arizona	2	1 (50)
Arkansas	4	2 (50)
Hawaii	2	1 (50)
Minnesota	6	3 (50)
Nebraska	2	1 (50)

State	# Hospitals	# HPCA[a](%)
New Mexico	2	1 (50)
West Virginia	2	1 (50)
California	34	19 (56)
Iowa	5	3 (60)
61%–80%		
Florida	20	13 (65)
North Carolina	26	17 (65)
Idaho	3	2 (67)
Massachusetts	3	2 (67)
Ohio	12	8 (67)
Virginia	3	2 (67)
Missouri	12	9 (75)
81%–100%		
New Jersey	1	1 (100)
Oregon	2	2 (100)
Utah	1	1 (100)
No public hospitals		
Delaware		
District of Columbia		
Maine		
Maryland		
Montana		
New Hampshire		
North Dakota		
Pennsylvania		
Rhode Island		
South Dakota		
Vermont		
Wisconsin		

[a]HPC, hospital palliative care.

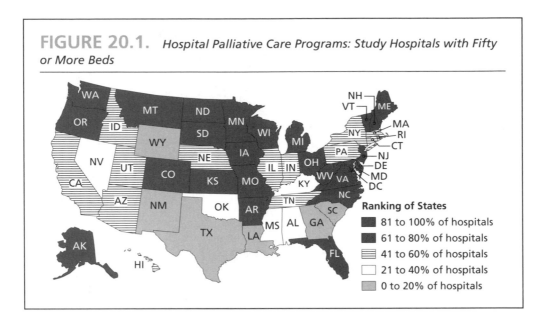

FIGURE 20.1. *Hospital Palliative Care Programs: Study Hospitals with Fifty or More Beds*

Ranking of States
- 81 to 100% of hospitals
- 61 to 80% of hospitals
- 41 to 60% of hospitals
- 21 to 40% of hospitals
- 0 to 20% of hospitals

Large hospitals constituted 2 to 46 percent of all hospitals in states across the country, with the exception of Wyoming (which had 0 large hospitals). State prevalence rates of hospital palliative care in large hospitals ranged from 0 percent in Nevada to 100 percent in twenty states, with a cumulative national average of 75.5 percent. Maps showing state ranks by prevalence of hospital palliative care in large hospitals are displayed in Figure 20.2.

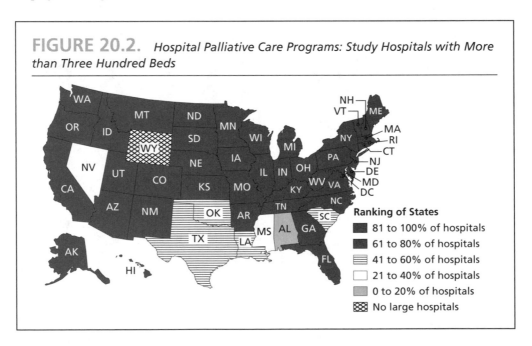

FIGURE 20.2. *Hospital Palliative Care Programs: Study Hospitals with More than Three Hundred Beds*

Ranking of States
- 81 to 100% of hospitals
- 61 to 80% of hospitals
- 41 to 60% of hospitals
- 21 to 40% of hospitals
- 0 to 20% of hospitals
- No large hospitals

Nationally, 40.9 percent (144/352) of public hospitals and 20.3 percent (84/413) of for-profit hospitals reported hospital palliative care. Among hospitals designated by Medicare as sole community providers, 160 of 554 hospitals (28.8 percent) reported palliative care services. State-by-state results for these subgroups can be found in Tables 20.3, 20.4, and 20.5.

Hospital, Geographic, and Regional Characteristics

Institution and community characteristics associated with the presence of hospital palliative care, stratified by bed size, are in Tables 20.1 and 20.2. Among institutions containing between 50 and 300 total facility beds (Table 20.1), hospitals located in the West and Midwest were significantly more likely to report hospital palliative care, after controlling for other variables (reference Northeast, odds ratio [OR] = 0.1.58; 95 percent confidence interval [CI], 1.1–2.27; $p = 0.01$ and OR = 2.16; CI, 1.56 to 3.01; $p < 0.0001$, respectively). For-profit hospitals were significantly less likely to report hospital palliative care, compared to not-for-profit institutions (OR = 0.21; CI, 0.15–0.29; $p < 0.001$). Variables found to be associated with the presence of hospital palliative care were institutions that owned a hospice program (OR = 1.82; CI, 1.44–2.3; $p < 0.0001$), status as an American College of Surgery (ACS)-approved cancer hospital (OR = 1.66; CI, 1.33–2.07; $p < 0.0001$), and the percent of persons in the county with a college education (reference below 70 percent; for 70 percent–90 percent, OR = 1.78; CI, 1.32–2.39; $p < 0.0001$; for 90 percent and up, OR = 2.43; CI, 1.58–3.75; $p < 0.0001$).

Among institutions containing more than 300 total facility beds (Table 20.3), for-profit and public hospitals were significantly less likely to report hospital palliative care when compared to not-for-profit hospitals (OR = 0.23; CI, 0.12–0.44; $p < 0.0001$ and OR = 0.25; CI, 0.14–0.43; $p < .0001$, respectively). Institutions that owned a hospice program (OR = 1.91; CI, 1.22–2.99; $p < 0.005$) and that were affiliated with a medical school (OR = 2.18; CI, 1.24–3.83; $p = 0.01$) were significantly more likely to report hospital palliative care.

Palliative Care Programs in Teaching Hospitals

Of the 121 allopathic medical schools in the United States, 116 were affiliated with hospitals that responded to the AHA survey. Of these 116 schools, 98 were affiliated with at least one hospital reporting hospital palliative care (national average, 84.5 percent). Thirty-eight of 43 (88.4 percent) private medical schools were affiliated with at least one hospital reporting hospital palliative care. The five private medical schools affiliated with hospitals not reporting hospital palliative care were Albany Medical College, Boston University School of Medicine, Meharry Medical College, Tufts University School of Medicine, and Yale University School of Medicine.

Sixty of 73 (82.2 percent) state-funded medical schools were affiliated with hospitals reporting hospital palliative care. The 13 schools not affiliated with a hospital palliative care were found in twelve states. While most of these states contained more than one state-funded medical school, four (33 percent) did not contain a medical school affiliated with a hospital palliative care program: Connecticut, Mississippi, Nebraska, and Nevada.

TABLE 20.3. **Prevalence of Palliative Care Programs in For-Profit Hospitals with Fifty or More Beds**

State	# Hospitals	# HPC[a](%)
0%–20%		
Alabama	13	0 (0)
Arizona	6	0 (0)
Georgia	15	0 (0)
Idaho	1	0 (0)
Illinois	2	0 (0)
Mississippi	17	0 (0)
Nebraska	1	0 (0)
Nevada	6	0 (0)
New Mexico	5	0 (0)
Oregon	2	0 (0)
Pennsylvania	9	0 (0)
Wyoming	1	0 (0)
Kentucky	8	1 (13)
South Carolina	16	2 (13)
Texas	85	12 (14)
Oklahoma	14	2 (14)
Utah	7	1 (14)
California	40	6 (15)
Louisiana	13	2 (15)
Massachusetts	5	1 (20)
21%–40%		
Arkansas	14	3 (21)
Tennessee	17	4 (24)
Florida	45	13 (29)
Missouri	12	4 (33)
41%–60%		
Ohio	3	3 (43)

State	# Hospitals	# HPC[a](%)
Kansas	7	1 (50)
New Hampshire	2	1 (50)
North Carolina	6	3 (50)
Virginia	10	5 (50)
West Virginia	6	3 (50)
Wisconsin	2	1 (50)
Indiana	11	6 (55)
61%–80%		
Washington	3	2 (67)
81%–100%		
Colorado	6	5 (83)
Alaska	1	1 (100)
Maryland	1	1 (100)
South Dakota	1	1 (100)
No for-profit hospitals		
Connecticut		
Delaware		
District of Columbia		
Hawaii		
Iowa		
Maine		
Michigan		
Minnesota		
Montana		
New Jersey		
New York		
North Dakota		
Rhode Island		
Vermont		

[a]HPC, hospital palliative care.

TABLE 20.4. **Hospital and Community Characteristics Associated with Hospital Palliative Care Programs for Institutions with Fifty to Three Hundred Beds**

	Odds Ratio	95% CI[a]	p Value
Region (reference: Northeast)			
Midwest	2.16	1.56, 3.01	<0.0001
South	1.19	0.85, 1.66	0.31
West	1.58	1.1, 2.27	0.01
Hospital ownership (reference is nonprofit)			
For-profit hospital	0.21	0.15, 0.29	<0.0001
Public hospital	0.58	0.43, 0.78	0.0004
Sole community providers	1.10	0.78, 1.54	0.60
Hospital owns hospice program	1.82	1.44, 2.3	<0.0001
American College of Surgery (ACS)–approved Cancer Program	1.66	1.33, 2.07	<0.0001
Percent > bachelor's degree in the county (reference: below 70%)			
90% and up	2.43	1.58, 3.75	<0.0001
70%–90%	1.78	1.32, 2.39	0.0001
Percentage white in the county (reference: below 40%)			
60% and up	1.09	0.78, 1.52	0.61
40%–60%	1.14	0.77, 1.7	0.52
Percentage age 65 and over in the county (reference: below 10%)			
15% and up	1.47	0.94, 2.31	0.09
10%–15%	1.17	0.85, 1.62	0.33
Percent below poverty level in the county (reference: below 10%)			
10% and up	1.09	0.84, 1.4	0.52
Medical school affiliation	1.04	0.39, 2.79	0.94

[a]CI: confidence interval.

TABLE 20.5. Hospital and Community Characteristics Associated with Hospital Palliative Care Programs for Institutions with More Than Three Hundred Beds

	Odds Ratio	95% CI[a]	p Value
Region (reference: Northeast)			
Midwest	1.67	0.84, 3.34	0.15
South	0.87	0.49, 1.54	0.63
West	1.69	0.83, 3.43	0.15
Hospital ownership (reference is nonprofit)			
For-profit hospital	0.23	0.12, 0.44	<0.0001
Public hospital	0.25	0.14, 0.43	<0.0001
Sole community providers	1.20	0.22, 6.4	0.84
Hospital owns hospice program	1.91	1.22, 2.99	0.0045
American College of Surgery (ACS)–approved Cancer Program	1.02	0.63, 1.67	0.92
Percent > bachelor's degree in the county (reference: below 70%)			
90% and up	2.27	0.94, 5.52	0.07
70%–90%	1.96	0.94, 4.08	0.07
Percentage white in the county (reference: below 40%)			
60% and up	1.09	0.63, 1.88	0.75
40%–60%	1.02	0.56, 1.85	0.95
Medical school affiliation	2.18	1.24, 3.83	0.0066

[a]CI: confidence interval.

Palliative Care and Health Care Utilization

There were significant correlations between state rankings of hospital palliative care penetration and state rankings of five of the six selected measures of health care utilization.

Greater state penetration of hospital palliative care was significantly correlated with lower Medicare hospital death rates ($R^2 = 0.028$, $p = 0.048$), fewer ICU/CCU admissions during terminal hospitalizations ($R^2 = 0.31$, $p = 0.03$), fewer ICU/CCU admissions per 1000 decedents in the last six months of life ($R^2 = 0.32$, $p = 0.02$), fewer ICU/CCU days per decedent in the last six months of life ($R^2 = 0.31$,

$p = 0.02$) and lower overall Medicare reimbursement/enrollee ($R^2 = 0.33$, $p = 0.02$). State ranking of the number of hospital admissions in the last six months of life was not significantly correlated with state ranking of hospital palliative care penetration ($R^2 = 0.25$, $p = 0.08$).

DISCUSSION

In this study, we have presented the most recent estimates to date of the prevalence of hospital palliative care programs in the United States. We found wide geographic variation in access to palliative care services, although factors predicting hospital palliative care have not changed markedly since our last report, in 2005.[3] Overall, we observed elevated rates of hospital palliative care in large hospitals (more than 300 beds, 75.5 percent) and decreased rates in small hospitals (fewer than 50 beds, 20.1 percent), with a national prevalence of hospital palliative care in study hospitals at 52.8 percent. A minority of public hospitals (40.9 percent), for-profit hospitals (20.3 percent), and sole-community-provider hospitals (28.8 percent) reported hospital palliative care. We observed that a majority of medical school–affiliated hospitals (84.5 percent) reported hospital palliative care.

Relationship to Prior Studies

There has been a steady increase in the number of U.S. hospitals reporting a palliative care program since we first examined prevalence rates of hospital palliative care in 2001[2] such that in 2006, 52.8 percent (1,294/2,452) of American hospitals reported a program. Using the inclusion and exclusion criteria used in this study, the yearly rates of hospital palliative care programs in the United States were 24.5 percent (658/2,686) in 2000, 30.4 percent (805/2,649) in 2001, 35.6 percent (946/2,658) in 2002, 40.4 percent (1,083/2,684) in 2003, 44.8 percent (1,151/2,570) in 2004, and 44.8 percent (1,151/2,570) in 2005.

Since our last report, in 2005,[3] which reflected data from 2003, the overall prevalence of hospital palliative care programs has increased 8.6 percent in the Northeast, 16.4 percent in the Midwest, 17.2 percent in the West, and 9.6 percent in the South. This growth has occurred largely in not-for-profit hospitals. In our examination of hospital subgroups, prevalence rates from 2003 to 2006 increased by 10 percent in public hospitals (30.9 percent to 40.9 percent) and 4.2 percent in for-profit hospitals (16.1 percent to 20.3 percent) while decreasing by 2.3 percent in sole-community-provider hospitals (31.1 percent to 28.8 percent).

Public Access

This study revealed important differences in access to hospital palliative care across this country. In the states of Vermont, Montana, and New Hampshire, seriously ill patients have access to palliative care services in nearly every hospital, whereas access to these services in Mississippi, Alabama, and Oklahoma is severely limited. In addition to notable disparities in geographic availability, we further observed strikingly low rates of hospital palliative care in public and sole-community-provider hospitals.

Public and sole-community-provider hospitals often serve as the only option for medical care for uninsured patients and geographically isolated communities, respectively. Thus our finding that the majority of these institutions lack palliative care services speaks to a disparity in access to comprehensive care for some of the sickest and most vulnerable patient populations. Indeed, based on our results, only 41 percent of public hospitals and less than 30 percent of sole-community-provider hospitals provide their patients with access to hospital palliative care. These data suggest that targeted efforts to enhance the development of palliative care programs in these environments are critically needed. The increasing data suggesting that palliative care programs not only improve quality of medical care for patients with serious illness[7-10] but do so with lower associated hospital costs than usual care[11-13] provide dual incentives for states, cities, and the federal government to promote the development of hospital palliative care programs in these settings while reducing hospital and patient cost during hospitalization. State legislatures can play an important role in this process by providing funding to hospitals to attend educational and technical assistance programs focused on promoting the development of palliative care programs, especially public and sole-community-provider hospitals. Additionally, state governments can further promote the development of palliative care through legislation that promotes palliative care education and training, as exemplified by the Palliative Care Education and Training Act recently passed in New York.[14,15] The New York legislation will support palliative care training programs for health care professionals, identify and fund the Centers for Palliative Care Excellence, and create the New York State Palliative Care Education and Training Council to guide state policies on palliative care.

Medical Training

While we found overall high rates of hospital palliative care in medical school teaching hospitals, complete penetration has not yet occurred in these institutions. Given that medical training is rooted in physician mentoring and role modeling, it is of critical importance that future physicians receive not only didactic training in palliative medicine but exposure to clinical practice and programs in their third and fourth years of undergraduate medical education. Although this study was unable to qualify or quantify the extent of exposure or formal education in palliative care in institutions reporting hospital palliative care, at the most basic level, palliative care services must be present within an institution before the opportunity for such education exists.

Health Care Utilization

States that ranked high in hospital palliative care penetration tended to rank low on a range of health care utilization measures, including number of hospital deaths, number of admissions during the terminal hospitalization, number of ICU/CCU admissions during the last six months of life, and total Medicare reimbursements. There are several reasons that may explain these findings. The underlying factors that result in lower health care utilization may also contribute to the development of palliative care programs. Second, underlying patient-related factors or community factors that promote the development of palliative care programs may also be associated with lower health care utilization. Finally, it is possible that the presence of hospital palliative care programs results in lower health care utilization and in improved quality for Medicare beneficiaries in the last six months of life. Future studies will need to address causal links between these findings.

Limitations

There are several limitations to this study that should be noted. First, the identification of hospital palliative care programs was based upon hospitals' self-reports to the American Hospital Association (AHA) Annual Survey and it is possible that hospitals' answers to the survey were inaccurate. As a result of anecdotal reports of inaccuracies in our last report, we conducted an additional survey providing hospitals with the opportunity to correct the AHA survey and, in particular, ensure that their hospital palliative care program was included in our results. Twenty percent of hospitals elected to respond to this survey. Of the nearly 900 hospitals that responded, over 80 percent agreed with the AHA's survey suggesting that the numbers that we report have strong validity.

Second, we have no information about the structure and quality of the programs that we identified. Specifically, using the data sources available to us, it was impossible to determine the administrative structure, size, and processes of care employed by these hospital palliative care programs and whether they were in compliance with the recently developed National Quality Forum Framework for palliative care. Third, for the purposes of this study we limited our primary study population to hospitals containing 50 or more facility beds, based upon the rationale that it is unlikely that smaller hospitals would have a patient population large enough to support a full interdisciplinary palliative care team, as recommended by the National Consensus Project.[16]

As a result of the limitations inherent in the AHA survey, we were unable to report on the prevalence of pediatric palliative care programs. The AHA reports the presence of hospital palliative care programs through a single variable and does not provide additional information on whether a pediatric palliative care program is also available at an institution. Separate analyses of children's hospitals are possible and should be addressed in the future.

Last, while we have chosen to exclude federal hospitals from all analyses because of their mandate to reach 100 percent penetration of palliative care programs,[6] we acknowledge the importance of the VA hospitals as clinical teaching sites for medical students across the country. However, VA hospitals typically do not serve as the primary clinical teaching site for any medical school in the United States and, as such, the presence of a palliative care program in a VA hospital does not ensure that all medical school students have access to a clinical palliative care program.

Despite these limitations, the data presented in this study represent the most recent estimates of access to hospital palliative care by patients and medical students reported in the literature to date.

CONCLUSION

We have identified significant disparities in public and educational access to hospital palliative care services. The ultimate goal of palliative care is improving the overall quality of care for patients with serious illness and their families. In order to do so, however, patients must be able to access these services in their local hospital, and medical trainees must receive training in and exposure to hospital palliative care. Future research needs to focus on efforts to promote the development of hospital palliative care programs in underrepresented hospitals (public, sole community provider, for profit), identifying barriers to the development of these programs, and on identifying the structures of existing programs and the care processes that they employ. Finally, the association between the prevalence of hospital palliative care programs and lower Medicare spending for the seriously ill is an intriguing finding that needs to be further studied.

ADDENDUM

Since this research was completed, Yale–New Haven Hospital has initiated a palliative care program.

REFERENCES

1. Meier DE. Palliative care in hospitals. *J Hosp Med.* 2006; 1: 21–28.

2. Pan CX, Morrison RS, Meier DE, Natale DK, Goldhirsch SL, Kralovec P, Cassel CK. How prevalent are hospital-based palliative care programs? Status report and future directions. *J Palliat Med.* 2001; 4: 315–324.

3. Morrison RS, Maroney-Galin C, Kralovec PD, Meier DE. The growth of palliative care programs in United States hospitals. *J Palliat Med.* 2005; 8: 1127–1134.

4. American FactFinder. U.S. Census Bureau. 2006. http://fact finder.census.gov (last accessed June 1, 2008).

5. *The Dartmouth Atlas of Health Care 2008.* www.dartmouth atlas.org (last accessed June 1, 2008).

6. VHA 2003–008, D. Palliative care consult teams. Veterans Health Administration February 4, 2003. www .ethosconsult.com (last accessed June 1, 2008).

7. Higginson IJ, Finlay I, Goodwin DM, Cook AM, Hood K, Edwards AG, Douglas HR, Normand CE. Do hospital-based palliative teams improve care for patients or families at the end of life? *J Pain Symptom Manage.* 2002; 23: 96–106.

8. Higginson IJ, Finlay IG, Goodwin DM, Hood K, Edwards AG, Cook A, Douglas HR, Normand CE. Is there evidence that palliative care teams alter end-of-life experiences of patients and their caregivers? *J Pain Symptom Manage.* 2003; 25: 150–168.

9. Finlay IG, Higginson IJ, Goodwin DM, Cook AM, Edwards AG, Hood K, Douglas HR, Normand CE. Palliative care in hospital, hospice, at home: Results from a systematic review. *Ann Oncol.* 2002; 13(suppl 4): 257–264.

10. Jordhoy MS, Fayers P, Loge JH, Ahlner-Elmqvist M, Kaasa S. Quality of life in palliative cancer care: Results from a cluster randomized trial. *J Clin Oncol.* 2001; 19: 3884–3894.

11. Smith TJ, Coyne P, Cassel B, Penberthy L, Hopson A, Hager MA. A high-volume specialist palliative care unit and team may reduce in-hospital end-of-life care costs. *J Palliat Med.* 2003; 6: 699–705.

12. Campbell ML, Guzman JA. Impact of a proactive approach to improve end-of-life care in a medical ICU. *Chest.* 2003; 123: 266–271.

13. Morrison RS, Chichin E, Carter J, Burack O, Lantz M, Meier DE. The effect of a social work intervention to enhance advance care planning documentation in the nursing home. *J Am Geriatr Soc.* 2005; 53: 290–294.

14. Palliative Care Education and Training Act. 2007 NY Acts A03016. January 22, 2007.

15. Palliative Care Education and Training Act. 2007 NY Acts S00597. January 5, 2007.

16. National Consensus Project. www.nationalconsensusproject.org (last accessed June 1, 2008).

ACKNOWLEDGMENTS

This study was supported by the National Palliative Care Research Center and the Center to Advance Palliative Care. Dr. Morrison is the recipient of a Mid-Career Investigator Award in Patient-Oriented Research from the National Institute on Aging (K24 AG022345). Mr. Goldsmith is a Doris Duke Clinical Research Fellow.

The Center to Advance Palliative Care and the National Palliative Care Research Center are supported by the Aetna, Brookdale, John A. Hartford, JEHT, Robert Wood Johnson, Emily Davie and Joseph S. Kornfeld, and Olive Branch Foundations.

AUTHOR DISCLOSURE STATEMENT

No conflicting financial interests exist.

DO PALLIATIVE CONSULTATIONS IMPROVE PATIENT OUTCOMES?

DAVID CASARETT, M.D., M.A., AMY PICKARD, B.A., F. AMOS BAILEY, M.D.,
CHRISTINE RITCHIE, M.D., M.P.H., CHRISTIAN FURMAN, M.D., M.P.H.,
KEN ROSENFELD, M.D., SCOTT SHREVE, M.D., M.B.A., ZHEN CHEN, PH.D.,
AND JUDY A. SHEA, PH.D.

This article originally appeared as Casarett D, Pickard A, Bailey FA, Ritchie C, Furman C, Rosenfeld K, Shreve
S, Chen Z, Shea JA. Do palliative care consultations improve outcomes? *J Amer Geriatr Soc*. 2008;56:593-599.

EDITORS' INTRODUCTION

A large survey of family members of veterans who died with and without palliative care services identified marked improvements in key patient and family-centered outcomes, including relief of pain and shortness of breath, and better communication, emotional and spiritual support, and well being and dignity among patients receiving palliative care. The earlier the palliative care service was received, the higher the likelihood of benefit, pointing to the importance of case finding and timely identification of patients and families likely to benefit from these services.

■ ■ ■

Over the past ten years, there has been a rapid growth in the number of palliative care consultation teams in U.S. hospitals. These teams generally consist of a physician and advanced practice nurse and often include a social worker, chaplain, and psychologist.[1,2] In keeping with the focus of palliative care on alleviating suffering and improving quality of life, teams participate in the care of hospitalized patients with life-threatening illnesses by providing advice about pain and symptom management, assistance with goal setting and advance care planning, emotional and spiritual support, hospice referral, and discharge planning.[3] Currently, well over one-quarter of hospitals have active palliative consultation teams.[4]

Previous studies have found that inpatient consultation teams frequently identify unrecognized problems (for example, symptoms) and unmet needs.[5-9] Consultations are also associated with less use of intensive care units,[10,11] a lower likelihood of dying in an intensive care unit,[12] and lower costs of care.[10,13] Finally, there is also growing evidence that consultations improve processes of care such as opioid prescribing and documentation of patients' goals.[8,14,15]

However, much less is known about whether inpatient palliative consultations improve the quality of care from the patient's or family's perspective. Although two controlled trials of palliative care have examined patients' or families' perceptions of care, they have focused on outpatient care management rather than inpatient consultations.[16,17] Finally, previous studies have tested high-intensity interventions in specific populations or settings, typically at a single site.[14,15]

Therefore, it is not known whether inpatient palliative consultations can improve patient- and family-focused outcomes of care in a population of patients who receive care in inpatient and outpatient settings. Nor is it known whether consultations have a greater effect on some domains of care than on others. Finally, it is not known whether consultations that are performed earlier in the patient's illness offer a greater benefit. The goal of this study was to determine whether palliative consultations improve patient- and family-focused outcomes of care in patients near the end of life.

METHODS

Setting and Description of Palliative Care Consultation Teams

This project was conducted in five VA Medical Centers and their affiliated nursing homes and clinics and was approved by each facility's institutional review board. These sites range in size from 114 to 980 beds and have between 2,850 and 7,050 admissions (acute care plus long-term care) per year. These teams rely primarily on physicians, nurse practitioners, or both, who contribute between 1.0 and 2.5 full-time equivalents to the consultation service. They also include nurses, social workers, chaplains, volunteers, and other disciplines on an as-needed basis (for example, physical therapists, occupational therapists, and psychologists).

Recruitment

Patient deaths between August 2006 and May 2007 were identified using the VA's electronic medical record (EMR) system, which in pilot testing identified more than 95 percent of veteran deaths within the recruitment window. Patients were included if they received any inpatient or outpatient care from a participating VA Medical Center in the last month of life. No exclusion criteria were used. During infrequent periods when the number of deaths exceeded the interviewers' capacity to conduct interviews, patients were selected at random for omission from the sample.

The following algorithm was used to identify potential respondents, in descending order: patient's next of kin, primary contact named in the EMR, individual holding durable power of attorney for health care. Because most potential respondents were related to the patient, they are referred to collectively as "family members." Four to six weeks after the patient's death, family members were sent a letter that described the study and provided a toll-free telephone number they could use to opt out. Approximately six weeks after the patient's death, interviewers made telephone calls to those who did not opt out. Interviewers made six attempts over four weeks, including at least one attempt after 5 P.M. local time. Family members who did not have a working telephone number, those who did not speak English, those with hearing impairment that precluded a telephone interview, and those who said they could not evaluate the care that the patient received in the last month of life were excluded.

Data Collection

Interviews were completed by telephone. After giving oral informed consent, family members provided demographic data about the patients and themselves. Next, they completed a survey that assessed their perceptions of the quality of the care that the patients and they themselves received during the patients' last month of life and after the patients' deaths. Family members who completed the interview received a

$30 check. Those who experienced any distress during the interview were offered an opportunity to speak with a counselor.

Interviews used the Family Assessment of Treatment at End-of-life (FATE) survey, which was developed using open-ended interviews and iteratively refined through expert panel input, cognitive interviewing, and psychometric testing.[18,19] The FATE has thirty-two items (Figure 21.1) that reflect key areas of palliative care outlined by current national guidelines.[1,2] All items evaluate outcomes by asking respondents for frequency ratings (for example, "How often did the patient's pain make him/her uncomfortable?") or yes/no responses (for example, "Do you think the patient died where he/she wanted to?"). In the validation study,[19] the FATE demonstrated good homogeneity (Cronbach alpha = 0.91), and all domains had a Cronbach alpha greater than 0.70, which is the generally accepted threshold for between-group comparisons.[20] The FATE is reproduced in full at http://www.caringforveterans.org.

Data Analysis

Items were coded as missing if respondents could not answer and as not applicable if they were not relevant to the patient's care (for example, for the "pain" item if a patient did not experience pain in the last month of life). Although it is possible that this coding strategy might have missed some patients whose symptoms were well controlled, it is likely that even the most aggressive symptom management regimen would permit occasional breakthrough symptoms over the course of a month. Those patients would have had some symptoms, and thus these items would have been applicable. To derive a score for each domain and the instrument, all "best possible" responses were summed and divided by the number of usable (that is, applicable and nonmissing) responses. Item, domain, and instrument scores were expressed as a percentage of usable responses for which family members gave the best possible response, with a possible range from 0 to 100.

Six domain scores encompass twenty-five of the FATE items: the patient's well-being and dignity (four items), adequacy of communication (five items), emotional and spiritual support (three items), care around the time of death (six items), access to home care services (four items), and access to benefits and services after the patient's death (three items). The remaining seven items are scored individually but contribute to the overall score.

Because patients who receive a palliative consultation may be different from those who do not, and because these differences may influence the outcomes measured, a propensity score was created to account for nonrandom assignment between the two groups. A propensity score provides a summary of the conditional probability of receiving a consultation based on all potential predictors, allowing efficient adjustment for those predictors.[21,22] To create the propensity score, potential predictors of palliative consultation were examined using variables in Table 21.1, as well as responses to FATE items that did not influence the score (for example, family did not want or need emotional support). Those with a P-value <.25 were considered for inclusion in a multivariable model.[23] Only those variables that a palliative consultation would not

FIGURE 21.1. *Family Assessment of Treatment at End-of-Life (FATE) Items and Domains*

Well-being and dignity[a]
Inpatient providers attended to the patient's personal care needs.
Inpatient providers handled the patient gently.
Inpatient providers supervised the patient closely enough.
Inpatient providers offered comfortable accommodations for family members.

Information and communication
Providers gave contradictory information.[b]
Providers spoke in an understandable way.
Providers listened to concerns.
Providers were available to talk to the patient/family.
Providers kept patient/family informed about the patient's condition and treatment.

Respect for treatment preferences
Patient received all desired medications or treatment.
Patient received unwanted medication or treatment.[b]

Emotional and spiritual support
Providers were kind, caring, and respectful.
Providers gave adequate spiritual support to patient/family prior to death.
Providers gave adequate emotional support to patient/family prior to death.

Management of symptoms
Shortness of breath made the patient uncomfortable.[b]
Pain made the patient uncomfortable.[b]
Confusion made the patient uncomfortable.[b]
Reexperiencing the stress and emotions of combat made the patient.
    uncomfortable (Post-Traumatic Stress Disorder–related symptoms).[b]

Choice of inpatient facility
The patient was admitted to the hospital facility of his/her choice.

Care around the time of death
Providers alerted family when the patient was close to death.
Providers explained the dying process.
The patient died where he/she wanted to.
The family understood the cause of the patient's death.
The family had enough warning one month prior to patient's death.
Providers gave the family enough emotional support after the patient's death.

Access to out patient services
The patient/family received enough help coordinating medical equipment.
The patient/family received enough care at home.
The VA provided enough assistance with the patient's transportation.
The VA provided enough reimbursement for the patient's transportation.

Access to benefits and services after the patient's death
The family received adequate information about benefits for spousest
    and dependents.
The family received adequate information about burial and memorial benefits.
The family received adequate help with funeral arrangements.

[a]Only applicable to patients who spent time in an inpatient facility in the last month of life.
[b]Affirmative responses reflect worse care; items were reverse-coded for scoring.

influence were considered, and the smallest number of variables that would yield a model with the highest possible area under the receiver operating characteristic (ROC) curve was selected. The Hosmer-Lemeshow goodness-of-fit test was used to test model fit,[24] and the area under the ROC curve was used to test model discrimination. The final model was applied to each patient in the sample, calculating his or her propensity score.

A linear regression model was then developed to examine the effect of palliative consultations on the FATE score (all thirty-two items), after adjusting for the propensity score and additional patient characteristics that were associated with the FATE score. Characteristics whose association with the FATE score had a P-value <.25 were considered for inclusion in a multivariable model.[23] Next, these variables (propensity score plus patient characteristics) were used in linear regression models to examine the independent effect of consultation on each of the six FATE domain scores. Finally, this procedure was repeated for the four symptom items (scored from 0 to 3) using ordinal logistic regression and for each of the three remaining items (scored 0/1) using logistic regression. For ease of interpretation, effect sizes were expressed as β coefficients for all models. Stata software (version 8.0, Stata Corp., College Station, TX) was used for all statistical analysis.

RESULTS

Patient and Family Characteristics

A total of 1,108 eligible patients were identified, of whom 67 (6 percent) were randomly selected for omission because of scheduling constraints. Of the remaining patients (n = 1,041), 345 (31 percent) were excluded because contact information for the patient's family was inadequate. Of family members who could be contacted (n = 696), 16 (2 percent) were excluded because they did not know enough about the patient's care, one (0.1 percent) because of hearing impairment, and one (0.1 percent) because the family member did not speak English. Of the remaining family members (n = 680), 524 completed an interview. Patients for whom an interview was completed are described in Table 21.1.

The response rate was 77 percent of all eligible family members with adequate contact information (524/680) and 50 percent of all eligible patient deaths (524/1,041). Most respondents were the patient's spouse or partner (265; 51 percent), child (135/524; 26 percent), sibling (65; 12 percent), or parent (24; 5 percent) and had a mean age of 63 (range 20–93). There was no difference between family members who consented and those who refused with respect to patient age, ethnicity, or use of a palliative care consultation.

Predictors of Consultation

Of the 524 patients in the sample, 296 (56 percent) received an inpatient palliative consultation in an acute care or long-term care setting. Most consultations occurred in the last weeks of life (mean and median fourteen days between consultation and death, interquartile range three to twenty-four days). There were several differences between

TABLE 21.1. **Patient Characteristics (N = 524)**

Patient Characteristic	All	Palliative Consultation (n = 296)	Usual Care (n = 228)	P-Value
Age, mean (range)	72 (26–100)	72 (27–93)	72 (26–100)	.62
Male, n (%)	513 (98)	292 (99)	221 (97)	.17
Ethnicity, n (%)				.59
White	395 (75)	227 (77)	168 (74)	
Nonwhite	126 (24)	69 (23)	57 (25)	
Previous hospitalization, n (%)	340 (65)	231 (78)	109 (48)	<.001
VA[a] facility, n (%)				<.001
1	72 (14)	26 (9)	46 (20)	
2	99 (19)	63 (21)	36 (16)	
3	76 (15)	31 (10)	45 (20)	
4	110 (21)	56 (19)	54 (24)	
5	167 (32)	120 (41)	47 (21)	
Site of death, n (%)				.12
Home	122 (23)	67 (23)	55 (24)	
VA nursing home	38 (7)	15 (5)	23 (10)	
VA acute care	318 (61)	185 (62)	133 (58)	
Other (non-VA inpatient)	46 (9)	29 (10)	17 (7)	
Diagnoses at the time of death, n (%)[b]				
Cancer	262 (50)	182 (61)	80 (35)	<.001
Heart failure	106 (20)	61 (21)	45 (20)	.81
Coronary artery disease	150 (29)	82 (28)	68 (30)	.59
Dementia	83 (16)	46 (16)	37 (16)	.83
Diabetes mellitus	162 (31)	79 (27)	83 (36)	.02
Human immunodeficiency virus or acquired immunodeficiency syndrome	8 (2)	4 (1)	4 (2)	.71
Presence of symptoms, n (%)				
Dyspnea	403 (77)	236 (80)	167 (73)	.27
Pain	424 (81)	251 (85)	173 (76)	.01
Confusion	344 (66)	216 (73)	128 (56)	<.001
Symptoms related to post-traumatic stress disorder	89 (17)	49 (17)	40 (18)	.71

[a]VA: Department of Veterans Affairs.
[b]Multiple diagnoses were coded for some patients.

patients who received a consultation and those who did not (Table 21.1), but families were similar with respect to age, ethnicity, and relationship to the patient.

In a multivariable logistic regression model, patients with cancer, patients who experienced an episode of confusion (per the family's report), and patients with a previous hospitalization were more likely to receive a consultation. Patients whose family members said that neither they nor the patient wanted emotional support from a health care provider were less likely to receive a consultation. Finally, there was significant intersite variability in the proportions of patients receiving a consultation (range of adjusted proportions: low, 0.34, 95 percent CI = 0.23–0.46; high, 0.74, 95 percent CI = 0.66–0.80).

This model had an acceptable fit (Hosmer-Lemeshow goodness-of-fit test Pearson $\chi^2 = 102$, with 107 covariate patterns; P = .35). The propensity score based on these variables had an ROC curve area of 0.82. This statistic indicates that the model's discrimination was high enough to allow balancing of the two groups but not so high (for example, >0.90) that the two groups were distinct.[25]

Consultation and Outcomes

In bivariate analysis, patients who received a consultation had significantly higher FATE scores than those who did not (64 versus 54; rank sum test P < .001). In a multivariable model that included consultation and the propensity score, ethnicity (white versus nonwhite) ($\beta = 0.053$; $P = .01$) and older age ($\beta = 0.02$; P = .001) were independently associated with higher FATE scores, so these variables were included in this and all subsequent models. Patients receiving a consultation had higher FATE scores after adjusting for the propensity score, age, and ethnicity (65, 95 percent CI = 62–66 versus 54, 95 percent CI = 51–56) (Table 21.2). This effect was significant for patients who died in the institution served by the palliative consultation team (n = 311; adjusted mean 65, 95 percent CI = 62–68 versus 56, 95 percent CI = 51–61; P < .001) and for those who died in other settings (n = 213; adjusted mean 61, 95 percent CI = 57–65 versus 51, 95 percent CI = 47–54; P < .001).

Patients who received a palliative consultation had significantly higher scores for five of the six domains: information and communication (P < .001), access to home care services (P = .007), emotional and spiritual support (P < .001), well-being and dignity (P = .001), and care around the time of death (P < .001) (Table 21.2). A trend toward higher scores for benefits and services provided to the family after the patient had died was not significant (P = .07) (Table 21.2). Scores for this domain showed a benefit of palliative consultations for patients who died in the facility served by the consultation team ($\beta = 0.10$; adjusted mean 67 versus 55; P = .047) but not for those who died in other settings ($\beta = 0.03$; adjusted mean 43 versus 45; P = .75).

In multivariable logistic regression models for single items, families of patients who received a consultation were more likely to say that the patient received all the treatment that he or she wanted (adjusted mean 76 versus 57; P < .001) and that the patient never received unwanted treatment (adjusted mean 84 versus 74; P = .002). Families were also more likely to say the patient was admitted to the inpatient facility that he or she would have chosen (adjusted mean 87 versus 79; P = .03) (Table 21.2).

TABLE 21.2. **Respondents' Perceptions of Care in the Last Month of Life**

Score	β Coefficient (95% Confidence Interval)[a]	Palliative Consultation Adjusted Score†	Usual Care Adjusted Score[b]	P-Value
Overall score	0.13 (0.09–0.17)	65	54	<.001
Domain scores				
Information and communication	0.17 (0.09–0.24)	67	56	<.001
Emotional and spiritual support	0.17 (0.09–0.25)	69	56	<.001
Care around the time of death	0.19 (0.14–0.24)	63	45	<.001
Access to benefits and services after the patient's death	0.07 (0.00–0.15)	61	52	.07
Access to home care services	0.09 (0.03–0.16)	72	64	.007
Well-being and dignity	0.14 (0.06–0.22)	65	52	<.001
Single-item scores				
Patient received the treatment he or she wanted	1.06 (0.60–1.51)	76	57	<.001
Patient never received unwanted treatment	0.77 (0.27–1.26)	82	74	.002
Patient was admitted to the facility of his or her choice	0.66 (0.07–1.24)	87	79	.03
Symptoms				
Pain	0.44 (0.02–0.86)	2.15	1.88	.04
Dyspnea	0.19 (−0.24–0.62)	1.03	0.87	.40
Confusion	0.35 (−0.13–0.83)	0.56	0.16	.17
Symptoms related to post-traumatic stress disorder	1.06 (0.15–1.98)	1.92	0.77	.02

[a]Linear regression models were used for the overall score and domain scores, logistic regression was used for dichotomous items, and ordinal logistic regression was used for symptom items. For all outcomes, β coefficients are presented for ease of interpretation.
[b]Higher scores indicate better outcomes. Adjusted for propensity score, patient age, and patient ethnicity.

To examine the effect of palliative consultation on symptoms, the full range of possible responses was used for each item (for example, the symptom "always," "most of the time," "sometimes," or "never" made the patient uncomfortable, scored from 0 to 3, respectively, with higher scores indicating better symptom management). In ordinal logistic regression models, adjusting for propensity score, age, and ethnicity, patients who received a consultation had better scores for pain (adjusted mean 2.15 versus 1.88; P = .04) and symptoms related to post-traumatic stress disorder (adjusted mean 1.92 versus 0.77; P = .02). There was no difference for confusion (adjusted mean 0.56 versus 0.16; P = .17) or dyspnea (adjusted mean 1.03 versus 0.87; P = .40) (Table 21.2).

Effect of Earlier Consultations

It was also desired to determine whether earlier palliative consultations were associated with better outcomes, so the time between consultation and death was calculated for patients who received a consultation (n = 296; 56 percent). In a multivariable regression model, time from consultation to death, site, and number of symptoms (possible range 0–4) were independently associated with better FATE scores (time: $\beta = 0.003$; P = .006). There was no evidence that any subgroup of patients (for example, according to age, diagnosis, or ethnicity) was more likely to benefit from earlier consultation. When domains and single items were examined as dependent variables, earlier consultations were associated with higher scores only for the communication ($\beta = 0.007$; P < .001) and the emotional support ($\beta = 0.007$; P < .001) domains.

DISCUSSION

Despite the rapid recent increase in the prevalence of inpatient palliative consultation teams, evidence to support their effect on outcomes has come from small, single-site studies of specific populations.[14,15] This study's results provide important evidence of the value of palliative care consultations across multiple settings. Three results in particular shed light on the value of palliative care consultation teams and should be useful in guiding future efforts to develop palliative care programs.

First, a clear effect of palliative consultation was found on families' perceptions of the care that patients received. This effect persisted after adjusting for predictors of receiving a consultation, as well as other confounders. The observed difference in adjusted scores (65 versus 54) indicates an 11 percent difference in the proportion of families who reported that a patient received the best possible care across all items. Moreover, a significant effect was found across almost all aspects of care. Together these results indicate that palliative care consultation services can improve the quality of end-of-life care.

Second, this study found that consultations may not improve all outcomes for all patients. For instance, an effect of consultations on families' perceptions of the benefits and services they received was found only if the patients died in the inpatient setting (hospital and nursing home) where the consultation service was located. Therefore, it is likely that a consultation service's effectiveness in this domain is limited to patients who die under its care.

Additionally, no effect of palliative consultations was found on dyspnea or confusion. This is surprising because management of these symptoms is an important part of palliative care.[1,2] It is possible that no effect was found because patients with more severe dyspnea or confusion were more likely to receive a consultation. This undetected referral bias would have led to greater symptom severity in patients who received a consultation, reducing the observed effectiveness of a palliative consultation. Although selective referral should also have reduced the observed effect of consultations on pain and symptoms related to post-traumatic stress disorder, it is possible that the effect of palliative care on these symptoms may have been large enough to overcome this source of bias. Further research is needed to define the effect of palliative consultations on symptoms and to define the mechanisms of that effect.

Third, this study provides novel evidence that earlier exposure to palliative consultations may be beneficial. Earlier consultations, and consequently more time between the initial consultation and the patient's death, were associated with better family perceptions of care as measured according to the overall FATE score. However, these results also suggest that benefits of earlier consultation may be most pronounced for communication and emotional support. This is not surprising, because one would expect a consultation team's effectiveness in these domains to depend on a close rapport with patients and families, which takes time to develop. Earlier consultations and potentially "case finding"[26] interventions may be particularly valuable for patients who need these services.

This study has two main limitations that should be noted. First, it was conducted in a VA population, whose demographic characteristics are atypical of the larger U.S. population, although it is reasonable to expect that palliative consultation teams outside the VA could have a similar effect on the outcomes reported here, assuming they have similar support and staffing.

Second, this study relied on families' perceptions of care rather than on direct assessments of patients' perceptions. However, retrospective surveys of family members have several important advantages over patient assessments. For instance, retrospective surveys can assess the care of patients whose prognosis is uncertain and who therefore might not be prospectively identified as "terminally ill." They also make it possible to examine the care of patients who are unable to respond to surveys or questionnaires, which is important because cognitive impairment is present in at least 50 percent of inpatients in the last weeks of life.[27] Retrospective surveys can also provide insights into the care that was delivered at the time of death, when prospective data collection from patients or families may be unacceptably intrusive. These surveys offer the only way to assess the care that is provided to the family after a patient's death. Therefore, although they should not be used as the sole source of data to evaluate outcomes, retrospective family surveys have been widely used to assess the quality of end-of-life care in a variety of health care settings.[27-34]

This study highlights the substantial benefits of palliative care consultations for patients near the end of life across virtually all domains of care. It also provides novel evidence of the potential effect of earlier consultations, particularly in improving communication and emotional support. Future research is needed to better understand the mechanisms and processes of care that contribute to consultations' effectiveness.

REFERENCES

1. *A National Framework and Preferred Practices for Palliative and Hospice Care Quality*. Washington, DC: National Quality Forum, 2006.

2. Clinical Practice Guidelines for Quality Palliative Care. National Consensus Project for Quality Palliative Care [on-line]. Available at http://www.nationalconsensusproject.org (accessed July 23, 2007).

3. Weissman DE. Consultation in palliative medicine. *Arch Intern Med*. 1997; 157:733–737.

4. Morrison RS, Maroney-Galin C, Kralovec PD et al. The growth of palliative care programs in United States hospitals. *J Palliat Med*. 2005; 8:1127–1134.

5. Abrahm JL, Callahan J, Rossetti K et al. The impact of a hospice consultation team on the care of veterans with advanced cancer. *J Pain Symptom Manage*. 1996; 12:23–31.

6. Bascom PB. A hospital-based comfort care team: Consultation for seriously ill and dying patients. *Am J Hosp Palliat Care*. 1997; 14:57–60.

7. Manfredi PL, Morrison RS, Morris J et al. Palliative care consultations: How do they impact the care of hospitalized patients? *J Pain Symptom Manage*. 2000; 20:166–173.

8. Bailey FA, Burgio KL, Woodby LL et al. Improving processes of hospital care during the last hours of life. *Arch Intern Med*. 2005; 165:1722–1727.

9. Kuin A, Courtens AM, Deliens L et al. Palliative care consultation in the Netherlands: A nationwide evaluation study. *J Pain Symptom Manage*. 2004; 27:53–60.

10. Penrod JD, Deb P, Luhrs C et al. Cost and utilization outcomes of patients receiving hospital-based palliative care consultation. *J Palliat Med*. 2006; 9:855–860.

11. Norton SA, Hogan LA, Holloway RG et al. Proactive palliative care in the medical intensive care unit: Effects on length of stay for selected high-risk patients. *Crit Care Med*. 2007; 35:1530–1535.

12. Elsayem A, Smith ML, Parmley L et al. Impact of a palliative care service on in-hospital mortality in a comprehensive cancer center. *J Palliat Med*. 2006; 9:894–902.

13. Smith TJ, Coyne P, Cassel B et al. A high-volume specialist palliative care unit and team may reduce in-hospital end-of-life care costs. *J Palliat Med*. 2003; 6:699–705.

14. Higginson I, Finlay I, Goodwin DM et al. Do hospital-based palliative care teams improve care for patients or families at the end of life? *J Pain Symptom Manage*. 2002; 23:96–106.

15. Higginson I, Finlay I, Goodwin DM et al. Is there evidence that palliative care teams alter end-of-life experiences of patients and their caregivers? *J Pain Symptom Manage*. 2003; 25:150–168.

16. Rabow MW, Dibble SL, Pantilat SZ et al. The comprehensive care team: A controlled trial of outpatient palliative medicine consultation. *Arch Intern Med*. 2004; 164:83–91.

17. Ringdal GI, Jordhoy MS, Kaasa S. Family satisfaction with end-of-life care for cancer patients in a cluster randomized trial. *J Pain Symptom Manage*. 2002; 24:53–63.

18. Casarett DJ, Pickard AP, Amos Bailey F et al. Important aspects of end-of-life care for veterans: Implications for measurement and quality improvement. *J Pain Symptom Manage*. 2007 Nov 27 [Epub ahead of print].

19. Casarett DJ, Pickard AP, Bailey FA et al. Preliminary results of a national system of quality measurement for end-of-life care. *J Palliat Med*, in press.

20. Nunnally JC. *Psychometric Theory*, 2nd Ed. New York: McGraw-Hill, 1978.

21. Rubin DB. Estimating causal effects from large data sets using propensity scores. *Ann Intern Med*. 1997; 127 (8 Part 2):757–763.

22. Rosenbaum PR, Rubin DB. The central role of the propensity score in observational studies for causal effects. *Biometrika*. 1983; 70:41–55.

23. Mickey J, Greenland S. A study of the impact of confounder-selection criteria on effect estimation. *Am J Epidemiol*. 1989; 129:125–137.

24. Hosmer DW, Lemeshow S. *Applied Logistic Regression*. New York: John Wiley and Sons, 1989.

25. Weitzen S, Lapane KL, Toledano AY et al. Principles for modeling propensity scores in medical research: A systematic literature review. *Pharmacoepidemiol Drug Safety*. 2004; 13:841–853.

26. Rosenfeld K, Rasmussen J. Palliative care management: A Veterans Administration demonstration project. *J Palliat Med*. 2003; 6:831–839.

27. Lynn J, Teno JM, Phillips RS et al. Perceptions by family members of the dying experience of older and seriously ill patients. SUPPORT investigators. *Ann Intern Med*. 1997; 126:97–106.

28. Baker R, Wu AW, Teno JM et al. Family satisfaction with end-of-life care in seriously ill hospitalized adults. *J Am Geriatr Soc*. 2000; 48:S61– S69.

29. Patrick DL, Engelberg RA, Curtis JR. Evaluating the quality of dying and death. *J Pain Symptom Manage*. 2001; 22:717–726.

30. Tolle SW, Tilden VP, Rosenfeld AG et al. Family reports of barriers to optimal care of the dying. *Nursing Res*. 2000; 49:310–317.

31. Somogyi-Zalud E, Zhong Z, Lynn J. Elderly persons' last six months of life: Findings from the hospitalized elderly longitudinal project. *J Am Geriatr Soc*. 2000; 48:S131– S139.

32. Hanson L, Danis M, Garrett J. What is wrong with end-of-life care? Opinions of bereaved family members. *J Am Geriatr Soc*. 1997; 45:1339–1344.

33. Connor SR, Tecca M, LundPerson J et al. Measuring hospice care: The national hospice and palliative care organization national hospice data set. *J Pain Symptom Manage*. 2004; 28:316–328.

34. Teno J, Clarridge B, Casey V et al. Family perspectives on end-of-life care at the last place of care. *JAMA*. 2004; 291:88–93.

ACKNOWLEDGMENTS

The views expressed here are those of the authors and do not represent the official position of the Department of Veterans Affairs.

CONFLICT OF INTEREST

The editor in chief has reviewed the conflict of interest checklist provided by the author and has determined that none of the authors have any financial or any other kind of personal conflicts with this article.

AUTHOR CONTRIBUTIONS

All listed authors made substantial contributions to the concept and design of the manuscript, acquisition and analysis of data, drafting and revision of the manuscript, and all approved the final version to be published.

SPONSOR'S ROLE

N/A.

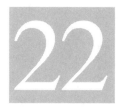

COST SAVINGS ASSOCIATED WITH U.S. HOSPITAL PALLIATIVE CARE CONSULTATION PROGRAMS

R. SEAN MORRISON, M.D., JOAN D. PENROD, PH.D., J. BRIAN CASSEL, PH.D., MELISSA CAUST-ELLENBOGEN, M.S., ANN LITKE, M.F.A., LYNN SPRAGENS, M.B.A., AND DIANE E. MEIER, M.D. FOR THE PALLIATIVE CARE LEADERSHIP CENTERS' OUTCOMES GROUP

Morrison RS, Penrod JD, Cassel JB, Caust-Ellenbogen M, Litke, A, Spragens L, Meier DE, for the Palliative Care Leadership Centers' Outcomes Group. Cost savings associated with United States hospital palliative care consultation programs. *Arch Intern Med.* 2008;168(16):1783–1790. Copyright © 2008, American Medical Association. All rights reserved. Reprinted with permission.

EDITORS' INTRODUCTION

Working with eight well-established hospital palliative care programs at a range of different hospital types and settings, this study found substantial cost savings among seriously ill patients receiving palliative care, as compared to similar patients getting "usual" care. Since 10 percent of patients with serious and complex illness drive 70 percent of health care costs in the United States, this evidence of more efficient and rational use of costly health care services associated with palliative care has major implications for health care reform.

■ ■ ■

Advances in disease prevention, disease-modifying therapies, and medical technology in combination with the aging of the population have resulted in a dramatic growth in the number of adults living with serious illness.[1] Despite enormous expenditures, patients with serious illness receive poor-quality medical care, characterized by untreated symptoms, unmet personal care needs, high caregiver burden, and low patient and family satisfaction.[2]

Palliative care is the interdisciplinary specialty that focuses on improving quality of life for patients with advanced illness and for their families through pain and symptom management, communication and support for medical decisions concordant with goals of care, and assurance of safe transitions between care settings.[3] Until a decade ago, palliative care in the United States was typically available only to patients living at home and enrolled in hospice. Now, palliative care programs targeting acutely ill patients are found increasingly in hospitals. As of 2005, 30 percent of U.S. hospitals and 70 percent of hospitals with more than 250 beds reported the presence of a palliative care program—an increase of 96 percent from 2000.[4] Unlike hospice, hospital palliative care is provided simultaneously with all other appropriate disease-directed treatments.[3]

Hospital palliative care programs have been shown to improve physical and psychological symptom management, caregiver well-being, and family satisfaction,[2,5-9] and small, single-site studies suggest that palliative care programs may reduce hospital and intensive care unit (ICU) expenditures by clarifying goals of care and assisting patients and families to select treatments that meet those goals.[10-15] This study was undertaken to estimate the effect of palliative care consultation programs on hospital costs.

METHODS

We used hospital administrative data to compare hospital costs of patients receiving palliative care consultation matched by propensity score[16-18] with patients receiving usual care from 2002 through 2004.

Sample

Eight geographically and structurally diverse hospitals representing low-, middle-, and high-cost markets served by six mature palliative care consultation teams (one team served three hospitals) were included (Table 22.1). For the main analyses, the patient sample included all patients eighteen years or older who had lengths of stay of seven to thirty days. We excluded patients with short lengths of stay because these patients were unlikely to receive palliative care consultation. Patients with lengths of stay of more than thirty days were excluded because they represented outliers that were unlikely to be generalizable. Patients receiving palliative care were identified through the palliative care consultation teams' administrative databases and billing records. The initial sample included 43,973 patients discharged alive and 4,726 patients who died in hospital.

Patient Factors

We used hospital databases to abstract patient characteristics. Medical comorbidities were determined using the Elixhauser algorithm that includes thirty categories of comorbid illnesses identified by secondary diagnosis codes and discharge diagnosis-related groups.[19]

Costs

Costs were abstracted from the hospitals' cost accounting systems. Each hospital used the same system, TSI (Transitions Systems, Inc., Boston, Massachusetts). TSI tracks all hospital resources and assigns cost (not charge) values to these resources. These estimates are based on direct acquisition costs for supplies and time-and-motion studies for labor costs.[20] Various procedures are also used to determine the proportion of other costs, such as plant costs (for example, lighting and heating), that should be applied to each resource. This approach is generally considered the most accurate method to estimate costs.[20] We abstracted direct and total costs for each subject for each hospital day and for the entire admission. Direct costs are costs that can be directly attributable to medications, procedures, or services. Indirect costs are the general costs of running a hospital that are not directly related to the test or service. Total costs are the sum of direct and indirect costs. We used Uniform Billing 92 codes to aggregate direct costs into specific categories that included the following: ICU, pharmacy and intravenous therapy, laboratory, and diagnostic imaging costs.[21] All costs were converted into 2004 U.S. dollars.

TABLE 22.1. Characteristics and Structures of Study Sites and Palliative Care Teams[a]

Variable	Hospital[b]							
	A	B	C	D	E	F	G	H
Hospital type	Com	Com	Acd	Com	Com	Com	Acd	Acd
No. of hospital beds	348	807	434	330	220	336	574	976
No. of admissions, y								
2002	13,342	27,379	19,921	17,645	14,916	22,463	20,302	38,849
2003	13,043	27,532	21,012	18,648	16,764	22,229	20,481	39,521
2004	12,905	27,423	22,564	22,618	19,280	20,787	22,096	40,730
No. of deaths, y								
2002	474	438	557	613	313	682	549	1,082
2003	406	397	547	614	351	691	527	1,063
2004	372	398	570	709	430	584	547	1,060
No. of Medicare admissions, y								
2002	7,871	6,078	6,693	5,927	2,958	6,593	7,308	15,153
2003	7,434	6,042	7,144	6,434	3,557	6,631	7,351	16,055
2004	7,355	6,158	7,672	7,542	3,961	6,202	7,950	16,815
Palliative care consultation team composition								
	1.0 MD	2.0 MD	3.0 MD	1.0 MD	1.0 MD	1.0 MD	1.0 MD	2.0 MD
	1.0 RN	1.5 ANP	3.0 RN	1.0 ANP	1.0 RNC	1.0 RNC	0.1 RN	2.0 NP
	1.0 SW	0.5 SW	1.0 Psych	0.1 SW	0.6 NP	0.1 SW	1.0 SW	1.0 SW
	1.0 Chapl	1.0 Chapl	3.0 MD		0.1 SW		0.1 PharmD	
							0.3 Chapl	

[a]Abbreviations: Acd, academic medical center; ANP, adult nurse practitioner; Chapl, chaplain; Com, community hospital; MD, doctor of medicine; Psych, psychologist; NP, nurse practitioner; PharmD, doctor of pharmacy; RN, registered nurse; RNC, registered nurse clinician; SW, social worker.
[b]A, Central Baptist Hospital, Lexington, Kentucky; B, University of Minnesota Medical Center, Fairview, Minneapolis; C, Froedtert Hospital, Milwaukee, Wisconsin; D, Mount Carmel Hospital East, Columbus, Ohio; E, Mount Carmel Hospital West, Columbus; F, Mount Carmel St Ann's Hospital, Columbus; G, UCSF Medical Center, San Francisco, California; H, Mount Sinai Hospital, New York, New York.

Analyses

Subjects were stratified by hospital site and then within each hospital into two strata comprising live discharges and hospital deaths. We computed propensity scores for each subject within each stratum.[16–18,22] Propensity scores were determined by regressing whether patients received palliative care consultation on all patient characteristics present at hospital admission listed in the hospital databases. These variables included patient age, sex, marital status, medical insurance, primary diagnosis, attending physician specialty, and Elixhauser comorbidity score. Within each stratum we matched each patient receiving palliative care consultation with one or more usual care patients whose logit of their propensity score was within ±0.05 standard deviations of the logit of the palliative care patient's score. Unmatched patients were excluded, and all subsequent analyses included matched live discharges and matched hospital deaths.

Bivariate comparisons of unadjusted per diem costs and patient demographics were examined using unpaired t tests and χ^2 tests as appropriate. Usual care patients' data were weighted to account for the one-to-many propensity score matching algorithm. Generalized linear models (GLMs) using normalized weighted data were estimated for total and direct costs per hospital admission and hospital day. In addition, we estimated GLMs for pharmacy, diagnostic imaging, laboratory test, and ICU direct costs for all usual care patients admitted to an ICU and for patients receiving palliative care consultation prior to ICU discharge. The GLMs were specified as having a gamma distribution and log link.[23,24] The dependent variable was cost, and the independent variables included patient age, principal diagnosis, comorbidity score, palliative care team, attending physician specialty, marital status, insurance type, hospital discharge site for live discharges, and the key independent variable, whether the patient received palliative care consultation. Each cost model was adjusted for clustering by hospital. The GLM was used to examine the effects of palliative care consultation on hospital length of stay in days, controlling for the aforementioned covariates.

Additional Confirmatory Analyses

We performed two additional confirmatory analyses. We matched usual care and palliative care patients by intensity of medical services before palliative care consultation to confirm that the palliative care and usual care groups were well matched. This analysis was performed by developing propensity scores using mean direct daily costs before consultation (palliative care patients) and before a corresponding reference day (usual care) as a regressor in the propensity score models. The reference day for usual care patients was hospital day six for patients with lengths of stay of ten days or less, day ten for those with lengths of stay of eleven to twenty days, and day eighteen for those with lengths of stay longer than twenty days. These reference days represented the average day of consultation for palliative care patients for lengths of stay within these three categories. The GLMs were used to estimate costs for the usual care and palliative care patients.

We also used the GLM to model costs up to the day before consultation for palliative care patients. We then used these models to predict hypothetical costs in the absence of a palliative care consultation for the remaining length of stay, assuming that the slope of the cost curves remained constant, as was actually observed for usual care patients. We compared these predicted costs to actual costs for palliative care patients.

All analyses were performed with Stata version 9.2 statistical software (StataCorp, College Station, Texas), and this study was approved by the institutional review boards of all sites.

RESULTS

Of the 2,966 patients who received palliative care consultation and who were discharged alive, 2,630 (89 percent) were matched to 18,427 usual care patients discharged alive, and of the 2,388 palliative care patients who died in hospital, 2,278 (95 percent) were matched to 2,124 usual care patients who died in hospital (Table 22.2 and Table 22.3). There were no statistically significant differences in length of stay between usual care and palliative care patients discharged alive (12.4 versus 13.1 days; $P = .12$) and those who died in hospital (13.9 versus 14.1 days; $P = .40$).

Costs for Patients Discharged Alive

Patients receiving palliative care consultation had significantly lower costs than usual care patients. For patients discharged alive, palliative care consultation was associated with adjusted net savings in total costs of $2,642 per admission ($P = .02$) and $279 per day ($P < .001$) compared with usual care. Adjusted net savings in direct costs associated with palliative care were $1,696 per admission ($P = .004$) and $174 per day ($P < .001$). These savings included significant reductions in laboratory costs ($424 per admission; $P < .001$) and ICU costs ($5,178 per ICU admission; $P < .001$) (Table 22.4). Including outlier patients—those with lengths of stay less than seven days and longer than thirty days—resulted in reductions in direct costs per day of $275 and $246, respectively, favoring palliative care.

Costs for Patients Who Died in Hospital

For patients who died in hospital, palliative care consultation was associated with adjusted net savings in total costs of $6,896 per admission ($P = .001$) and $549 per day ($P < .001$). Adjusted net savings in direct costs were $4,908 per admission ($P = .003$) and $374 per day ($P < .001$). These reductions in direct costs included significant reductions in pharmacy costs ($1,544 per admission; $P = .04$), laboratory tests ($926 per admission; $P < .001$), and ICU costs ($6,613 per ICU admission; $P < .001$) (Table 22.4). Including outlier patients—those with lengths of stay less than seven days and longer than thirty days—resulted in reductions in direct costs per day of $559 and $370, respectively, favoring palliative care.

TABLE 22.2. Demographics and Characteristics of Patients Discharged Alive from the Hospital[a]

Variable	Weighted Value			Nonweighted Value
	Usual Care Patients (n = 18,427)	Matched Palliative Care Patients (n = 2,630)	P Value	Unmatched Palliative Care Patients (n = 306)
Age, mean (range), y	68.07 (18-106)	68.2 (18-104)	.78	71.2 (18-99)
Men, %	41.8	41.19	.90	47.1
Married, %	42.0	41.7	.52	41.3
Insurance, %				
Medicare	69.4	69.4		73.9
Medicaid	9.7	11.2		7.8
Managed care	16.4	15.7	.21	14.2
Indemnity plan	3.2	2.4		1.0
Other	1.4	1.3		3.2
Principal diagnosis, %				
Cancer	28.4	28.9		36.8
Infection	4.4	4.3		3.3
Cardiovascular	18.9	18.6		17.8
Pulmonary	15.8	15.4	.90	16.8
Gastrointestinal	6.7	7.2		6.2
Genitourinary	4.4	3.8		4.1
Other	21.4	21.9		15.2
Comorbidities, mean (range), No.	2.6 (0-10)	2.6 (0-11)	.86	3.0 (0-9)
Physician specialty, %				
Internal medicine	69.4	67.0		74.2
Oncology	12.7	14.9		13.9
Surgery	12.7	12.9	.96	7.7
Other	5.2	5.2		4.3
Admitted to ICU, %	38.6	37.5	.43	50.3
Discharge destination, %				
Home	67.4	56.3		58.2
Nursing home	25.7	38.1	<.001	37.5
Other	6.9	5.6		4.3
Hospital, %[b]				
Hospital A	12.6	12.6		3.4
Hospital B	6.8	6.8		1.7
Hospital C	13.0	13.0		5.3
Hospital D	14.3	14.3	.99	85.6
Hospital E	18.2	18.3		1.3
Hospital F	9.3	9.3		1.4
Hospital G	2.3	2.3		0.7
Hospital H	23.5	23.5		0.5
Days receiving palliative care, mean (range)	NA	6.5 (1-29)	NA	7.2 (1-28)

[a]Abbreviations: ICU, intensive care unit; NA, not applicable.
[b]For a description of hospitals, see Table 22.1, note a.

TABLE 22.3. **Demographics and Characteristics of Patients Who Died in the Hospital**

| Variable | Weighted Value | | *P* Value | Nonweighted Value |
	Usual Care Patients (n = 2,124)	Matched Palliative Care Patients (n = 2,278)		Unmatched Palliative Care Patients (n = 110)
Age, mean (range), y	71.7 (18-103)	71.6 (19-104)	.82	68.8 (19-100)
Men, %	48.4	48.1	.79	47.1
Married, %	43.9	44.0	.97	50.0
Insurance, %				
Medicare	74.9	75.6		69.0
Medicaid	8.6	8.4		7.3
Managed care	12.6	12.2	.99	7.3
Indemnity plan	2.8	2.8		4.4
Other	1.0	1.0		11.8
Principal diagnosis, %				
Cancer	19.3	19.0		23.5
Infection	11.5	11.3		2.0
Cardiovascular	24.8	24.3		27.9
Pulmonary	17.6	18.3	.99	16.0
Gastrointestinal	9.0	9.0		8.8
Genitourinary	3.7	3.9		4.4
Other	14.2	14.2		16.1
Comorbidities, mean (range), No.	2.9 (0-9)	2.9 (0-10)	.98	2.5 (0-7)
Physician specialty, %				
Internal medicine	74.8	74.8		32.0
Oncology	8.8	8.8		10.0
Surgery	13.2	13.0	.96	8.0
Other	3.2	3.4		50.0
Admitted to ICU, %	74.2	68.3	<.001	60
Hospital, %[b]				
Hospital A	5.4	5.4		0
Hospital B	3.0	3.0		4.4
Hospital C	11.4	11.4		11.8
Hospital D	19.7	19.7	.99	39.7
Hospital E	18.0	18.0		20.6
Hospital F	11.1	11.1		5.9
Hospital G	10.1	10.0		5.9
Hospital H	21.3	21.3		11.8
Days receiving palliative care, mean (range)	NA	4.8 (1-28)	NA	3.9 (0-15)

[a]Abbreviations: ICU, intensive care unit; NA, not applicable.
[b]For a description of hospitals, see Table 22.1, note a.

TABLE 22.4. Adjusted Costs for Live Discharges and Hospital Deaths[a]

Cost	Live Discharges				Hospital Deaths			
	Usual Care (95% CI), $	Palliative Care (95% CI), $	Net Δ	P Value	Usual Care (95% CI), $	Palliative Care (95% CI), $	Net Δ	P Value
Total costs admission	19,379 (18,984-19,773)	16,737 (15,546-17,927)	-2,642	.02	37,391 (34,952-39,830)	30,494 (28,414-32,575)	-6,896	.001
Total costs per day	1,450 (1,430-1,470)	1,171 (1,082-1,260)	-279	<.001	2,468 (2,332-2,603)	1,918 (1,787-2,050)	-549	<.001
Direct costs per admission	11,140 (10,884-11,395)	9,445 (8,761-10,126)	-1,696	.004	22,674 (20,871-24,477)	17,765 (16,201-19,330)	-4,908	.003
Direct costs per day	830 (815-846)	656 (588-723)	-174	<.001	1484 (1391-1577)	1,110 (1,029-1,191)	-374	<.001
Laboratory costs	1,227 (1,185-1,268)	803 (712-893)	-424	<.001	2,765 (2,443-3,086)	1,838 (1,588-2,088)	-926	<.001
ICU costs	7,096 (5,801-8,390)	1,917 (1,646-2,187)	-5,178	<.001	14,542 (13,685-15,399)	7,929 (7,181-8,676)	-6,613	<.001
Pharmacy costs	2,190 (2,116-2,265)	2,001 (1,821-2,180)	-190	.12	5,625 (4,890-6,361)	4,081 (3,530-4,632)	-1,544	.04
Imaging costs	890 (868-913)	949 (884-1,014)	58	.52	1,673 (1,563-1782)	1,540 (1,433-1,646)	-133	.21

[a]Abbreviations: CI, confidence interval; ICU, intensive care unit.

Confirmatory Analyses

Including mean cost per day before palliative care consultation and before the reference day for usual care subjects in the propensity score models as a surrogate for intensity of medical services resulted in qualitatively similar results (that is, the parameter estimates were contained within the 95 percent confidence intervals of the estimates of the primary analyses) across all major cost categories, albeit with fewer matched subjects (78 percent of palliative care patients discharged alive could be matched to a usual care patient, and 92 percent of palliative care patients who died could be matched to a usual care patient).

Figure 22.1 displays mean daily direct costs for live discharges and hospital deaths. For palliative care patients, we plotted the six days before and after palliative care consultation (day zero). For usual care patients, day six was the reference day established for the confirmatory analyses previously described. There were no significant differences observed between the cost curves' slopes or the mean daily direct costs for palliative care and matched usual care groups before the day of consultation (palliative care patients) or the reference day (usual care patients). Whereas the slope of the usual care cost curve approached zero following the reference day, palliative care consultation was associated with a significant reduction in hospital costs twenty-four to forty-eight hours after consultation. For patients discharged alive (Figure 22.1A), mean direct costs per day decreased from $843 for the forty-eight hours before palliative care consultation to $605 for the forty-eight hours after consultation ($P = .001$) and from $1,163 for the forty-eight hours before consultation to $589 for the forty-eight hours after consultation ($P = .003$) for patients who died (Figure 22.1B).

We projected what the adjusted direct costs per admission for palliative care patients would have been if they had not received palliative care consultation. Projected direct costs per admission were $11,787 for patients discharged alive and $22,301 for patients who died in hospital. These projected costs were not significantly different from the costs actually observed in the usual care group ($11,140 [$P = .26$] for live discharges and $22,674 [$P = .44$] for deceased patients).

Finally, to explore the question of whether the recommendations of the palliative care consultation teams reduced hospital costs or were simply a marker of changes in treatment plans already implemented by the primary care team, we plotted mean direct costs for each day of admission for usual care patients and for patients receiving palliative care consultation on hospital days seven, ten, and fifteen for patients who died (Figure 22.2). Costs for patients who received palliative care were no different from those in the usual care group until twenty-four to forty-eight hours after palliative care consultation, at which time costs in the palliative care group started to decrease. A similar pattern was observed for patients discharged alive (data not shown).

COMMENT

Studies have consistently demonstrated that patients with life-threatening illness experience untreated pain and other symptoms, lengthy hospitalizations involving unwanted, often low-yield and costly medical treatments, and low overall family

FIGURE 22.1.

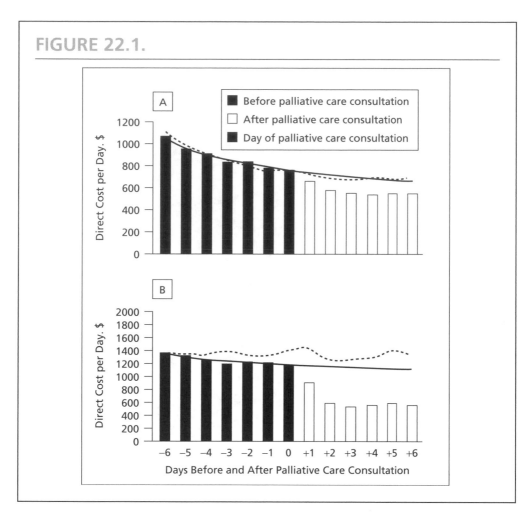

Mean direct costs per day for palliative care patients who were discharged alive (A) or died (B) before and after palliative care consultation. The solid line represents the regression curve of actual costs before palliative care consultation (day0) and estimated costs (days 1-6) assuming that palliative care consultation had not occurred. The dashed line represents direct costs per day for usual care patients for the 6 days before and after hospital day 6 (patients with lengths of stay ≤ 10 days), hospital day 10 (for patients with lengths of stay of 11-20 days), or hospital day 18 (for patients with lengths of stay of >20 days).

satisfaction.[2,9,25–27] Hospital palliative care consultation programs have been associated with reductions in symptoms and higher family satisfaction with overall care, and greater emotional support as compared with usual care.[2,6,28,29] Although others have postulated that palliative care programs could substantially reduce hospital costs,[26,30] this study is the first, to our knowledge, to empirically evaluate the actual effect of palliative care on U.S. hospital costs, using a sample size sufficient to assure reliable results, using propensity-score–matched control patients, and enrolling patients from eight diverse hospitals serving low-, medium-, and high-cost markets, thus enhancing

FIGURE 22.2.

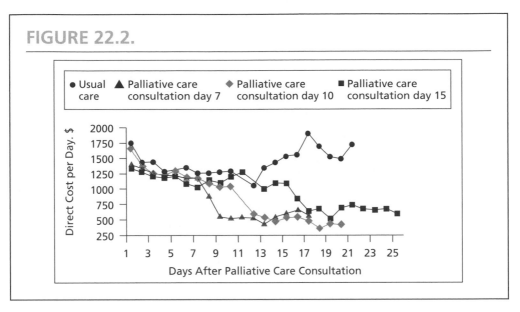

Mean direct costs per day for patients who died and who received palliative care Consultation on hospital days 7, 10, and 15 compared with mean direct cost for usual care patients matched by propensity score. Hospital day 1 is the first full day after the day of admission.

the generalizability of our results. Our finding that palliative care consultation is associated with significant reductions in hospital costs has important implications for hospitals and policy makers.

Other Factors That Could Account for the Observed Savings

It is possible that the cost saving observed might have occurred spontaneously without the palliative care consultation team's intervention, due to unmeasured confounding variables that we were unable to obtain from administrative data. Specifically, it is possible that before the palliative care consultation, physicians recommended and patients agreed to forgo some therapies and that the palliative care team enacted a previously decided-on care plan. Data suggest that this is unlikely. Although this study was a retrospective analysis, three of the participating palliative care teams have reported that most palliative care consultations are requested to help address goals of care and to discuss with patients all treatment options, including that of forgoing treatments that will not meet their goals or prolong life in a meaningful fashion.[12,31,32] Other studies lend credence to this argument. The Study to Understand Prognoses and Preferences for Outcomes and Risks of Treatments (SUPPORT), which included more than nine thousand seriously ill adults, demonstrated that patient preferences and physicians' knowledge of patients' preferences and prognoses did not have a measurable effect on hospital costs and treatments.[25]

Our data suggest that it was the actions of the palliative care teams that resulted in cost reductions. First, we found no significant differences in the palliative care and usual care groups across all observable patient characteristics, suggesting that the two groups were well matched. Second, as shown in Figure 22.1 and Figure 22.2, the decrease in costs consistently occurred forty-eight hours after consultation—no matter when the consultation occurred—and no corresponding decline was observed in the usual care group at any point in their hospital stay. If palliative care was only a marker for change, we would have expected the cost curves to drop before or at the time of consultation rather than be delayed for forty-eight hours, as was observed. Finally, our confirmatory analyses replicated our main findings. Specifically, including mean cost per day before palliative care consultation or the equivalent reference day for usual care patients as a surrogate for intensity of medical services in the propensity score analyses resulted in almost identical results. A comparison of the actual costs for palliative care patients after palliative care consultation with estimated costs in the case that palliative care consultation had hypothetically not occurred also resulted in almost identical savings.

What Accounts for the Cost Savings?

While it may appear self-evident that discontinuing costly nonbeneficial interventions among seriously ill patients reduces hospital costs, such a fundamental shift in the usual hospital care pathway is neither a simple nor straightforward process, given the highly patterned treatment culture of the U.S. hospital, which is structured to prolong life and avert death at all costs. In this context, the fact that palliative care consultation appeared to consistently influence this process is an important finding. Indeed, prior studies have definitively demonstrated that even when seriously ill patients' preferences for treatments focused solely on comfort are documented and known by their physicians, these patients continue to receive low-yield, burdensome, and high-cost tests and treatments, including prolonged ICU stays—a probable result of highly ingrained physician and hospital practice patterns and prevailing hospital culture.[25] Our data suggest that palliative care consultation fundamentally shifts the course of care off the usual hospital pathway and, in doing so, significantly reduces costs. This shift is likely accomplished by establishing clear treatment goals, reviewing current treatments to establish their concordance with these goals, and recommending and legitimizing discontinuation of treatments or tests that do not meet established goals.

Relationship to Other Studies

Our data confirm and extend previously published small single-site studies. Two studies performed at Department of Veterans Affairs (VA) medical centers reported reduced health care utilization and costs associated with palliative care programs.[10, 11] Outside the VA, Cowan[33] reported reduced charges associated with a palliative care consultation team in a community hospital; Elsayem and colleagues[13] reported reduced charges associated with a palliative care inpatient unit in a cancer hospital; and Campbell and Frank[34] and Norton and colleagues[14] demonstrated reductions in ICU resource utilization associated with an ICU-based palliative care team. Two single-site studies have looked at non-VA overall hospital costs. Smith and colleagues[12] found significantly lower costs for patients who died in an inpatient palliative care unit, compared with matched controls who died in other hospital units, and Ciemens and colleagues[15] observed similar findings associated with a palliative care consultation service.

Our study has several strengths compared with these studies. We included data from eight geographically and structurally diverse hospitals but with similarly structured palliative care consultation teams—now the standard of palliative care practice in U.S. hospitals—thus enhancing the generalizability of our results. Prior studies used highly variable models of care and interventions that are neither comparable nor replicable. We used hospital costs rather than charges and thus our results reflect true rather than estimated savings. Finally, our estimates of savings per day may be conservative because the main analyses did not include patients with a length of stay longer than thirty days. The inclusion of outliers resulted in even greater savings.

Implications

Our results provide strong fiscal incentives for hospitals and policy makers to develop or expand palliative care consultation programs—programs that have already been demonstrated to improve quality and patient and family satisfaction. The most medically complex patients, such as the patients enrolled in this study, account for a growing proportion of admissions, bed days, and use of hospital resources. The median operating margin for a hospital is 2 percent ($27–$40 per day);[35] thus the $174-per-day savings in direct costs for live discharges associated with palliative care consultation in this study could have a significant impact on hospital performance, particularly as the proportion of older, complex, and chronically ill admissions increases over the coming years. Whether a hospital is paid on a diagnosis-related group or a per diem basis, they benefit from the lower costs. As the proportion of discounted-fee-for-service patients continues to dwindle, this is of increasing importance.[36]

Hospital palliative care programs are also likely to help reduce Medicare expenditures. Five percent of Medicare enrollees with the most serious illness account for over 43 percent of Medicare expenditures, with the top 25 percent of enrollees accounting for 85 percent of the costs.[37] Three-quarters of these 25 percent of "highest cost" enrollees have at least one hospital admission per year, and approximately 60 percent of total Medicare health care expenditures are for hospital care.[37,38] Expansion of palliative care consultation programs to adequately serve the complex patient base of hospitals reduces cost pressures between hospitals and Medicare. Discharge orders and care plans resulting from palliative care consultations may also reduce ongoing care costs in the outpatient arena.

Limitations

This was not a randomized trial, and it is possible that the cost differences resulted from unmeasured differences between the two groups. We used several design and analytic measures to limit bias and confounding. First, we included subjects with a defined length of stay, to eliminate the effects of outliers. Second, we stratified our sample both by site and by vital status prior to propensity score matching, to minimize unobserved confounders. Third, we used propensity score methods to match patients based on patient characteristics, to balance observed covariates, and cannot draw conclusions about unmatched patients. However, the numbers of unmatched palliative care patients were relatively small (11 percent of patients discharged alive and 5 percent of patients who died). Finally, we used appropriate multivariable techniques to control for nonpatient-based characteristics. Thus, although possible, we believe that it is unlikely that the magnitude of the effects noted here could be due to persistent unobserved confounders such as patient or physician preferences. Specifically, if patient preferences or another unmeasured variable were confounding our results, the parameter estimate would need to be several orders of magnitude larger than that observed in SUPPORT for us to have obtained these results, given the effects sizes observed in our models.[25]

CONCLUSIONS

This study found that palliative care consultation was associated with a reduction in direct hospital costs of almost $1,700 per admission ($174 per day) for live discharges and of almost $5,000 per admission ($374 per day) for patients who died. For an average 400-bed hospital containing an interdisciplinary palliative care team seeing 500 patients a year (300 live discharges and 200 hospital deaths), these figures translate into a net savings of $1.3 million per year, after adding physician revenues ($240,000) and subtracting personnel costs ($418,000).[39] This study adds to the growing literature on the benefits of palliative care consultation by demonstrating that, in addition to improved clinical care and patient, family, and physician satisfaction, these programs are associated with considerable reductions in hospital costs. The growth of the number of adults living with advanced and complex chronic illnesses, the documented inadequacies in care quality, and the increases in expenditures highlight the need for efficient models, such as palliative care consultation teams, that deliver quality services to complex patient populations.

REFERENCES

1. Field MJ, Cassel CK, eds. *Approaching Death: Improving Care at the End of Life*. Washington, DC: National Academy Press; 1997.

2. Teno JM, Clarridge BR, Casey V, et al. Family perspectives on end-of-life care at the last place of care. *JAMA*. 2004; 291(1):88–93.

3. Morrison RS, Meier DE. Clinical practice: palliative care. *N Engl J Med*. 2004; 350 (25):2582–2590.

4. American Hospital Association. *AHA Hospital Statistics*. Chicago, IL: American Hospital Association; 2007.

5. Higginson IJ, Finlay IG, Goodwin DM, et al. Is there evidence that palliative care teams alter end-of-life experiences of patients and their caregivers? *J Pain Symptom Manage*. 2003; 25(2):150–168.

6. Jordhøy MS, Fayers P, Loge JH, Ahlner-Elmqvist M, Kaasa S. Quality of life in palliative cancer care: results from a cluster randomized trial. *J Clin Oncol*. 2001; 19(18):3884–3894.

7. Ringdal GI, Jordhøy MS, Kaasa S. Family satisfaction with end-of-life care for cancer patients in a cluster randomized trial. *J Pain Symptom Manage*. 2002; 24(1):53–63.

8. Christakis NA, Iwashyna TJ. The health impact of health care on families: a matched cohort study of hospice use by decedents and mortality outcomes in surviving, widowed spouses. *Soc Sci Med*. 2003; 57(3):465–475.

9. Casarett D, Pickard A, Bailey A, et al. Do palliative consultations improve patient outcomes? *J Am Geriatr Soc*. 2008; 56(4):593–599.

10. Back AL, Li Y-F, Sales AE. Impact of palliative care case management on resource use by patients dying of cancer at a Veterans Affairs medical center. *J Palliat Med*. 2005; 8(1):26–35.

11. Penrod JD, Deb P, Luhrs C, et al. Cost and utilization outcomes of patients receiving hospital-based palliative care consultation. *J Palliat Med*. 2006; 9(4):855– 860.

12. Smith TJ, Coyne P, Cassel B, Penberthy L, Hopson A, Hager MA. A high-volume specialist palliative care unit and team may reduce in-hospital end-of-life care costs. *J Palliat Med*. 2003; 6(5):699–705.

13. Elsayem A, Swint K, Fisch MJ, et al. Palliative care inpatient service in a comprehensive cancer center: clinical and financial outcomes. *J Clin Oncol*. 2004; 22(10):2008–2014.

14. Norton SA, Hogan LA, Holloway RG, Temkin-Greener H, Buckley MJ, Quill TE. Proactive palliative care in the medical intensive care unit: effects on length of stay for selected high-risk patients. *Crit Care Med*. 2007; 35(6):1530–1535.

15. Ciemins EL, Blum L, Nunley M, Lasher A, Newman JM. The economic and clinical impact of an inpatient palliative care consultation service: a multifaceted approach. *J Palliat Med*. 2007; 10(6):1347–1355.

16. Rubin DB. Estimating causal effects from large data sets using propensity scores. *Ann Intern Med*. 1997; 127(8, pt 2):757–763.

17. Rubin DB. Using propensity scores to help design observational studies: application to the tobacco litigation. *Health Serv Outcomes Res Methodol*. 2001; 2(3– 4):169–188.

18. Rubin DB, Thomas N. Matching using estimated propensity scores: relating theory to practice. *Biometrics*. 1996; 52(1):249–264.

19. Elixhauser A, Steiner C, Harris DR, Coffey RM. Comorbidity measures for use with administrative data. *Med Care*. 1998; 36(1):8–27.

20. Pronovost P, Angus DC. Cost reduction and quality improvement: it takes two to tango. *Crit Care Med*. 2000; 28(2):581–583.

21. Birkenshaw C. *UB-92 Handbook for Hospital Billing, with Answers, 2005 Edition*. Chicago, IL: American Hospital Association; 2005.

22. Rubin DB. The design versus the analysis of observational studies for causal effects: parallels with the design of randomized trials. *Stat Med*. 2007; 26(1):20–36.

23. Blough DK, Madden CW, Hornbrook MC. Modeling risk using generalized linear models. *J Health Econ*. 1999; 18(2):153–171.

24. Manning WG, Mullahy J. Estimating log models: to transform or not to transform? *J Health Econ*. 2001; 20(4):461–494.

25. The SUPPORT Principal Investigators. A controlled trial to improve care for seriously ill hospitalized patients: the study to understand prognoses and preferences for outcomes and risks of treatments (SUPPORT). *JAMA*. 1995; 274 (20):1591–1598.

26. Hamel MB, Phillips R, Teno J, et al. Cost effectiveness of aggressive care for patients with nontraumatic coma. *Crit Care Med*. 2002; 30(6):1191–1196.

27. Hogan C, Lunney J, Gabel J, Lynn J. Medicare beneficiaries' costs of care in the last year of life. *Health Aff (Millwood)*. 2001; 20(4):188–195.

28. Jordhøy MS, Fayers P, Saltnes T, Ahlner-Elmqvist M, Jannert M, Kaasa S. A palliative-care intervention and death at home: a cluster randomised trial. *Lancet*. 2000; 356(9233):888–893.

29. Higginson IJ, Finlay I, Goodwin DM, et al. Do hospital-based palliative teams improve care for patients or families at the end of life? *J Pain Symptom Manage*. 2002; 23(2):96–106.

30. Emanuel EJ. Cost savings at the end of life: what do the data show? *JAMA*. 1996; 275(24):1907–1914.

31. Manfredi PL, Morrison RS, Morris J, Goldhirsch SL, Carter JM, Meier DE. Palliative care consultations: how do they impact the care of hospitalized patients? *J Pain Symptom Manage*. 2000; 20(3):166–173.

32. Santa-Emma PH, Roach R, Gill MA, Spayde P, Taylor RM. Development and implementation of an inpatient acute palliative care service. *J Palliat Med*. 2002; 5(1):93–100.

33. Cowan JD. Hospital charges for a community inpatient palliative care program. *Am J Hosp Palliat Care*. 2004; 21(3):177–190.

34. Campbell ML, Frank RR. Experience with an end-of-life practice at a university hospital. *Crit Care Med*. 1997; 25(1):197–202.

35. Appleby J. Hospitals' profit margin hits 6-year high in 2004. *U.S.A Today*. January 4, 2006. http://www.usatoday.com/news/health/2006-01-04-hospital-profits-usat _x.htm (accessed June 3, 2008).

36. Garber KM, ed. *The U.S. Health Care Delivery System: Fundamental Facts, Definitions and Statistics*. Chicago, IL: American Hospital Association; 2006.

37. Congressional Budget Office. High-cost Medicare beneficiaries. http://www.cbo.gov/ftpdocs/63xx/doc6332/05-03-MediSpending.pdf (accessed August 13, 2007).

38. Center for Medicare and Medicaid Services. Hospital care and physician and clinical service expenditures by source of payment: 1990–2004. http://www.census.gov/compendia/statab/tables/07s0127.xls (accessed November 15, 2007).

39. Center to Advance Palliative Care. Building a hospital-based palliative care program. http://www.capc.org/building-a-hospital-based-palliative-care-program (accessed January 17, 2008).

CORRESPONDENCE

R. Sean Morrison, M.D., Hertzberg Palliative Care Institute of the Brookdale Department of Geriatrics, Mount Sinai School of Medicine, Box 1070, One Gustave L. Levy Place, New York, NY 10029; sean.morrison@mssm.edu.

AUTHOR CONTRIBUTIONS

Dr. Morrison had full access to all of the data in the study and takes responsibility for the integrity of the data and the accuracy of the data analysis.

STUDY CONCEPT AND DESIGN

Morrison, Penrod, Cassel, Caust-Ellenbogen, Spragens, and Meier.

ACQUISITION OF DATA

Morrison, Caust-Ellenbogen, Litke, and Spragens.

ANALYSIS AND INTERPRETATION OF DATA

Morrison, Penrod, Cassel, Caust-Ellenbogen, Litke, and Spragens.

DRAFTING OF THE MANUSCRIPT

Morrison, Penrod, Cassel, Spragens, and Meier.

CRITICAL REVISION OF THE MANUSCRIPT FOR IMPORTANT INTELLECTUAL CONTENT

Morrison, Penrod, Cassel, Caust-Ellenbogen, Litke, and Meier.

STATISTICAL ANALYSIS

Morrison, Penrod, Cassel, and Litke.

OBTAINED FUNDING

Morrison and Meier.

ADMINISTRATIVE, TECHNICAL, AND MATERIAL SUPPORT

Litke, Spragens, and Meier.

STUDY SUPERVISION

Morrison and Meier.

THE PALLIATIVE CARE LEADERSHIP CENTERS' OUTCOMES GROUP

Center to Advance Palliative Care, New York, New York
Jessica Dietrich, M.P.H., Bradley Griffith, M.B.A., Amber Jones, M.Ed., Catherine Maroney, M.P.H., and Carol Sieger, J.D.

Hospice and Palliative Care of the Bluegrass, Lexington, Kentucky
Janet Braun, R.N., M.S.P.H., and Terence Gutgsell, M.D.

Medical College of Wisconsin, Milwaukee
David Weissman, M.D.

Fairview Health Services, Minneapolis, Minnesota
Andrea Brandt, B.A., Carolyn Ceronsky, M.S., A.P.R.N., and Mark Leenay, M.D.

Mount Carmel Health System, Columbus, Ohio
Philip Santa-Emma, M.D., and Mary Ann Gill, M.A., R.N.

University of California, San Francisco
Kathleen Kerr, B.A., and Steven Z. Pantilat, M.D.

FINANCIAL DISCLOSURE

None reported.

FUNDING/SUPPORT

This project was supported by the Center to Advance Palliative Care, by the National Palliative Care Research Center, and by a Mid-Career Investigator Award in Patient-Oriented Research (K24 AG022345) from the National Institute on Aging (Dr. Morrison). The Center to Advance Palliative Care and the National Palliative Care Research Center are supported by the Aetna, Brookdale, John A. Hartford, JEHT, Robert Wood Johnson, Emily Davie and Joseph S. Kornfeld, and Olive Branch Foundations.

CARE GIVING

Carol Levine, "The Loneliness of the Long-Term Care Giver"

Ezekiel J. Emanuel, Diane L. Fairclough, Julia Slutsman, Linda L. Emanuel, "Understanding Economic and Other Burdens of Terminal Illness: The Experience of Patients and Their Caregivers"

THE LONELINESS
OF THE LONG-TERM
CARE GIVER

CAROL LEVINE, M.A.

EDITORS' INTRODUCTION

Carol Levine has done more than anyone in this country to focus attention on our society's abandonment of the chronically ill and their overwhelmed family caregivers. Telling the story of her own experience with the care of her husband, she brings the problem powerfully to life.

■ ■ ■

I am standing at a bank of phones, desperately punching in codes and numbers. Each time, the line goes dead. "Why can't I get through to anyone?" I think. "I must be doing something wrong."

I wake up. This time it's only a dream. But the dream originated in a real experience. On the icy morning of January 15, 1990, my husband lay comatose in the emergency room of a community hospital after an automobile accident. Uninjured but dazed, I stood at a bank of hospital phones trying to reach people who could help me transfer him to a major medical center. I was unaware that, by a malevolent coincidence, most of the phones in the region were not working.

The dream recurs, and it has now taken on a new meaning. In the nine years since the accident, and especially in the eight years I have struggled to take care of my husband at home, I have frequently despaired: "Why can't I get through to anyone?" Only in the past few years have I realized that I am not doing anything wrong. It is the health care system that is out of order.

Since I have spent twenty years as a professional in the fields of medical ethics and health policy, it is hardly surprising that I should reach such a conclusion. A recent series of articles in the *Journal* made clear the increasing fragmentation and inequities in the current market-driven health care economy.[1] But my personal experience as a family care giver has given me a different perspective. I see the health care system through everyday encounters with physicians, nurses, social workers, receptionists, vendors, ambulette drivers and dispatchers, administrators, home health aides, representatives of my managed-care company, and a host of other "providers." The attitudes, behavior, and decisions of specific individuals make the system work or fail for me.

There are of course critical links between the behavior of individual persons and the system's structural and financial incentives and rewards. Health policy makers and analysts rarely consider the impact of these incentives on the twenty-five million unpaid, "informal" care givers in the United States, who get little from the system in return for the estimated $196 billion a year in labor they provide.[2] Family care givers are largely invisible, as individuals and as a labor force.

When my journey began, no one told me what to expect. There is no process of informed consent for family care givers. On that unforgettable January day, I knew that I must ask, "Is my husband brain-dead?" And I knew what to do if the answer was yes. "No," said the neurosurgeon at the community hospital, "but he has suffered a severe brain-stem injury. At his age [then sixty-two] it is unlikely that he will survive." The neurosurgeon at the medical center disagreed. "He will walk out of here 100 percent, but it will take some time." "How long?" I asked. "Weeks," he replied, "maybe months."

My husband did survive, a testament to one of American medicine's major successes—saving the lives of trauma patients. But he will never walk, and he is far from 100 percent. While he was in a coma, I read to him, played his favorite music, and showed him family pictures. After four months he gradually emerged from the coma, his thinking chaotic. After many more months of relearning basic words and concepts, he recovered many cognitive functions, and there were occasional flashes of his old intelligence and humor. But he is not the same person in any sense.

Although I worried most about his mental functioning, it is his body that has recovered least. He is totally disabled and requires twenty-four-hour care. He is incontinent of bladder and bowel. He is quadriparetic, with mobility limited to the partial use of his left hand. (His right forearm was amputated as a result of an iatrogenic blood clot that failed to respond to surgery and drug treatment.) Even so, the most difficult aspect of his care is his changed personality and extreme emotional lability. Antipsychotic drugs now generally control his violent outbursts, but there are still unpredictable rages and periods of withdrawal.

As a rehabilitation inpatient he had physical therapy, occupational therapy, speech therapy, cognitive therapy, psychological counseling, nerve blocks, injections of botulinum toxin, hydrotherapy, recreational therapy, and therapeutic touch. He benefited to some degree, but nothing restored true function. He has undergone numerous operations, including placement of a shunt after a blood clot formed in his leg, tendon releases in both legs, removal of a kidney stone, and, most recently, removal of a pituitary tumor. He has undergone oral surgery and extensive dental work.

During my nine-year odyssey, I stopped being a wife and became a family care giver. In the anxious weeks when my husband was in the intensive care unit, I was still a wife. Doctors and nurses informed me of each day's progress or setbacks and treated me with kindness and concern. At some point, however, when he was no longer in immediate danger of dying, and as the specialists and superspecialists drifted out of the picture, I became invisible. Then, when the devastating and permanent extent of his disabilities became clear to clinicians, I became visible again.

At that point, I was important only as the manager and, it was expected, the hands-on provider of my husband's care. In retrospect, I date my rite of passage into the role of family care giver to the first day of my husband's stay in a rehabilitation facility, a place I now think of as a boot camp for care givers. A nurse stuck my husband's soiled sweat pants under my nose and said, "Take these away. Laundry is your job." A woman whose husband had been at the same facility later told me the same story—different nurse. The nurse's underlying message, reinforced by many others, was that my life from now on would consist of performing an unrelieved series of nasty chores.

The social worker assigned to my husband's case had one goal: discharge. I was labeled a "selfish wife," since I refused to take him home without home care. "Get real," the social worker said. "Nobody will pay for home care. You have to quit your job and 'spend down' to get on Medicaid." Eventually I got the home care I needed— temporarily. Despite a written agreement to pay for it, the insurance company later cut off the benefit retroactively, without informing me, leaving me with an $8,000 bill from a home care agency. The agency, which had failed to monitor its own billing, sued me. We settled for less.

When I brought my husband home, he had undiagnosed severe sleep apnea (which caused nighttime screaming), undiagnosed hearing loss, and poorly treated major depression. The first few months at home were nightmarish. Since the problems had not been diagnosed correctly, much less treated, I did not know where to turn. Yet a single home visit by a psychiatrist and a specially trained home care nurse, arranged by a sympathetic colleague who treats patients with cancer, gave me enough information, advice, and referrals to begin to master the situation.

In addition to holding a full-time job, I manage all my husband's care and daily activities. Being a care manager requires grit and persistence. It took me ten days of increasingly insistent phone calls to get my managed-care company to replace my husband's dangerously unstable hospital bed. When the new bed finally arrived—without notice, in the evening, when there was no aide available to move him—it turned out to be the cheapest model, unsuitable for a patient in my husband's condition. In these all too frequent situations, I feel that I am challenging Goliath with a tiny pebble. More often than not, Goliath just puts me on hold.

Being a care manager also takes money. I now pay for a daytime home care aide and serve as the night nurse myself. My husband's initial hospitalization and rehabilitation were paid for by his employer-based indemnity insurance plan. He is now covered by my employer-based managed-care company, which pays for hospital and doctors' bills and, with a $10 copayment, for prescription medicines. Home care aides, disposable supplies, and most forms of therapy are not covered, because they are "not medically necessary." My husband recently needed a new customized wheelchair, which cost $3,700; the managed-care company paid $500. Medicare, his secondary payer, has so far rejected all claims. No one advocates on my husband's behalf except me; no one advocates on my behalf, not even me.

I feel abandoned by a health care system that commits resources and rewards to rescuing the injured and ill but then consigns such patients and their families to the black hole of chronic "custodial" care. I accept responsibility for my husband's care. Love and devotion are the most powerful motives, but there are legal and financial obligations as well. My income would be counted toward his eligibility for Medicaid, should we ever come to that.

The broader issue of a family's moral responsibility to provide or pay for care is much more complex.[3] Why should families be responsible for providing such demanding, intensive care? Should this be a social responsibility? American society places a high value on personal and family responsibility. The thin veneer of consensus that supported some sense of communal responsibility in the past is cracking. This is not a uniquely American problem, however. Even with national health insurance, Australian, Canadian, and British care givers report similar problems of isolation and unmet financial and other needs.[4] Only the Scandinavian countries assume that the community as a whole is primarily responsible for long-term care. Even so, the Swedish Social Services Act specifies some spousal responsibility.[5]

Widely held concepts of family responsibility derive from religious teachings, cultural traditions, community expectations, emotional bonds, or gratitude for past acts. Care givers rarely sort out their mixed feelings. From a policy perspective, there are historical antecedents and financial realities that encourage looking first to families for care. Perhaps the most important justification is that most families, or some members, want this responsibility. Many derive spiritual or psychological rewards from care giving. Taking care of each other comes with being a family. This is an especially strong value among recent immigrants or tightly knit ethnic communities who distrust the formal system but who often have too few resources to cope on their own.

The problem is not that public policy looks first to families but that it generally looks only to families and fails to support those who accept responsibility. The availability of family care givers does not absolve policy makers of their own responsibility to make sure that their actions assist rather than destroy families. Family members should not be held to a level of moral or legal responsibility that entails jeopardizing their own health or well-being.

Given the complexity of the health care system, what changes would make a difference for family care givers? The automatic answer tends to be: Whatever they are, we can't afford them. Or, whatever we can afford is not worth doing. Many family care givers have serious financial problems. Nevertheless, a single-minded focus on money, based on an unsubstantiated assumption that most care givers want to be replaced by paid help, diverts attention from other critical needs.

The reaction to the Clinton administration's January proposal for assistance for the elderly and family care givers is an instructive example of the differing worldviews of health policy analysts and family care givers. Most professionals focused on the proposed tax credit of $1,000 and found it wanting. The credit would not apply to people who pay no taxes, nor would it make a dent in the heavy costs of full-time paid care. The proposal does not do anything to create a coherent long-term care policy.[6] All these observations are true. On the other hand, family care givers and organizations that represent their interests have been largely positive about the proposal. The tax credit is a tangible benefit that will help many middle-class families. Equally important, the proposal puts family care giving on the national agenda and gives states money and incentives to develop resource centers. These points are also all true.[7]

In my professional role, I know that much more is needed, including a restructuring of Medicare to better meet the long-term needs of the elderly and disabled and the creation of a more flexible range of options for home and community-based care.[8] I also know that change will take a long time and will be determined by the interests of the major players and by political considerations. As a family care giver, I will take whatever help I can get when I need it, and that is right now.

Clinicians as well as policy makers have responsibilities toward family care givers. Care givers say they want better communication with professionals, education and training, emotional support, and advocacy to obtain needed services for their relatives and themselves. They want help in negotiating the impenetrable thicket of financing mechanisms, the frequent denials of services or reimbursements, and the inconsistent interpretations of policies and eligibility. They want respite, too, but through services that they can tailor to their needs. These are modest requests—too modest, perhaps—but unfulfilled nonetheless.

Care givers in the focus groups convened by the United Hospital Fund's Families and Health Care Project reported a lack of basic information about the patient's diagnosis, prognosis, and treatment plan, the side effects of the patient's medication, the symptoms to watch for at home, and whom to call when problems occur.[9] Sometimes care givers reported that they were given conflicting information.

Managed care did not create this problem, but it seems to have exacerbated it. Often, professionals convey information in such a hurried, technical way that anxious care givers cannot absorb it. Hospital staff members may assume, erroneously, that a home care agency will instruct the care giver. There are costs to these lapses. Failures in communication can lead to serious problems with the care of patients, including unnecessary hospital readmissions. Some families, however, become experts on the conditions of their relatives and the specifics of their care. Yet professionals frequently ignore this expertise, because it comes from laypersons.

Family care givers also want to be involved in decision making that affects the patient and themselves. Elsewhere, Connie Zuckerman and I have described some of the reasons clinicians have difficulties with family members, especially with respect to decisions about acute care.[10] In my husband's case, I alone made the only important decision, which was to transfer my husband to a medical center on the day of the accident. After that there were never any clear-cut decisions, no discussions about the goals of care, and certainly no long-term planning. Although I repeatedly asked to attend a team meeting to discuss his prognosis and care, I was never given that opportunity. Nor was there ever any follow-up at home, a common complaint among care givers.

Care givers want education and training that recognizes their emotional attachment to the patient. Professionals seldom appreciate how much fear and anxiety complicate the learning of new tasks. Learning how to operate a feeding tube or change a dressing or inject a medication is hard enough for a layperson; care givers learn how to perform these procedures for the first time on a person they love. Fearful of making a mistake or simply upset by the idea of having to perform unaccustomed and unpleasant tasks, care givers may resist or fail, or persist at great emotional cost.

Months before my husband was ready to go home, a nurse insisted that I learn how to put on my husband's condom catheter. "I don't need to know this yet," I protested, "and besides, maybe he won't need it later." Ignoring our emotional state at the time, she forced me to do it (badly) until both my husband and I burst into tears. Later, when I complained to her supervisor, I was told, "We just wanted to break through your denial."

Families need emotional support. They frequently bring a patient home to a living space transformed by medical equipment and a family life constrained by illness. Privacy is a luxury. Every day must be planned to the minute. The intricate web of carefully organized care can unravel with one phone call from an aide who is ill, an ambulette service that does not show up, a doctor's office that cannot accommodate a wheelchair, an equipment company that does not have an emergency service. There are generally no extra hands to help out in a crisis and no experienced colleagues to ask for advice. Friends and even family members fade away.

Programs that train and support family care givers can be based in hospitals, community agencies, schools and colleges, home care agencies, managed-care companies, or other settings. The United Hospital Fund's Family Caregiving Grant Initiative is funding several such projects.

If family care givers need education, professionals need it just as much. Education for doctors, nurses, and social workers should include understanding the needs of family care givers. Ideally, all professionals should have the experience of seeing firsthand what is really involved in home care. Inservice programs can educate health care professionals about family dynamics as well as build communication and negotiating skills.

Family care givers must be supported, because the health care system cannot exist without them. And there is another compelling reason: Care givers are at risk for mental and physical health problems themselves. Exhausted care givers may become care recipients, leading to a further, often preventable, drain on resources. Does my managed-care company realize, for instance, that during the past year it paid more for my stress-related medical problems than for my husband's medical care?

No single intervention will change the system, but small steps taken together can cover a long distance. As I enter my tenth year as a family care giver, it is hard to believe I have come this far. Today is a reasonably good day. But what about tomorrow? And next week? Hello? Is anyone listening?

REFERENCES

1. Angell M. The American health care system revisited—a new series. *N Engl J Med.* 1999; 340:48.

2. Arno PS, Levine C, Memmott MM. The economic value of informal caregiving. *Health Aff (Millwood).* 1999; 18:182–188.

3. Levine C. Home sweet hospital: the nature and limits of private responsibilities for home health care. *J Aging Health.* 1999; 11(3):341–59.

4. Schofield H, Booth S, Hermann H, Murphy B, Nankervis J, Singh B. *Family caregivers: disability, illness and aging.* St. Leonards, Australia: Allen & Unwin, 1998.

5. Barusch AS. Programming for family care of elderly dependents: mandates, incentives, and service rationing. *Soc Work.* 1995; 40:315–322.

6. Graham J. Halfway measures. *Chicago Tribune.* January 17, 1999.

7. Statement by Suzanne Mintz, President, National Family Caregivers Association, Kensington, Md., January 6, 1999.

8. Cassel CK, Besdine RW, Siegel LC. Restructuring Medicare for the next century: what will beneficiaries really need? *Health Aff (Millwood).* 1999; 18:118–131.

9. Levine C. *Rough crossings: family caregivers' odysseys through the health care system.* New York: United Hospital Fund, 1998.

10. Levine C, Zuckerman C. The trouble with families: toward an ethic of accommodation. *Ann Intern Med.* 1999; 130:148–152.

UNDERSTANDING ECONOMIC AND OTHER BURDENS OF TERMINAL ILLNESS: THE EXPERIENCE OF PATIENTS AND THEIR CAREGIVERS

EZEKIEL J. EMANUEL, M.D., PH.D., DIANE L. FAIRCLOUGH, D.PH.,
JULIA SLUTSMAN, B.A., AND LINDA L. EMANUEL, M.D., PH.D.

This article originally appeared in Emanuel EJ, Fairclough DL, Slutsman J, Emanuel LL. Understanding economic and other burdens of terminal illness: the experience of patients and their caregivers. *Ann Intern Med.* 2000;132(6):451–459. Copyright © 2000, American College of Physicians–American Society of Internal Medicine. All rights reserved. Reprinted with permission.

EDITORS' INTRODUCTION

Ezekiel J. Emanuel and his colleagues have conducted consistently influential research on the salient medical ethical issues of our time, including this demonstration of the enormous economic burdens of serious illness on patients, all of whom had medical insurance, and their families. The study identifies the adverse consequences of these financial pressures, including patients' desire for physician-assisted suicide or euthanasia to protect their families from economic devastation.

■ ■ ■

Serious illness has an adverse effect on patients, family, and friends. Previous studies have demonstrated that caregivers of patients with cancer and dementia have increased health problems and psychosocial stress.[1-7] For example, studies have reported that up to one-third of spouses of patients with terminal cancer have depressive symptoms.[8,9] Families of terminally ill patients also experience adverse economic effects. The Study to Understand Prognoses and Preferences for Outcomes and Risks of Treatment (SUPPORT) reported that families of seriously ill patients experienced substantial economic losses. In 20 percent of families, a family member had to stop working; 31 percent of families lost most of their savings.[7]

Data on the cause of these adverse effects are scarce. The SUPPORT investigators stated, "Although our results document substantial burdens to family members of seriously ill patients, they do not explain the mechanism of these burdens. . . . Our results highlight the need for future research efforts to examine the mechanism of these burdens."[7] In addition, without understanding the cause of these burdens, it is difficult to identify interventions that could meet the care needs of terminally ill patients without imposing additional hardships on their families and friends.

To determine the cause of economic and other burdens, and to identify some potential interventions that could mitigate them, we studied the experiences of 988 terminally ill patients with different illnesses and their 893 caregivers.

METHODS

Recruitment

Our methods have been described in detail elsewhere[10] and are outlined in Figure 24.1. Briefly, patients were recruited on the basis of physician determination of terminal status. Because many terminally ill patients are no longer admitted to hospitals and do not die in hospitals, we recruited through outpatient settings. Similarly, because SUPPORT found that patients' six-month survival rates determined by physicians were almost as accurate as those determined by using formal medical criteria[11] and because in routine practice, such as hospice referral, physicians determine terminal illness without using formal criteria, we relied on physician determination of patients' terminal status.

Site Selection

We divided all fifty states into four census regions: Northeast, South, Midwest, and West. The Group Health Association of America issued a report on the proportion of the insured population that was enrolled in health maintenance organizations (HMOs) in the fifty-four largest metropolitan statistical areas (MSAs).[12] According to this report, we classified MSAs as having high or low managed care penetration. High penetration was defined as HMO enrollment of 20 percent or more of the population in 1991, the last year for which managed care penetration data were available before site selection. In each of the four regions, one MSA with high HMO penetration was randomly selected: Worcester, Massachusetts; St. Louis, Missouri; Tucson, Arizona; and Birmingham, Alabama. Among the MSAs with low penetration, one site was selected: Brooklyn, New York. To represent the 24 percent of the U.S. population that resides in rural areas, one site was randomly selected among all non-MSA primary sampling units (that is, all non-MSA counties or collections of counties): Mesa County, Colorado.

Physician Identification

At each site, lists of physicians were obtained from state boards of medical registration, medical societies, and specialty societies. From these lists, physicians were selected by simple random sampling that aimed for the same patient sample size in each site. At the rural site, however, all physicians were selected because of small numbers. Selected physicians were mailed a letter stating that the purpose of the study was to "learn about how these patients [with significant illness] experience health care" and that patient and caregiver interviews would be done in person. Physicians were asked to identify all of their patients who had "a significant illness [except HIV infection or AIDS] and a survival time of six months or less, in your opinion." The physicians used their own discretion to decide whether to discuss the study with patients before identifying them. A total of 383 physicians referred patients, whom we then interviewed.

Patient Selection

No patient or caregiver was paid to participate in the study. Patients were eligible to participate if they had any substantial illness, excluding HIV infection or AIDS; had an estimated survival time of less than six months, as determined by their physician; spoke English; had no hearing difficulty; and were able to arrange an interview time and place and sign a consent form. Patients were not randomly selected; instead, all patients identified by physicians were sent a letter that explained the study and included a postage-paid "opt-out" card. The letter stated that the study aimed to understand "the attitudes of patients with a significant illness and their caregivers towards the quality of the patient's health care." Patients were informed that the interview would be conducted

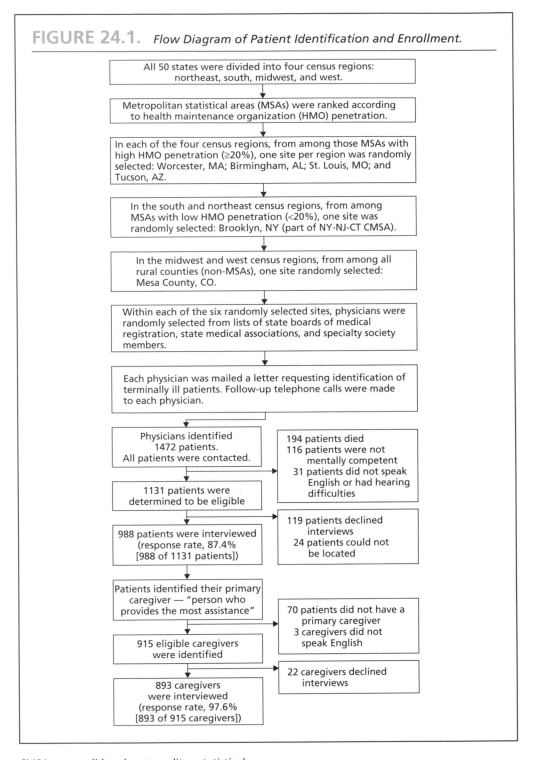

FIGURE 24.1. *Flow Diagram of Patient Identification and Enrollment.*

All 50 states were divided into four census regions: northeast, south, midwest, and west.

Metropolitan statistical areas (MSAs) were ranked according to health maintenance organization (HMO) penetration.

In each of the four census regions, from among those MSAs with high HMO penetration (≥20%), one site per region was randomly selected: Worcester, MA; Birmingham, AL; St. Louis, MO; and Tucson, AZ.

In the south and northeast census regions, from among MSAs with low HMO penetration (<20%), one site was randomly selected: Brooklyn, NY (part of NY-NJ-CT CMSA).

In the midwest and west census regions, from among all rural counties (non-MSAs), one site randomly selected: Mesa County, CO.

Within each of the six randomly selected sites, physicians were randomly selected from lists of state boards of medical registration, state medical associations, and specialty society members.

Each physician was mailed a letter requesting identification of terminally ill patients. Follow-up telephone calls were made to each physician.

Physicians identified 1472 patients. All patients were contacted.

194 patients died
116 patients were not mentally competent
31 patients did not speak English or had hearing difficulties

1131 patients were determined to be eligible

119 patients declined interviews
24 patients could not be located

988 patients were interviewed (response rate, 87.4% [988 of 1131 patients])

Patients identified their primary caregiver — "person who provides the most assistance"

70 patients did not have a primary caregiver
3 caregivers did not speak English

915 eligible caregivers were identified

22 caregivers declined interviews

893 caregivers were interviewed (response rate, 97.6% [893 of 915 caregivers])

CMSA = consolidated metropolitan statistical area.

in person. If the opt-out card was not received within two weeks, the patient was contacted to arrange an interview.

Physicians identified 1,472 patients, of whom 341 were ineligible (194 died and 116 became mentally incapacitated before being interviewed; 31 did not speak English or had hearing limitations that precluded interviews). Of the 1,131 eligible patients, 119 declined to participate, 24 could not be located, and 988 completed interviews (response rate, 87.4 percent).

Caregiver Selection

Patients were asked to identify their primary caregiver, who was specified as the family member, friend, or other person who provided the most assistance. Caregivers were ineligible if they could not speak English, had hearing limitations that prevented them from understanding questions, or were not able to arrange an interview time and place or sign a consent form. Seventy of 988 patients reported that they did not have caregivers. Three caregivers did not speak English, and 22 caretakers declined to participate. Therefore, 893 caregivers were interviewed (response rate, 97.6 percent).

Survey Development

Survey development was guided by a conceptual framework that has been outlined elsewhere.[13] In conjunction with the Center for Survey Research and the National Opinion Research Center, we developed survey instruments after (1) performing a literature search, (2) conducting fifteen focus groups that included patients, caregivers, elderly persons, and health care providers, (3) conducting six in-depth interviews with terminally ill patients and caregivers, (4) creating the survey instruments, (5) conducting cognitive, behavioral, and reliability pretest, (6) submitting the survey instruments for review by an expert panel, and (7) refining the final survey. Eighteen patients and 15 caregivers in Cleveland, Ohio, and Dallas, Texas, pretested the survey instruments.

The patient survey contained 135 questions, and the caregiver survey contained 118 questions. Questions focused on health status and symptoms, social supports, communication with health care providers, personal and spiritual meaning, care needs, end-of-life care plans, economic burdens, sociodemographic characteristics, euthanasia and physician-assisted suicide, and interview-related stress.

Survey questions on symptoms were adapted from the Wisconsin Brief Pain Questionnaire,[14] the Medical Outcomes Study 36-Item Short-Form Health Survey,[15, 16] and the Eastern Oncology Cooperative Group performance measure.[17] Questions on social supports were adapted from the Medical Outcomes Study social support survey.[18] Using questions from Siegel and colleagues,[4] Rice and coworkers,[19] and SUPPORT,[7, 20] we asked patients and caregivers about their need for assistance in four areas: transportation, nursing care, homemaking, and personal physical care. Questions determined the degree of assistance needed in each area, the person who provided assistance, the use of home health care or hospice services, and any unmet needs for additional assistance. Questions regarding economic burdens and financial expenditures on health care were taken from Epstein and colleagues[21] and Covinsky and coworkers.[7] Some questions on physician-patient communication were adapted from SUPPORT.[20] Questions on euthanasia and physician-assisted suicide were adapted from Emanuel and colleagues.[22] Some of the questions on physician-patient communication, personal meaning, advance care planning, and economic burdens of care were newly developed. The instruments are available from the authors.

Interview Process

Twenty-four interviewers from the National Opinion Research Center who were trained to interview terminally ill patients conducted all interviews in person between March 1996 and March 1997.

Human Subjects Approval

The protocol, letters, survey instruments, and consent documents were approved by the institutional review boards at Harvard Medical School and the Dana-Farber Cancer Institute (Boston, Massachusetts) as well as at 38 medical institutions in the six study sites. The patient identification and selection procedures were approved as being consistent with the recommendations of the institutional review board guidebook.[23] We ensured that participants had no emotional contraindications to study involvement by asking physicians to recommend appropriate patients. The investigators kept patients' personal information confidential and did not use it for any commercial purposes. The identifying information did not include data on extremely sensitive matters, such as history of drug abuse, sexually transmitted diseases, or psychiatric illness. Patients were able to decline participation through the opt-out card, when they were contacted to arrange an interview, when the interviewer arrived to conduct the interview, and at any point during the interview.

Statistical Analysis

Each patient was asked to rate the amount of assistance he or she needed in four areas—transportation, nursing care, homemaking, and personal care—on a 4-point scale, ranging from "none at all" to "a lot." Scores from the four areas were summed and rescaled so that the scores had a range of 0 to 10, with 10 being the greatest need for care. High care needs were defined as a score of more than 7.5, moderate care needs were defined as a score of 5.1 to 7.5, some care needs were defined as a score of 2.5 to 5.0, and low or no care needs were defined as a score less than 2.5. Substantial care needs were defined as moderate or high care needs (a score of 5.0 to 10). Similarly, each patient was asked to rate his or her unmet needs for nursing care and homemaking. Scores were summed and rescaled in the same manner.

Univariate tests of association between levels of care needs and patient characteristics used the Mantel-Haenszel chi-square statistic for ordered categorical outcomes. To retain efficiency and power, and because none of the outcomes had bimodal distributions, the outcomes were divided at the median unless an obvious division was dictated

by the meaning of the responses. Multivariate logistic regression was used to identify the characteristics that were independently associated with substantial care needs.
Statistically significant groups of factors were first identified from potential explanatory variables in five groups. The five groups were patient demographic characteristics
(age, sex, marital status, income, ethnicity, education, indicators of religious affiliation,
and geography), health-related symptoms (performance status, pain, depressive symptoms, shortness of breath, and incontinence), diagnostic factors (diagnosis of cancer,
heart disease, or chronic obstructive pulmonary disease; length of illness; and hospitalization in the previous six months), economic factors (insurance status, out-of-pocket
expenses for health care [excluding insurance premiums] of more than 10 percent of
income, subjectively perceived economic hardship, and use of home care or hospice),
and communication factors (trust in physician, availability of clear information from
the provider, and the ability to talk freely about the end of life).

To minimize the type I errors associated with the exploratory nature of the analysis,
and to minimize statistically significant but clinically insignificant factors, the α value
was set at 0.05 for the type I error rate of each group of explanatory variables—that
is, the criteria for the likelihood ratio test for all factors from the group. If statistical
significance ($P < 0.05$) was observed for the group, the α value was set at 0.01 for the
selection criteria for each explanatory variable. The final model was developed from
the factors that were the strongest explanatory variables from each group, as determined
by the highest chi-square value. The model was determined to be clinically meaningful
if the results were consistent with the previously available data, if the direction of
association did not change when going from the univariate tests of association to the
multivariate model, and if no unreasonable assumptions had to be made about the
outcomes.

Association between level of care needs and the patient's or caregiver's burden
were tested by using the Mantel-Haenszel chi-square statistic for ordered categorical
outcomes. Computations were performed by using Proc Logistic, version 6.12 (SAS
Institute, Cary, North Carolina).

RESULTS

Characteristics of Terminally Ill Patients

The sociodemographic characteristics of the 988 terminally ill patients are comparable
to those seen in the U.S. population and SUPPORT (Table 24.1). (SUPPORT data were
provided by R. Phillips and J. Soukup, personal communication.) In our study, the mean
age of the terminally ill patients was 66.5 years (range, 22 to 109 years), and 59.4 percent
of patients were at least 65 years of age. The leading causes of terminal illness were
cancer (51.8 percent), heart disease (18.0 percent), and chronic obstructive pulmonary
disease (10.9 percent). Among all patients, 50.2 percent experienced substantial pain,
17.5 percent were bedridden for more than 50 percent of the day, 70.9 percent had
shortness of breath while walking one block or less, 35.5 percent had urinary or fecal
incontinence, and 16.8 percent had depressive symptoms. In the previous six months,
33.5 percent of the patients had not been hospitalized, 36.8 percent had undergone a

surgical procedure, and 22.3 percent had required a hospital stay involving a period in the intensive care unit.

Care Needs of Terminally Ill Patients

Overall, 16.3 percent of terminally ill patients had high care needs for transportation, nursing care, homemaking, and personal care. An additional 18.4 percent had moderate care needs, 26.0 percent had some care needs, and 39.2 percent had little or no care needs. Of patients who had high or moderate care needs, 62.0 percent needed transportation assistance, 28.7 percent needed nursing care, 55.2 percent needed homemaking assistance, and 26.0 percent needed personal care. In addition, 18.2 percent of patients had unmet needs for nursing care and 23.1 percent had unmet homemaking needs.

Predictors of Substantial Care Needs and Unmet Needs

In univariate analysis, terminally ill patients with poor physical function, pain, incontinence, shortness of breath while walking one block, or depressive symptoms had significantly greater care needs ($P \leq 0.001$). For example, 36.7 percent of patients with shortness of breath but only 25.6 percent of patients without shortness of breath had substantial care needs ($P < 0.001$). Similarly, 75.0 percent of patients who were bedridden for more than 50 percent of the day but only 26.2 percent of those who were not had substantial care needs ($P < 0.001$).

In addition, univariate analysis showed significant disparities in care needs according to sex, ethnicity, age, and income but not according to marital or insurance status. For example, 42.0 percent of African American persons required assistance with nursing care but only 27.8 percent of white persons and 16.1 percent of Hispanic persons required such assistance ($P < 0.001$). Similarly, 31.4 percent of patients 65 years of age and older required assistance with personal care needs but only 17.5 percent of patients younger than 65 years of age required such assistance ($P < 0.001$). Among patients whose yearly incomes were less than $15,000, 38.4 percent required nursing care; however, only 23.5 percent of those with higher incomes required such care ($P < 0.001$).

In multivariate logistical analysis, four factors were independently associated with substantial care needs: poor physical function (odds ratio, 2.77 [95 percent CI, 2.32 to 3.32]); age 65 years or older (odds ratio, 1.95 [CI, 1.38 to 2.77]); fecal or urinary incontinence (odds ratio, 1.88 [CI, 1.33 to 2.63]); and income less than $15,000 per year (odds ratio, 1.81 [CI, 1.29 to 2.54]). Other factors, such as sex, ethnicity, education, marital status, religion, pain, depressive symptoms, cancer, length of illness, hospitalization in the previous six months, and managed care insurance, were not independently associated with substantial need for assistance. Three factors were independently associated with unmet care needs: substantial care needs (odds ratio, 4.93 [CI, 3.52 to 6.91]), female sex (odds ratio, 1.98 [CI, 1.34 to 2.93]), and African American ethnicity (odds ratio, 2.37 [CI, 1.48 to 3.79]).

TABLE 24.1. **Characteristics of Terminally Ill Patients Compared with the U.S. Population and the Study to Understand Prognoses and Preferences for Outcomes and Risks of Treatment Sample[a]**

Characteristic, %	Overall Patient Cohort			Patients 65 Years of Age and Older		
	Current Study	U.S. Population	SUPPORT	Current Study	U.S. Population	SUPPORT
Sex						
Male	48.5	48.2	43.7	53.5	41.1	54.6
Female	51.5	51.8	57.3	46.5	58.9	45.4
Ethnicity						
White	78.9	75.2	79.4	82.5	84.7	85.0
African American	13.7	11.2	15.3	12.6	8.0	12.0
Hispanic	3.2	9.6	3.2	1.7	4.9	1.6
Other	4.2	4.1	2.1	3.1	2.4	1.4
Education						
8th grade or less	14.0	7.2	16.4	20.4	18.8	22.7
Some high school	18.9	11.4	28.1	19.8	15.7	27.6
High school	27.4	33.4	27.7	24.6	34.3	25.4
Some college	21.8	19.4	15.8	17.2	12.9	13.3
College graduate	11.5	21.7	6.8	11.2	12.9	6.3
Graduate school	6.3	6.9	5.2	6.7	5.4	4.7
Religion						
Protestant	61.8	58.0	52.0	61.8	NA	48.4
Catholic	25.4	25.0	27.9	25.3	NA	28.8
Jewish	4.3	2.0	8.5	5.0	NA	13.1
Other	8.4	15.0	11.7	8.0	NA	9.7
Yearly income[b]						
<$15,000	38.4	20.3	55.9	41.9	37.8	62.4
$15,000–$24,999	21.1	15.4	20.5	23.1	23.4	23.1
$25,000–$49,999	24.9	30.0	15.2	23.6	24.7	9.0
≥$50,000	15.6	34.3	8.4	11.4	14.1	5.4
Marital status						
Married	59.7	59.6	53.4	57.4	55.6	52.2
Widowed	20.3	7.0	20.1	29.6	33.4	32.9
Divorced	9.0	9.9	15.2	4.9	6.8	9.7
Other	10.8	23.5	11.4	8.1	4.2	6.1

[a]Participants in our study ranged in age from 22 to 109 years. Figures for the U.S. population in 1997 include only persons older than 18 years except for the figures for education, which include persons older than 25 years of age. Percentages may not equal 100 because of rounding. Data on U.S. population are taken from reference 24. Data on SUPPORT cohorts were provided by R. Phillips and J. Soukup (personal communication). NA = not available; SUPPORT = Study to Understand Prognoses and Preferences for Outcomes and Risks of Treatment.
[b]In SUPPORT, income is recorded as less than $11,000 or as $11,000 to $25,000. Consequently, the categories do not precisely match U.S. population data or data from our study.

Burdens of Substantial Care Needs

Substantial need for care was strongly associated with economic and other burdens (Figure 24.2). Terminally ill patients with moderate or high care needs were significantly more likely than those with low care needs to report that "the cost of [their] illness and medical care was a moderate or great economic hardship" for their family (44.9 percent compared with 35.3 percent; difference, 9.6 percentage points [CI, 3.1 to 16.1 percentage points]; $P = 0.005$); that 10 percent of their household income was spent on health care costs other than health insurance premiums (28.0 percent compared with 17.0 percent; difference, 11.0 percentage points [CI, 4.8 to 17.1 percentage points]; $P \leq 0.001$); and that they or their families had to sell assets, take out a loan or mortgage, or obtain an additional job to pay for health care costs (16.3 percent compared with 10.2 percent; difference, 6.1 percentage points [CI, 1.4 to 10.6 percentage points]; $P = 0.004$). Among patients requiring substantial assistance, 14.9 percent had seriously thought about or discussed euthanasia or physician-assisted suicide; however, only 8.2 percent of patients with few care needs had done so ($P = 0.001$).

Similarly, caregivers of patients with substantial care needs were significantly more likely than caregivers of patients with low care needs to have depressive symptoms (31.4 percent compared with 24.8 percent; difference, 6.6 percentage points [CI, 0.4 to 12.8 percentage points]; $P = 0.01$) and to report that their role as caregiver was

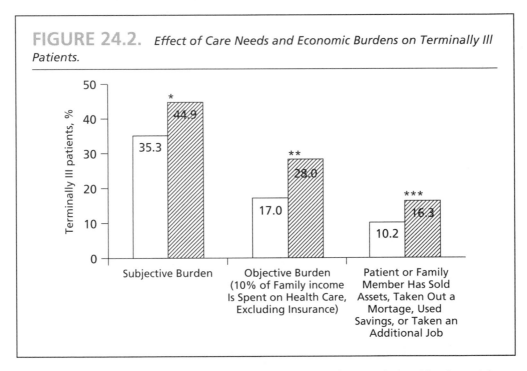

FIGURE 24.2. *Effect of Care Needs and Economic Burdens on Terminally Ill Patients.*

White bars indicate patients with few care needs; striped bars indicate patients with substantial care needs. *$P = 0.005$; **$P = 0.001$; ***$P = 0.004$

"interfering with [their] family or personal life" (35.6 percent compared with 24.3 percent; difference, 11.3 percentage points [CI, 5.0 to 17.7 percentage points]; $P = 0.001$) (Figure 24.3).

Interventions to Ameliorate the Burdens of Care Needs

Caregivers of patients with substantial needs who reported that the physicians they dealt with listened to "the needs and opinions [of the caregiver] about the patient's illness or

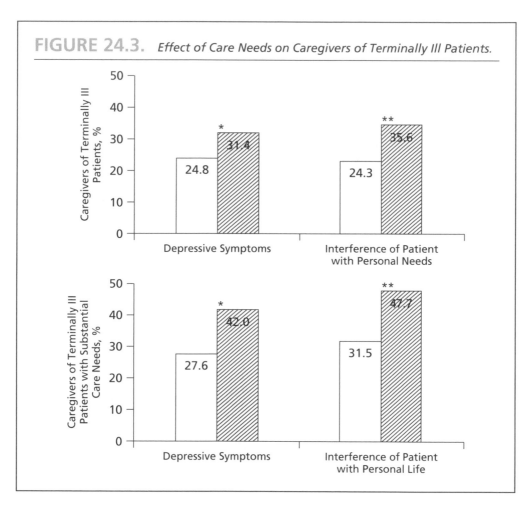

FIGURE 24.3. *Effect of Care Needs on Caregivers of Terminally Ill Patients.*

Top: Relation between patients' care needs and caregivers' psychosocial burdens. White bars indicate caregivers of patients with few care needs; striped bars indicate caregivers of patients with substantial care needs. *$P = 0.01$; **$P = 0.001$

Bottom: Relation between the empathy of patients' physicians and the psychosocial burdens of caretakers of patients with substantial care needs. White bars indicate caregivers of patients with empathetic physicians; striped bars indicate caregivers of patients with nonempathetic physicians. *$P = 0.005$; **$P = 0.015$

medical treatment" were significantly less likely to be depressed than caregivers who dealt with physicians who did not listen (27.6 percent compared with 42.0 percent; difference, 14.4 percentage points [CI, 2.5 to 26.3 percentage points]; $P = 0.005$) and to report that their role as caregiver interfered with their personal lives (31.5 percent compared with 47.7 percent; difference, 16.2 percentage points [CI, 4.1 to 28.4 percentage points]; $P = 0.015$) (Figure 24.3).

DISCUSSION

Our study suggests a model that illuminates the previously unknown mechanism by which terminally ill patients and their families experience economic, psychosocial, and other burdens (Figure 24.4). Although the data presented here cannot prove causality, a plausible model based on the data suggests that terminally ill patients with physical symptoms experience substantial care requirements and, in turn, economic and other burdens.

The model generalizes the results of previous work that was limited to patients with cancer and applies them to patients with all terminal illnesses; it indicates that poor physical function, incontinence, older age, and low income are associated with greater care needs.[4,25,26] More important, the model provides a plausible and coherent explanation of data from SUPPORT[7] and other studies,[4] which indicate that physical functioning status and low income are associated with economic burdens: Economic hardships arise from the high care needs of terminally ill patients. Similarly, the model provides an explanation for previous data[1–6,8,9] that document the psychosocial burdens,

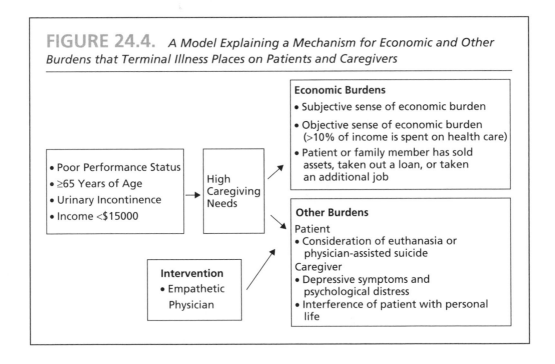

FIGURE 24.4. *A Model Explaining a Mechanism for Economic and Other Burdens that Terminal Illness Places on Patients and Caregivers*

such as depression, experienced by caregivers of terminally ill patients: The need to provide substantial assistance to dying patients generates psychosocial stresses on the caregivers.

However, the underlying factors that are associated with significant care needs and economic burdens in this model—older age, low income, poor physical function, and incontinence—are not readily modifiable or amenable to medical interventions. There is no way to change a patient's age, and no interventions can reliably and effectively improve physical function or prevent incontinence. This may severely limit or make more remote the possibility of alleviating economic and other burdens on terminally ill patients and their families. The only interventions that may be able to reduce burdens will probably be directed at attending to patients' care needs. Implementing interventions that provide assistance for patients' needs without imposing additional cost or effort on the caregiver may be the best way to ease the economic burdens of terminal illness. Additional hospice or home care services, especially unskilled home care services, may be useful only if they do not impose additional costs through high copayments. Unskilled care is frequently not considered a covered health benefit but may help address many care needs that are generated by poor physical function and incontinence, such as transportation, homemaking, and personal care. By performing these services, unskilled caregivers can provide relief for primary caregivers, allowing them to offer emotional and other support to the patient.

It is important to note that our data suggest a mechanism to ameliorate some of the psychosocial burdens on caregivers without requiring additional health care resources. It seems that physicians can reduce caregivers' depression simply by listening well. One effective way to improve physicians' empathy and ability to listen to patients and caregivers may be the implementation of more formalized and structured instruction during medical school, internships, and residency training.

Previous surveys of physicians who have received requests for euthanasia or physician-assisted suicide indicate that patients' fear of being a burden is a primary motivation for such inquiries.[27,28] Our data indicate a link between patients' reports of substantial care needs and consideration of euthanasia or physician-assisted suicide.

Our study has several limitations. First, our patient sample may be biased because physicians may have selectively referred patients who had fewer symptoms and problems. However, other studies of dying patients have required the consent of patients' physicians because of the sensitivity of interviewing terminally ill patients.[7,20,22,29] It is important to note that this bias did not seem to be considerable in these studies. The characteristics of the patients in our study mirror those seen in the U.S. population and in SUPPORT. Furthermore, physicians did not exclude patients who were experiencing substantial pain, functional debility, incontinence, depression, or care needs. In addition, physicians who referred patients did not know the hypotheses of our study and could not have anticipated the kinds of analyses of care needs that would be performed.

Second, 21 percent of the referred patients (310 of 1,472) died or became mentally incapacitated before being interviewed. Patients with only days to live may have different needs and characteristics than terminally ill patients with a few months to live.

Third, more than 50 percent of the patients in our study had cancer, and 23 percent of decedents die of cancer. This is not unusual, because cancer is the leading cause of predictable deaths.[13,30] Deaths from heart disease, stroke, and other diseases are often sudden or occur after years of exacerbations and recoveries. Physicians may be more comfortable identifying patients with cancer as terminally ill. Consequently, our patient sample probably accurately reflects the attitudes and needs of patients who are known to be dying and situations in which interventions can facilitate a "good death."[13,30]

Our study suggests that substantial care needs are a key mechanism that generates economic and psychosocial burdens on terminally ill patients, their families, and their caregivers. It also suggests that empathetic physicians who listen to patients and caregivers can reduce some of the burdens on caregivers. Training physicians to listen and increasing coverage of additional home care services—especially unskilled assistance—without increasing patients' and families' expenses could effectively relieve economic and other burdens.

REFERENCES

1. Cantor MH. Strain among caregivers: a study of experience in the United States. *Gerontologist*. 1983; 23:597–604.[Medline]

2. George LK, Gwyther LP. Caregiver well-being: a multidimensional examination of family caregivers of demented adults. *Gerontologist*. 1986; 26:253–9.[Medline]

3. Pruchno RA, Potashnik SL. Caregiving spouses. Physical and mental health in perspective. *J Am Geriatr Soc*. 1989; 37:697–705.[Medline]

4. Siegel K, Raveis VH, Houts P, Mor V. Caregiver burden and unmet patient needs. *Cancer*. 1991; 68:1131–40.[Medline]

5. Patrick C, Padgett DK, Schlesinger HJ, Cohen J, Burns BJ. Serious physical illness as a stressor: effects on family use of medical services. *Gen Hosp Psychiatry*. 1992; 14:219–27.[Medline]

6. Berkman BJ, Sampson SE. Psychosocial effects of cancer economics on patients and their families. *Cancer*. 1993; 72:2846–9.[Medline]

7. Covinsky KE, Goldman L, Cook EF, Oye R, Desbiens N, Reding D, et al. The impact of serious illness on patients' families. SUPPORT Investigators. Study to Understand Prognoses and Preferences for Outcomes and Risks of Treatment. *JAMA*. 1994; 272:1839–44.[Abstract]

8. Kissane DW, Bloch S, Burns WI, McKenzies D, Posterino M. Psychosocial morbidity in the families of patients with cancer. *Psycho-Oncology*. 1994; 3:47–56.

9. Greer DS, Mor V, Morris JN, Sherwood S, Kidder D, Birnbaum H. An alternative in terminal care: results of the National Hospice Study. *J Chronic Dis*. 1986; 39:9–26.[Medline]

10. Emanuel EJ, Fairclough DL, Slutsman J, Alpert H, Baldwin D, Emanuel LL. Assistance from family members, friends, paid care givers and volunteers in the care of terminally ill patients. *N Engl J Med*. 1999; 341:956–63.[Abstract/Free Full Text]

11. Knaus WA, Harrell FE, Lynn J, Goldman L, Phillips RS, Connors AF. The SUPPORT prognostic model. Objective estimates of survival for seriously ill hospitalized adults. Study to Understand Prognoses and Preferences for Outcomes and Risks of Treatment. *Ann Intern Med*. 1995; 122:191–203.[Abstract/Free full text]

12. Group Health Association of America. *National Directory of HMOs*. Washington, DC: Group Health Association of America; 1992.

13. Emanuel EJ, Emanuel LL. The promise of a good death. *Lancet*. 1998; 351:SII21– SII29.

14. Daut RL, Cleeland CS, Flanery RC. Development of the Wisconsin Brief Pain Questionnaire to assess pain in cancer and other diseases. *Pain*. 1983; 17:197–210.[Medline]

15. Ware J. *SF-36 Health Survey: Manual and Interpretation Guide*. Boston: The Health Institute, New England Medical Center; 1993.

16. Berwick DM, Murphy JM, Goldman PA, Ware JE, Barsky AJ, Weinstein MC. Performance of a five-item mental health screening test. *Med Care*. 1991; 29:169–76.[Medline]

17. Zubrod C, Scheiderman M, Frei E, Brindley C, Gold GL, Shnider B, et al. Appraisal of methods for the study of chemotherapy of cancer in man: comparative therapeutic trial of nitrogen mustard and triethylene thiophosphoramide. *J Chron Dis*. 1960; 11:7–33.

18. Sherbourne CD, Stewart AL. The MOS social support survey. *Soc Sci Med*. 1991; 32:705–14.

19. Rice DP, Fox PJ, Max W, Webber PA, Lindeman DA, Hauck WW, et al. The economic burden of Alzheimer's disease care. *Health Aff (Millwood)*. 1993; 12:164–76.[Abstract]

20. The SUPPORT Principal Investigators. A controlled trial to improve care for seriously ill hospitalized patients. The Study to Understand Prognoses and Preferences for Outcomes and Risks of Treatments (SUPPORT). *JAMA*. 1995; 274:1591–8.[Abstract]

21. Epstein AM, Seage G, Weissman JS, Cleary PD, Fowler FJ, Gatsonis C, et al. Costs of medical care and out-of-pocket expenditures for persons with AIDS in the Boston Health Study Inquiry. 1995; 32:211–21.[Medline]

22. Emanuel EJ, Fairclough DL, Daniels ER, Clarridge BR. Euthanasia and physician-assisted suicide: attitudes and experiences of oncology patients, oncologists, and the public. *Lancet*. 1996; 347:1805–10.[Medline]

23. Office for Protection from Research Risks. *Protecting Human Research Subjects: Institutional Review Board Guidebook*. Washington, DC: U.S. Government Printing Office; 1993:4–19– 4–20.

24. Bureau of the Census. *Statistical Abstract of the United States, 1998*. 118th ed. Washington, DC: U.S. Government Printing Office; 1998.

25. Houts PS, Yasko JM, Harvey HA, Kahn SB, Hartz AJ, Hermann JF, et al. Unmet needs of persons with cancer in Pennsylvania during the period of terminal care. *Cancer*. 1988; 62:627–34.[Medline]

26. Mor V, Guadagnoli E, Wool M. An examination of the concrete service needs of advanced cancer patients. *Journal of Psychological Oncology*. 1987; 5:1–17.

27. Meier DE, Emmons CA, Wallenstein S, Quill T, Morrison RS, Cassel CK. A national survey of physician-assisted suicide and euthanasia in the United States. *N Engl J Med*. 1998; 338:1193–201. [Abstract/Free full text]

28. Van Der Maas PJ, Van Delden JJ, Pijnenborg L, Looman CW. Euthanasia and other medical decisions concerning the end of life. *Lancet*. 1991; 338:669–74.[Medline]

29. Ganzini L, Johnston WS, McFarland BH, Tolle SW, Lee MA. Attitudes of patients with amyotrophic lateral sclerosis and their care givers toward assisted suicide. *N Engl J Med*. 1998; 339:967–73.[Abstract/Free full text]

30. Field MJ, Cassel CK. *Approaching Death: Improving Care at the End of Life*. Washington, DC: National Academy Pr; 1997.

ACKNOWLEDGMENTS

The authors thank Drs. DeWitt Baldwin, Marion Danis, Lee Goldman, and Russell Phillips for critical review of the manuscript. They also thank Erica Omundsen for research assistance and Alma Kuby and the National Opinion Research Council for conducting the patient and caregiver interviews.

GRANT SUPPORT

In part by grants from the Commonwealth Fund and the Nathan Cummings Foundation.

CONCEPTION AND DESIGN

E. J. Emanuel, D. L. Fairclough, L. L. Emanuel.

ANALYSIS AND INTERPRETATION OF THE DATA

E. J. Emanuel, D. L. Fairclough, L. L. Emanuel.

DRAFTING OF THE ARTICLE

E. J. Emanuel, D. L. Fairclough, J. Slutsman, L. L. Emanuel.

CRITICAL REVISION OF THE ARTICLE FOR IMPORTANT INTELLECTUAL CONTENT

E. J. Emanuel, D. L. Fairclough, L. L. Emanuel.

FINAL APPROVAL OF THE ARTICLE

E. J. Emanuel, D. L. Fairclough, J. Slutsman, L. L. Emanuel.

STATISTICAL EXPERTISE

D. L. Fairclough.

OBTAINING OF FUNDING

E. J. Emanuel, L. L. Emanuel.

ADMINISTRATIVE, TECHNICAL, OR LOGISTIC SUPPORT

J. Slutsman.

COLLECTION AND ASSEMBLY OF DATA

E. J. Emanuel, J. Slutsman.

THE ENDS OF MEDICINE AND SOCIETY

Stephen J. McPhee, Michael W. Rabow, Steven Z. Pantilat, Amy J. Markowitz, and Margaret A. Winker, "Finding Our Way: Perspectives on Care at the Close of Life"

FINDING OUR WAY

Perspectives on Care at the Close of Life

STEPHEN J. MCPHEE, M.D., MICHAEL W. RABOW, M.D.,
STEVEN Z. PANTILAT, M.D., AMY J. MARKOWITZ, J.D.,
AND MARGARET A. WINKER, M.D.

This article originally appeared as McPhee SJ, Rabow MW, Pantilat SZ, Markowitz AJ, Winker MA. Finding our way—perspectives on care at the close of life. *JAMA.* 2000;284(19):2512–2513. Copyright © 2000, American Medical Association. All rights reserved. Reprinted with permission.

EDITORS' INTRODUCTION

This article launched a bimonthly series in the *Journal of the American Medical Association* on practical, case-based approaches to handling common palliative care challenges. The series, edited by the authors, is aimed at the practicing physician and makes clinical evidence and nuts-and-bolts recommendations easily accessible to doctors and their patients.

■ ■ ■

Hope does not lie in a way out, but in a way through.
Robert Frost

Dying is inevitable; there is no escape, no way out. Despite an ideal vision of the end of life, in which people die peacefully and comfortably at home, surrounded by supportive family and friends, many individuals die in hospitals, and many are in pain and alone.[1] Increasingly, clinicians are recognizing the difficulties that arise when caring for dying patients.[2] Perceiving death as a personal defeat or professional failure despite its being a natural event,[3,4] clinicians caring for patients at the close of life may feel lost in a foreign land without a map. Clinicians sometimes fear that recognizing the imminence of death may remove a patient's hope. They also may have little confidence in their ability to manage severe pain, dyspnea, and other terminal symptoms. The intense emotions that patients and their families display, and the equally strong emotions that clinicians experience, can be uncomfortable and troublesome. Too frequently, clinicians feel out of place negotiating the complexities of a family's dynamics at a time when the integrity of the family is most at stake. When spiritual questions and longings arise, clinicians may feel ill equipped to help patients in their search for meaningful answers. Even years of experience caring for dying patients does not lessen the challenge of confronting the deaths of friends and family or, ultimately, oneself.

These challenges to clinicians should not be surprising. Several studies have documented that end-of-life care is inadequately taught during medical school and residency training.[5-7] In 1995, only 26 percent of residency programs in the United States offered a course on care at the end of life as part of the curriculum, and 15 percent of programs offered no formal training.[8] The very personal reactions students have to interacting with dying patients and their families are frequently unexamined. Students have found few role models to help them handle end-of-life care, leaving them at an unfortunate remove from the richness the experience could otherwise bring.[9] Compounding this problem is the lack of information about good palliative care in mainstream textbooks to which physicians and nurses turn for information about patient care.[10-12] Furthermore, while the medical literature contains a wealth of information about palliative care, much of it is in specialty journals or textbooks unlikely to be seen by most clinicians. Journals geared to experts in the field frequently focus on important research concerns, but consequently may not always offer practical, clinically useful information. Moreover, these issues are compounded by a society constantly yearning for perpetual youth and longer life while denying and trying to avoid death.

There is hope, however. Clinicians' deficits of knowledge and patients' dissatisfactions with the quality of care have led both the medical profession and the public to devote increasing attention to palliative care. This attention has led to a series of major initiatives to improve palliative care education for both clinicians and the public, including the Education for Physicians in End-of-life Care Program of the American Medical Association, the Faculty Scholars in End-of-Life Care Program of the Department of Veterans Affairs, the Improving Residency Training in End-of-Life Care Program of the American Board of Internal Medicine, the Project on Death in America of the Soros Foundation, and the Last Acts Program of the Robert Wood Johnson Foundation.

In this issue, *JAMA* adds to the educational resources available to physicians, nurses, and other clinicians by launching a new bimonthly series devoted to caring for patients who are near or at the end of life. Titled "Perspectives on Care at the Close of Life," the series was developed after discussions with Steven Schroeder, M.D., Rosemary Gibson, M.Sc., and Merry Wood of the Robert Wood Johnson Foundation and is produced with the generous support of the foundation. This column will present a series of case-based discussions of challenging problems in caring for patients with end-stage, serious illness. The series is coordinated and edited by a team at the University of California, San Francisco, led by Stephen J. McPhee, M.D., and at *JAMA* by section editor Margaret Winker, M.D. The column is case-driven, just as the "Clinical Crossroads" series in *JAMA* has been.[13,14]

The goal of each article is to present practical, clinically useful, authoritative recommendations to clinicians in various specialties who care for patients at the end of life. The articles will examine common, difficult-to-manage issues in end-of-life care, including treating distressing symptoms, addressing psychological issues, and meeting spiritual needs. The articles will be based on available evidence and, where objective evidence does not exist, on clinical expertise. Cases will reflect the epidemiology, ethnicity, and disease pathways of serious illness and will be drawn from the inpatient, outpatient, and nursing home settings. Articles in this first year will trace the trajectory of end-of-life care from opening the discussion about death and dying with the patient through grief and bereavement.

The creation of each article for this column begins with identifying a topic important to care at the end of life and a discussant expert on that topic. A patient is identified who faces this issue at the end of life, and who, along with the patient's caregiver(s) and primary care physician, is willing to be interviewed and consents to share his or her perspective with an international audience. The interviews are then provided to the discussant, who weaves elements of the interviews throughout the discussion to illustrate the issues faced by the patient, family and caregivers, and the primary care physician. The discussion is peer reviewed and revised, but the interviewees' insights remain in their own voices. In the context of the patient's and caregivers' concerns, the articles will present evidence-based discussions of common issues raised by the patient's story. Like "Clinical Crossroads," "Perspectives on Care at the Close of Life" will provide follow-up of each case, completing the patient's story and ultimately presenting thoughts and reflections of family members and clinicians after the patient's death. In this issue of THE JOURNAL, the inaugural article by Quill[15] explores broaching end-of-life issues with patients and their families. The article is based on interviews with an eighty-one-year-old man with advanced pulmonary fibrosis, his son, and his primary care physician. As noted by Quill, patients, their families, and their clinicians frequently collude to avoid mentioning death or dying, even when suffering is severe and prognosis is poor. To address this problem, Quill provides practical suggestions about initiating end-of-life discussions, including the who, what, when, why, and how of such interactions. The article illustrates how conducting such discussions earlier and more systematically can allow patients to make more informed choices, achieve better palliation of symptoms, and have more opportunity to work on issues of life closure.

We hope this new column will engage readers in the process of improving care for patients at the end of life. Individuals interested in contributing cases or who have suggestions regarding topics or the section overall should contact the series editors.

Death is inevitable, and while there is no way out, there is a way through. Caring for patients at the close of life is one of the greatest challenges most clinicians ever face, yet it can be one of the most appreciated and personally rewarding experiences. Listening to the rich and varied perspectives of these dying patients, their families, and their clinicians, and learning from these authors and from one another, will help meet this challenge, and help find a way through. At the close of life, clinicians can learn to attend to patients' hopes to have their symptoms controlled, their emotions understood, their relationships supported, and their spiritual concerns addressed. One of the greatest gifts in confronting death is the perspective it offers about living life. Perhaps we too can achieve some perspective and understanding of how to share fully in the lives of those we love, all of whom will inevitably die, and how to live our own lives well in the time we have.

REFERENCES

1. A controlled trial to improve care for seriously ill hospitalized patients: the Study to Understand Prognoses and Preferences for Outcomes and Risks of Treatments (SUPPORT). *JAMA*. 1995; 274:1591–1598.

2. Block SD, Sullivan AM. Attitudes about end-of-life care: a national cross-section study. *J Palliat Med*. 1998; 1:347–355.

3. McCue J.D. The naturalness of dying. *JAMA*. 1995; 273:1039–1043.

4. Kane RS. The defeat of aging versus the importance of death. *J Am Geriatr Soc*. 1996; 44:321–325.

5. Holleman WL, Holleman MC, Gershenhom S. Death education curricula in U.S. medical schools. *Teach Learn Med*. 1994; 6:260–263.

6. Billings JA, Block S. Palliative care in undergraduate medical education: status report and future directions. *JAMA*. 1997; 278:733–738.

7. Weissman DE, Ambuel B, Norton AJ, Wang-Cheng R, Schiedermayer D. A survey of competencies and concerns in end-of-life care for physician trainees. *J Pain Symptom Manage.* 1998; 15:82–90.

8. Hill TP. Treating the dying patient: the challenge for medical education. *Arch Intern Med.* 1995; 155: 1265–1269.

9. Barzansky B, Veloski JJ, Miller R, Jonas HS. Education in end-of-life care during medical school and residency training. *Acad Med.* 1999; 74(10 suppl):S102– S104.

10. Carron AT, Lynn J, Keaney P. End-of-life care in medical textbooks. *Ann Intern Med.* 1999; 130:82–86.

11. Ferrell B, Virani R, Grant M, Juarez G. Analysis of palliative care content in nursing textbooks. *J Palliat Care.* 2000; 16:39–47.

12. Rabow MW, Hardie GE, Fair JM, McPhee SJ. End-of-life care content in 50 textbooks from multiple specialties. *JAMA*. 2000; 283:771–778.

13. Lynn J. An 88-year-old woman facing the end of life. *JAMA*. 1997; 277:1633–1640.

14. Foley K. A 44-year-old woman with severe pain at the end of life. *JAMA*. 1999; 281:1937–1945.

15. Quill, TE. Initiating end-of-life discussions with seriously ill patients: addressing the "elephant in the room." *JAMA*. 2000; 284:2502–2507.

THE EDITORS

DIANE E. MEIER, M.D., FACP, is director of the Center to Advance Palliative Care (CAPC), a national organization devoted to increasing the number and quality of palliative care programs in the United States. She is also director of the Lilian and Benjamin Hertzberg Palliative Care Institute as well as professor of geriatrics and internal medicine and Catherine Gaisman Professor of Medical Ethics at Mount Sinai School of Medicine in New York City. A recipient of numerous awards—including a MacArthur Fellowship in 2008, the Open Society Institute Faculty Scholar's Award of the Project on Death in America, the Founders Award of the National Hospice and Palliative Care Organization, and the Alexander Richman Commemorative Award for Humanism in Medicine—she is the principal investigator of an NCI-funded five-year multisite study on the outcomes of hospital palliative care services in cancer patients. Meier received her B.A. from Oberlin College and her M.D. from Northwestern University Medical School. She completed her residency and fellowship training at Oregon Health Sciences University in Portland. She has been on the faculty of the Department of Geriatrics and Adult Development and Department of Medicine at Mount Sinai since 1983.

STEPHEN L. ISAACS, J.D., is a partner in Isaacs/Jellinek, a San Francisco–based consulting firm, and president of Health Policy Associates, Inc. A former professor of public health at Columbia University and founding director of its Development Law and Policy Program, he has written extensively for professional and popular audiences. His book *The Consumer's Legal Guide to Today's Health Care* was reviewed as "the single best guide to the health care system in print today." His articles have been widely syndicated and have appeared in law reviews and health policy journals. He also provides technical assistance internationally on health law, civil society, and social policy. A graduate of Brown University and Columbia Law School, Isaacs served as vice president of International Planned Parenthood's Western Hemisphere Region, practiced health law, and spent four years in Thailand as a program officer for the U.S. Agency for International Development.

ROBERT G. HUGHES, PH.D., is a vice president of the Robert Wood Johnson Foundation and its chief learning officer. Since joining the Foundation in 1989 as director of program research, and then vice president, Hughes has played an instrumental role in program development and management in tobacco control, children's health insurance, tracking health systems change, and community health projects. Hughes is currently responsible for the Pioneer Portfolio, the component of the Foundation dedicated to promoting fundamental breakthroughs in health and health care through innovative projects, including those from nontraditional sources and fields. Before joining the Robert Wood Johnson Foundation, Hughes was an assistant dean at Johns Hopkins University. He also taught at the University of Washington School of Public Health and Community Medicine and at the Arizona State University College of Business. Hughes received a B.A. from DePauw University, an M.A. from Ohio State University, a Ph.D. in behavioral sciences from Johns Hopkins University, and a Pew postdoctoral fellowship in health policy at the University of California, San Francisco.

Index